A PSYCHIATRIC ODYSSEY

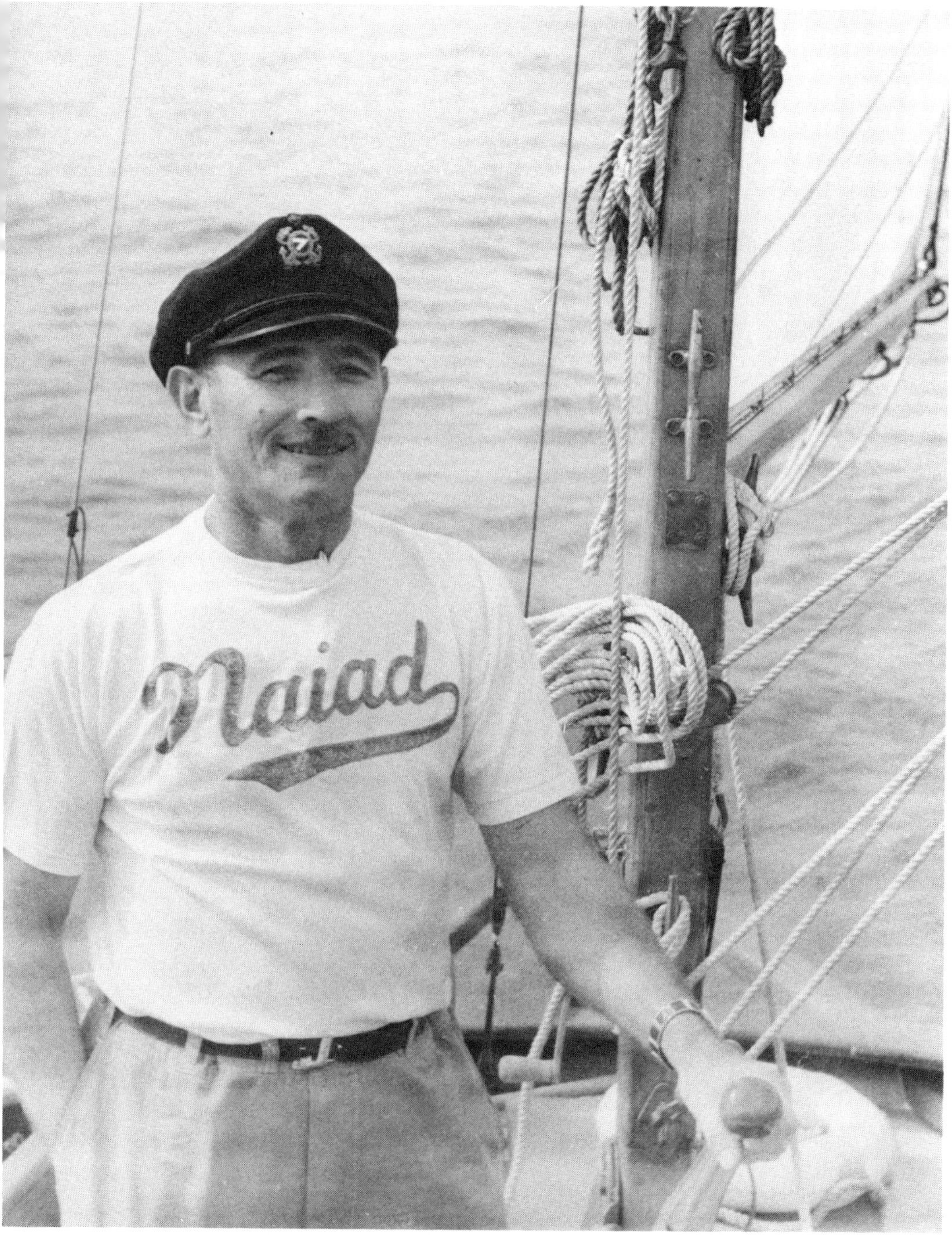
Naiad

A PSYCHIATRIC ODYSSEY

Jules H. Masserman, M. D.

Science House

New York

The publisher and author wish to acknowledge use of material from the following:
L. Wolberg, *Short-term Psychotherapy.* New York: Grune & Stratton, 1965. Copyright © 1965, Grune & Stratton.
J. H. Masserman, ed., *Current Psychiatric Therapies,* Vol. VIII. New York: Grune & Stratton, 1968. Copyright © 1968, Grune & Stratton.
———, ed., *Youth: A Transcultural Approach.* New York: Grune & Stratton, 1969. Copyright © 1969, Grune & Stratton.
———, "Faith and Delusion in Psychotherapy." *American Journal of Psychiatry* 110: 324-333, 1953. Copyright © 1953, The American Psychiatric Association.
———, Review of Stein's *Contemporary Psychotherapists. Archives of General Psychiatry* 12: 461, 1962. Copyright © 1962.
———, Review of Frank's *Persuasion and Healing. American Journal of Psychiatry* 118: 659-661, 1962. Copyright © 1962, The American Psychiatric Association.

Library of Congress Catalog Number: 76-110255
Standard Book Number: 87668-030-9

Manufactured by Haddon Craftsmen, Inc.
Scranton, Pennsylvania

CONTENTS

PROLOGUE

This is a curious book.

It began a year ago in my sanctum at the Center for Advanced Study in the Behavioral Sciences at Stanford. With my office hi-fi playing the deeply reflective Mozart D minor Quartet in soft *obligato,* I sat gazing dubiously at San Francisco Bay across a desk piled high with old files of letters, comments, reviews and other literary bric-a-brac that recorded forty years of a strenuous, traumatic, ecstatic, peripatetic and partially fulfilling professional life now drawing to a close. I wondered whether, if I recollected these *ex-periences*, would they, as the latter Latin derivative would have it, "pierce through" to another reader? Would anyone else sense, or care, about my puzzlement, patience, pain and pride in trying to pass from scholastic to scholar, from invest-igator to re-searcher, from physiologist to physician, from in-structor to pro-fessor, from writer to author? Indeed, was there actually anything unique in my asymptotic search for scientific integration and personal integrity . . . ?

But then I reflected further: during those forty years, had I not also wished that my own teachers and mentors would have disclosed how *they* had striven toward these goals? Would I not have learned much about their vicissitudes and victories from their recall of crucial conversations, the letters they wrote, their abandoned as well as published manuscripts, and other intimate memorabilia that would have served as guideposts for those that would follow—and mayhap take a few hopeful steps beyond?

It was this recollection—and perhaps also a wish to stay the kaleidoscope of past existence and view once more some of its individually colored patches of memory before they whirled into the grey blur of Lethe—that led to the assembly of this volume. Just possibly, after reading it, the colleagues who are the multiple *dramatis personae* in this account would like to compare their views of events with mine, or younger behavioral scientists could plan their own multifaceted careers more wisely. Perhaps, also, inquisitive and thoughtful non-professionals—and this book is not addressed to the uncurious and unintelligent—may wish to learn how one becomes a doctor, a psychoanalyst, an author, and eventually even a half-willing draftee of the academic and professional Establishment.

Out of respect for this prospective coterie of communicants, I shall not recount the events of the last four decades by the usual modes of wishfully colored retrospection. Instead, after only the briefest of autobiographical introductions, I shall reproduce, with no attempts to gloss their grammar, let alone their gaucheries or grandiosities, the letters, reports, and commentaries precisely as written during contemporary moments of illusory conviction. Whenever it would not violate ethics to do so, I shall also quote verbatim corresponding communications from my protagonists; at other times, I shall try, necessarily in my own words, to present their versions of the dialogues as fairly as possible.

Here, then, are forty years of the vagaries, vices, vicissitudes and vicarious victories of a vagrant psychiatrist.

J.H.M.

1. ORIGINS

I was born in Chudnov, a rural hamlet perennially shuttled by politics and militarism between Russia and Poland, but not worth the trouble in either modality. My father emigrated to America just before the birth of my only brother, then sent for us when I was five years old. I can vaguely remember our tiny stucco cottage with its thatched roof, the dark attic retreat above the clay bake oven, the single muddy street off the village square, and the mounted Cossacks who seemed to delight in clattering down on small children. Later, I see myself with mother, aunt and brother in a dark steerage cubicle over a stormy sea, a chimera terminating in a vivid image of mother with me in tow, carrying our bundles and my infant brother through long immigrant lines at Ellis Island and trying desperately to convey in broken Russian to whomever would listen that we wished to get to my father in Michigan—a village she supposed was just a few *versts* from New York.

Father Abram met us dispassionately at the train station in Detroit and escorted us to our new home: three rented rooms over his tailor shop in a marginal slum section of the city. Since father had always professed to be a scholar and philosopher, it was mother who had to learn American ways as rapidly as possible and help mind the family business as well as wash, cook, mend, keep house and save enough money to assure a proper education for her precious sons. Mostly because of her diligence, after a few years we were able to move to our own home close to a school. But even though I supplemented the family income by working at the earliest permissable age of thirteen, family finances ever remained a problem until I graduated medicine and brother Ted was admitted to the bar. Soon after that our parents decided to terminate a quarter century of variably overt incompatibility in a divorce, after which father moved to another city and remarried. I rarely saw him again until his death a decade later, but I continued to revere and honor my mother—and to support her financially when she finally had to permit it—as the most gentle, modest, intelligent and kindest human being I have ever known.

One of my few memories of the 1890 model grammar school I attended in southeast Detroit concerns my early disillusionment about a third-grade teacher, who could not herself understand an assigned arithmetic lesson which stated that 2+ stood for all fractions between 2 and 2½, whereas 3- included all between 2½ and 3. After-hours parochial school was enjoyed until our progressive young instructor was fired because he had taught us to converse in Hebrew, and was replaced by a bearded disciplinarian who demanded rote learning of prayer-book chants and litanies. But I clearly recall the joy of discovering, this time under my father's guidance, that the local branch of the public library would, almost unbelievably, lend me two books to read every other week; I also remember the librarian's surprise when, as I began my survey of her store of riches beginning with stack A, I chose an illustrated tome on Old Stone Age man for my first borrowed treasure. Once home, I read it continuously in utter fascination until mother, on some midnight mission, saw the light under my bedroom door and summarily confiscated the volume until after I washed the dinner dishes and finished my regular schoolwork the next day. Other books followed in rapid and often indiscriminate succession, and perhaps still provide the odd bits of information that I include, with some trepidation, in my lectures and, after necessary confirmation, in my writings.

High school years were a round of routine uninspired classes and hurried half-hours of violin or viola practice: mother never gave up the notion that I could also be a virtuoso "if I only practiced more," whereas father, in one of his not infrequent rages against an unappreciative and discordant world, once splintered my viola. Three evenings a week and all summer "vacations" were spent clerking in drugstores to earn school expenses and, supposedly, to help prepare me for the ultimate study of medicine. This dubious notion also led to my taking a six-week intensive summer course at a cram school and passing the Michigan State Boards for licensure as a registered pharmacist—a step that increased my summers' income, but only confused later studies of medical pharmacology. Concurrently, music developed into a life-long love, and it became another source of needed savings when I grew adept enough to play for pay and to teach beginning students how to hold a violin and draw a bow so as to delight their uncritical parents. But all this left little time for more than an occasional Sunday morning game of tennis, and what little peer life I had was further impaired by the agonies of a persistent adolescent acne. Social confidence and sexual experiences came late, and subsequent over-compensations, along with a retained avidity for long hours of intensive work, study and recreation, have made for a full but strenuous life.

My high school and junior college studies produced class standings sufficiently distinctive to qualify me for admission to the Detroit College of Medicine—a marginal school with dilapidated lecture and laboratory facilities and matching faculty and curriculum, but the only one geographically and financially available. Nor were my initial impressions of medical education improved when, in his welcoming address, the Dean, with evident relish, predicted that one in every three or four of us would be found wanting in our first or second year and then be eliminated forever from medicine. With this warning and with little explanation as to the relevance of what we were learning, we plunged into what were essentially exercises in memorizing minute details of bone anatomy, the structure of cell nucleoli, the formulae of bacterial culture media and other such transient trivia of the "pre-clinical sciences." And throughout the year it was repeatedly made ominously clear that should anyone fail even one of these "basic courses" his career was irretrievably ended. This led to one of the most stressful episodes of my life which I recall as follows:

Our then professor of physiology, a pompous Ph.D. with a patronizing Bostonian accent and an I.Q. of about 95, had droned through two semesters of lectures, the contents of which could only be guessed at by those of us who had discovered the obscure and outmoded British textbook from which he had cribbed them. I had retained a fairly high class rating, mainly by turning in for the required bi-monthly inspection my "lecture notes" (including his perennial errors), neatly outlined in red and black ink. Nevertheless, whether I passed or flunked the course—and therefore whether I would ever become a physician—depended on surmounting two all-important high hurdles that had wrecked the careers of many former aspirants: to wit, the dreaded written and "practical" final examinations in physiology. Inasmuch as I had learned the miniscule content of our professor's repetitious lectures by heart and had good reasons to believe that he knew nothing else to inquire about, I had little fear of the written test. However, since the "practical" dealt only marginally with either knowledge or skill, and a grade below 75% meant inevitable failure and expulsion from school, it remained a prospect of unpredictable horror. The circumstances were these:

Throughout two semesters we had had weekly laboratory sessions in which pairs of students conducted a total of thirty so-called experiments purportedly designed to illustrate various physiologic functions. The methods employed ranged from the simple recording of a lab partner's pulse and breathing by tying rubber diaphragms around his wrist and chest, through various observations of exposed frog hearts and intestines, to highly complex procedures involving hours of coordinated and specialized efforts. At the final "practical examination," the instructor pinned the names of various "experiments" on slips of paper face down on a board, which was passed to the students seated at isolated desks; each student picked a slip and then was required to conduct successfully whatever "experiment" fell to his lot within the required ninety minutes. Everyone knew that at least two of the procedures—the ones on reciprocal innervation in a frog and decerebration of a pigeon—almost inevitably meant sudden death both for the animal and the hopes of the human victim, since only a quarter of the students even when paired had succeeded in completing either experiment in the regular two-and-a-half-hour lab period. But then, as our placid professor perennially put it, "That's the kind of fate that made me a perfessor and you just students."

And as kind fate had it, when I unfolded the slip it was my turn to pick, it read, "Reciprocal Innervation in a Frog." This meant that alone and in only the ninety minutes allowed for the practical examination in laboratory physiology I had to:

1. Smoke a three-foot roll of recording paper and mount it on a pair of revolving kymograph drums (minimum time required, 5 minutes).
2. Obtain a frog from the storeroom (minimum, 5 minutes).
3. Anesthetize the frog by "pithing," i.e., destroying its upper spinal cord (minimum, 3 minutes).
4. Fix the frog to an operating board, dissect out the opposing muscles of one leg, tie their tendons individually with fine threads under a warm saline drip to counterbalanced levers adjusted to write on the recording paper along with a half-second timer, and set the whole assemblage, creaking from many years of abuse, to working in proper order (minimum time required if every step goes perfectly, 45 minutes).
5. Arrange a Harvard inductorium so that properly placed electrodes stimulate a flexor muscle to show that its opposite muscle would simultaneously extend. Reverse the procedure and record all the tracings, properly timed, on the revolving drums. Thirty percent credit on interim inspection by a lab monitor (12 minutes).
6. Demonstrate the same effects from electrical stimulation of the lower spinal cord. Thirty percent credit (5 minutes).
7. Disconnect the inductorium and show that a drop of acetic acid on the frog's crotch would, by stimulating its skin, also produce reciprocal reflex effects on its leg muscles. Thirty percent credit (5 minutes, including obtaining the bottle of acid from the supply room).
8. Finally remove, mark, shellack and dry the smoked paper and bring it to the examiner's desk for check-in along with a write-up of the experiment. Final "bonus" of ten percent (10 minutes).

Miraculously, and despite my initial panic, the experiment went far better in steps one through six than it ever had for any two students during the year: the frog stayed alive, the muscles did not dry out, the tendons and threads did not tear, the levers duly went in opposite directions when the muscles and spinal roots were stimulated and the ancient kymographs creaked along steadily and recorded it all. Indeed I had fully 20 minutes left to obtain the bottle of acid from the laboratory, put a drop on the frog's skin, record the final muscular responses and be on my joyful way to the Nobel Prize in Medicine—when paralysis struck: there were no muscular responses whatever to the acid, no matter how liberally I applied it. The explanation soon became obvious: when I put a drop of the stuff on my own skin it showed no redness; a drop on my tongue produced no taste; in my eye, no burn! Obviously, the acid, too, had been kept in laboratory stock so long that it had become neutral and ineffective—a point I tried to demonstrate to the professor himself on his next round of inspection by desperately repeating the skin, tongue and eye tests in his presence—only to be told haughtily that if I didn't make the acid experiment work properly as required in the 10 minutes remaining, the most I could get on the lab test even if all else was perfect was the failing grade of 70%.

This left only one course open: to cheat—nor have I for a moment since then regretted that I did so. As inconspicuously as possible I fixed fine electrodes to the frog's back and connected them through a foot switch concealed beneath the desk to a stimulator hidden in a wooden drawer. I then humbly recalled our Bostonian savant, apologized for not having conducted the last part of the experiment efficiently, again placed an innocuous drop of "acid" on the frog's skin, surreptitiously stepped on the foot switch and demonstrated that indeed under these circumstances the opposing mucles twitched dramatically in opposite directions. In the remaining five minutes I wrote my notes, but since the shellacked paper was not quite dry when I turned it in, I got only a 95% grade for the "Practical" and, therefore, rated only second in physiology in the freshman class of sixty-five.

The following summer was again devoted to working in a pharmacy, playing occasionally in a radio quartet and reading in preparation for my second year in medical school. Somewhat better-taught sophomore courses in pathology, neurology and medicine began opening entrancing vistas of the vast science of medicine. But then overwork took its toll. Bloody urine and excruciating backaches brought me to a urologist who, after various injections of dyes and x-ray studies, informed me with professional somberness that both kidneys were definitely tuberculous, that one had to be removed, and that if the other did not heal I had about six months to live. Fatalistically—since life did not otherwise seem worth living—I returned to classes for the week before surgery. My left kidney was indeed removed, and after four subsequent weeks of stormy convalescence, I resumed my studies—but again in vain. The operative wound refused to heal, and the persistent drainage and debility finally necessitated my leaving school. Mother took me, pale and weak, for a nine months' sojourn in southern California where, providentially, the right kidney resumed function and the wound began to close, although troublesome drainage and fatiguability persisted well into my internship.

I returned to medical school in 1927 to repeat my sophomore year, now made easier by the circumstance that I had spent much of my convalescence writing a long, hand-illustrated, extravagantly referenced monograph on the pathology of thyroid diseases, secretly subtitled, in the idiom of the day, "Getting Gerty's Goitre." The work was accorded a Sophomore Prize Thesis by Dr. Elmer Davis, Professor of Pathology, one of the few truly dedicated and inspiring teachers I encountered in my pre-clinical years. This also earned me an assistantship in the animal surgical laboratory where, after some now dubious research on supposed "inguinal sphincters," I wrote two articles on a questionable new technique of hernia repair. The articles were promptly published by the Professor of Surgery under his own name. Since I had the good sense not to object, I was offered a permanent Assistantship in Pathology and was assured it would lead to a faculty appointment on graduation. But I declined what then seemed a fantastic opportunity for a secure academic career because I had already resolved to graduate in medicine for only one purpose: to become a neurologist and psychiatrist.

After forty years of reflection, I still do not know how that resolution took form and direction. I had always been interested in all aspects of what are now called the behavioral sciences; readings in evolution, biology, anthropology, and psychology, however indiscriminate and poorly understood, had ever been preferred to fiction; I avidly consumed review books *about* art, history and philosophy, largely because the original tomes of the truly great historians, theologians or philosophers would have taken time then not available. However much I delighted in discovering Mark Twain in my teens, I preferred his *Innocents Abroad* or his acrid commentaries on Christian Science to the smooth fictional flow of *Huck Finn.* In high school and pre-medical studies I admired the logical precision of physics and mathematics, but regarded them as intellectual games much like chess rather than as gateways to engineering or any other technical career. So also, courses in chemistry and biology were fascinating only when they touched on the universals of life, but onerous when they dealt merely with sterile descriptions and artificial classifications. As already noted, in medical school I felt tested and martyred rather than adequately instructed when I was made to study dry bones, dissect variable venules and nerve filaments in the skin of a cadaver, look at mummified cells under a microscope, produce sugar precipitates or fatty acids in test tubes, or record the metabolic agonies of anesthetized dying animals. Indeed it was not until the junior year of medical school that we were allowed to deal with living patients—and it was then also that we had our first lecture in psychiatry.

That was many years ago but I remember it well: Dr. Harry August, a mere clinical instructor on the faculty roster, talked to us of how intense anxiety, which could be re-evoked by the stresses of adult life from latencies in the forgotten frustrations of childhood, could produce transient or permanent deviations of body functions and behavior—a thesis he illustrated by citing case histories of patients in his private practice whom he had "cured by psychotherapy alone." In subsequent lectures he demonstrated group hypnosis on the entire class, and in general succeeded despite the sly snickers and winks of the few inevitable cynics. He then went on to inform us about the current classifications of "mental disorders" and to discuss the psychiatric theories of the day, from the genetic-constitutional concepts of Kraepelin and Bleuler through Watsonian behaviorism to the speculations of Freud, Adler, Jung and Sullivan. It is a whimsical commentary that, a full decade later, he and Louis Schwartz, the only other psychiatrist who occasionally lectured us, decided to commute weekly from Detroit to join me in training at the Chicago Psychoanalytic Institute, and thereafter abandoned their former eclectic breadth to become almost completely stultified by psychoanalytic orthodoxy; nevertheless, during my medical school days they fitted my concepts of broadly humanitarian psychiatrists and strengthened my resolve—if strengthening were needed—to emulate their examples and acquire their knowledge and skills. Thus my junior and senior years in medical school gradually became filled with what I had always sought: contacts with human beings whom I could examine medically, begin to understand personally and, with or without supervision, try to help comprehensively.

Social self-confidence increased in and out of school although a prolonged sex liaison with a compliant schoolmate tapered off when she dropped medicine and extended her favors elsewhere. In the summer between my junior and senior years I served as a medical extern in a Catholic hospital, and there began to learn about the seamy side of medicine. A Supervising Sister refused to let me give emergency aid to a slum child with third-degree burns until her distraught parents paid for the treatment in advance, and when the entire family could not muster enough cash, the Sister sent them and the child away. I protested this cold outrage to the Mother Superior to no avail, and after another such episode two weeks later quit the hospital in what I felt was righteous indignation—with the result that my "defalcation from duty" was reported to my medical school in terms that led an assistant dean to threaten me with expulsion if I "let the affair get into the papers, or ever got out of line that way again."

I married Jeanette, the gentle, unassuming sister of a friend, but remained so immersed in my studious self-importance that I did not adequately appreciate her quiet devotion. I was readmitted to the senior year, graduated with honors, and departed for an internship in San Diego, leaving Jeanette in Detroit on the plea—only liminally justified—that I could not support her in California on my stipend of twenty-five dollars a month and that in any case we would have very little time together. As usual, she accepted this arrangement without protest and returned to live with her family. She died of a previously undiagnosed internal cancer nine months later, and left a dark cloud of pity and remorse I shall never eradicate from my conscience. Apart from any altruism, perhaps some of my intense dedication to work and service since then has been partly in expiation.

2. INTERN AND PSYCHIATRIC RESIDENT

On my graduation from the Detroit College of Medicine I wanted to get as far away as possible from that flat grimy city to new environmental and medical horizons. San Diego, California seemed the most distant and pleasantly situated prospect, and it listed a general hospital which, to my astonishment, accepted me for internship. The advanced duties with which I was entrusted could hardly have been anticipated: I assisted in brain surgery, performed intricate podalic versions in obstetrics and I was the principal physician for many difficult medical and surgical patients. On the occasional half days or partial weekends off, I revelled in San Diego's then crystal air, the nearby mountain vistas, and the clean beaches. I bought a teredo-infested catboat for thirty dollars, sailed with three other intern friends to the Coronado Islands off the coast of Mexico, got becalmed, and navigated back to our mooring two days late—completely unnoticed by the half dozen local ships of the U. S. Navy that had been sent on a rescue mission to search (as I learned later) for what the local papers had headlined as "Four Hospital Doctors Lost at Sea!"

I was loath to leave San Diego in June, 1931, and had I never done so, may have had a considerably more serene life.

However, the offer of a Residency in Psychiatry and Neurology at the prestigious Stanford University in San Francisco could not be refused. In my year there I learned that the faculty and attending staff in both psychiatry and neurology were too preoccupied with sexual liaisons and academic rivalries to have time for teaching residents, but that one could nevertheless learn much from books and patients. I also found, to my disillusioned astonishment, that I could publish articles on such obvious inventions as a binaural stethoscope for application to opposite points of a patient's chest to detect momentary delay in the breath sounds of a diseased lung, or a mechanical device for modifying spinal puncture techniques to minimize post-puncture headaches. I had another lesson in the stringencies of academic subservience when I made a factual entry in a patient's chart without anticipating that it would later contradict a Professor of Medicine's opinion, which he offered as an "expert witness" in a court case; for this cardinal sin I was officially reprimanded, this time by the dean himself. This episode resolved any uncertainty I may still have felt about leaving Stanford to accept a Chief Residency in Psychiatry at the Baltimore City Hospitals, with opportunities for training under the world famous Adolf Meyer at the Phipps Psychiatric Clinic of the Johns Hopkins Hospital.

The Baltimore Psychiatric Hospital turned out to be a prison-like institution housing some 300 patients strictly segregated by sex and color, but otherwise thrown together without regard to age, circumstance, or psychiatric status. I was entrusted with their medical care and I was responsible for admitting from ten to twenty new patients each week, conducting two staff rounds daily, and maintaining mountainous records. And yet so interesting was the work and so profitable were my concurrent studies at Hopkins that I twice applied for, and was granted, yearly renewals of my residency.

The latter years furnished adequate time for fairly intensive investigations of spinal fluid dynamics and the use of intravenous injections of sucrose to diminish intracranial pressure. In the first attempt on record to determine the latter effect, I injected a 10% solution of grape sugar into my own veins, with the result that my diuresis that evening was so prolonged and urgent that I had time to hear only every third aria at an opera I attended. I again found that my reports of this research were readily accepted for publication in leading professional journals, and thus cultivated a penchant for writing that has since, *mea culpa,* produced twenty score articles, thirty books, the plethora of material sampled in this volume and other scribblings more appropriately relegated to files or wastebaskets. During my residency at Baltimore this urge took another bent: the composing of music and poetry and the writing of short stories derived from my daily experiences at the hospital. I only recently discovered the latter handwritten, yellowed and almost illegible manuscripts in an old, forgotten folder perhaps a sampling may illuminate something of Baltimore—and of myself—nearly forty years ago:

Maria

When she was fourteen, Maria Boccini—to all practical purposes—was raped.

How do we know? Take her mother's word for it: Hadn't Maria for months been making eyes at that blond gardener boy on the Duncan Estate? Hadn't the *sfrenata,* contrary to admonitions in fluent Italian, persisted in going over to "play with him?" Hadn't Maria returned from one of these excursions with a story of how, after he had chased her through a particularly boisterous romp, Sven had become irritated and ordered her away, decreeing that he no longer wanted any Wop girls hanging around? Hadn't Maria come home sobbing, her dress muddy, and her underthings blood-smeared? And hadn't a quick maternal examination revealed conclusively where the blood was coming from? Likely story the girl told! Her mother (remembering certain of her own girlhood experiences) knew better: Maria had been raped.

Take the paternal Boccini's word for it. Not, surely, that he hadn't raised both his daughters to be good girls, respectful of the Trinity and the rod. But Maria was still only a child. She had fallen an easy victim to that bully Sven Erickson who, being a Swede and a Protestant, was by nature capable of any iniquity. Besides, hadn't Mrs. Boccini's examination revealed the awful truth? No doubt about it: his Maria had been raped!

Take the word of Maria's elder sister: Helene had been concerned about the actions of that hare-brained little tramp for some time and had, she now frankly admitted, predicted Maria's disgrace. Italian girls mature early; Helene knew. Even nice boys like Sven, she pointed out, could be provoked beyond endurance. Rape indeed! Put the blame where it belonged . . .

It mattered not that both Sven and Maria at first didn't understand the accusations, then rather dazedly denied them. It mattered not that Mrs. Boccini, after an ignorant and prejudiced examination, had overlooked the fact that Maria had reached an age when soiled stockings were to become a temporarily unpredictable if periodic occurrence. No physician, of course, was called to confirm a fact so apparent: Maria had been raped.

Mr. Boccini carried the matter directly to Sven's father, butler on the Duncan Estate. Mr. Erickson listened gravely, solemnly conferred with his son, then unhurriedly but convincingly ushered the gesticulating Mr. Boccini out of the house. The neighbors—to whom the Erickson integrity was a byword—likewise showed an unmistakable tendency to disbelieve Mr. Boccini's protestations, and, later, became actually suspicious of the motives of Maria's family. The police too had had previous dealings with the mercurial Boccinis, and proved similarly hard to convince of the great wrong *filia* had suffered.

Nothing, then, for the Boccinis to do but swallow their injured pride and comfort poor Maria.

Day in and weary day out Maria was comforted, sympathized with, reassured, heartened, until the bewildered girl, numbed by the veiled implications, actually came to believe herself in some way guilty of some awful transgression that doomed her to perdition. Nor were the effects of that belief long delayed. Tacitly labeled fallen, Maria conceived herself to have little reputation to uphold. She became sensitive . . . resentful . . . suspicious of her former friends. Too young and high-spirited to maintain a self-enforced social seclusion, Maria made new, less finicky acquaintances in an Italian stratum she had heretofore ignored. Why save the shreds of self-respect that remained? Maria learned to drink, to flirt. . . .

At seventeen, she was committed to the State Home for Delinquent Girls. Maria's family bewails Maria's ruin and continues to blame her seducer, Sven Erickson.

When she was fourteen Maria—to all practical purposes—was raped.

Black on White

My telephone tinkles. My telephone and I being old friends, it had of late gotten to anticipate what my calls would be about, and to inform me in advance. This time it seemed to have a peculiarly merry ring, so I answered promptly with the curt self-importance of a two-term Chief Psychiatric Resident, "Dr. Masserman! Yes?"

An ominously ingratiating female voice answered, "Oh, Dr. Masserman, so glad I caught you in! (a gratuitous remark, since she knew I was on twenty-four-hour weekend duty). This is Miss Reeves at the State Mental Office speaking. We've got quite a problem, and I'm sure you can help us. Won't you?"

I already knew that all Baltimore County social workers' days are divided into twenty-four equal segments, each filled with sixty equally serious problems, so I replied, "Of course. How can I?"

"It's at the Crown Point State Hospital for the Colored Insane. Seems like one of their top attendants got all excited and started beating up his wife at their home. Then the two of them got arrested, and the attendant was so violent that the police doctor made out papers calling him insane and bound him over for commitment. And now we're stuck."

The difficulty, however, seemed not immediately apparent. I also knew that all Maryland state hospital administrative attendants were white, and that Crown Point State Hospital was reserved for "the Negro Insane." But the man could easily be sent to one of the three other state hospitals exclusively dedicated to serving the Master Race. Ergo: "But why 'stuck,' Miss Reeves? Send the man to Spring Grove. It's only a few miles from here, and he certainly doesn't belong in the Baltimore City Hospital unless there are very special circumstances."

More consternation. "But there are, Dr. Masserman. He was arrested with his wife, and she is colored! And she insists that he's colored too, and has just been passing as white all this time!"

"But then they can admit him at Crown Point."

"But they can't do that either. You see, they have him on their books as a white man; it must be that way, or he couldn't be on the payroll. And worst of all—and I'm sure you'll keep this confidential—it seems he is a first cousin of a State Senator. And the Senator has got wind of the affair and threatens that if the man is sent to Crown Point he'll have me fired. And he can, too. And so you see . . . oh, Dr. Masserman, your hospital is the only one in the State that takes both white and colored. And you don't have to classify him publicly. Can't you take him, *please?*"

As a firm believer in preventive psychiatry, my obvious duty was to prevent bloody conflicts among the two state hospital superintendents, Mrs. Reeves, and our worthy State Senator. I admitted the attendant, treated his delirium tremens and in a week he was back at work, recertified as white, on a less sensitive post office job also secured for him by his senatorial cousin.

Marguerite

Marguerite Maglia's father was a cruel man. Nor did he ever realize how terribly cruel he had been to Marguerite.

Mrs. Maglia had died in childbirth, leaving two-year-old Marguerite and her new-born sister Helene to the mercies of their irresponsible, alcoholic father. Somehow, the children survived the four months that preceded Maglia's remarriage. The second Mrs. Maglia was kind, but proved no more able than the first to withstand abuse, and within three years followed her predecessor to the city cemetery.

No woman in the Sicilian colony of a Baltimore suburb cared to volunteer as a third victim. Maglia *signor,* deprived of a sexual partner, resorted to other makeshift outlets. As these closed to him he turned to his maturing daughters. Since he was now sexually impotent, Maglia found vicarious physical satisfaction in inflicting manual "punishments" on the helpless girls for the slightest real or imagined infraction of his unpredictable discipline.

Marguerite, at fourteen, was the first to bear the brunt of

her father's inescapable perversions. With the first sotted gleam in his eyes, the ritual would begin: her clothes would be totally removed, and her body beaten about the breasts and hips until her father fell drunk and exhausted. . . .

And yet, as time went on, Marguerite's initial pain and horror became tinctured with a strange fascination, and her flagellant sufferings became colored with sensuous ecstasies. Marguerite soon ceased to fear her father's sudden "anger"; instead, she often did precisely what she had learned would induce him to whip her. And as the significance of their encounters became covertly clear, a strange attachment between father and daughter arose and grew ever stronger.

In contrast, the younger Helene, who greatly resembled her father both in appearance and character, felt nothing but dread for her father's cruelty and despised Marguerite's misunderstood docility. At fifteen, Helene acceded to the propositions of a wandering Italian herb-mendicant and, without warning, disappeared from home. Marguerite, with a filial devotion that was the marvel of the Sicilian colony, remained with her father, continued to care for his rapidly failing health, and deeply mourned his death two years later.

At this point, the faithful Marguerite's lonely helplessness touched the heart of a childless, well-to-do Sicilian widow, a Mrs. Vanzetti, who adopted her. Marguerite was given the advantages of a comfortable home, a parochial education and derived a social prestige that obliterated her own genealogy. The girl reached marriageable age with the charms of her wistful beauty and unassuming virtues enhanced by the prospects of the Vanzetti dowry. None of the colony's local finest, however, seemed to arouse in Marguerite more than a passing interest until, at twenty-four Marguerite chose Giuseppe, a youth whose low forehead, brutish eyes and stocky stature were remarkably reminiscent of the paternal Maglia, but who also had talent enough to qualify as a violist in the Baltimore Symphony. The match was approved in formal Sicilian council by Mrs. Vanzetti and Mr. Chiappi, Giuseppe's father, and a wedding satisfactory to all concerned was arranged. Mrs. Vanzetti thereupon called the groom into private conference and (as she later recalled the interview for me) told him: "Giuseppe, you know all about Marguerite's bad time she have when young with her *padre,* how bad he treated her and how he used to beat her. But I give her nice home, and treat her good, because she good girl. Giuseppe, when you marry Marguerite you both live with me. I got lots money, and I treat you good too. But you got treat Marguerite same. You got be nice, you got be kind when marry. You make Marguerite happy, and I take care you both."

Giuseppe, who was already devoted to Marguerite and had hardly dreamed of making so favorable a match, was doubly delighted. The couple went to live with Mrs. Vanzetti, and under the latter's watchful eye Giuseppe, a tender soul at heart, evolved into what most Sicilian wives would consider a model husband. Love-making was gentle, drinking moderate, scolding infrequent, beatings banned; in no way did Giuseppe fulfill his resemblance to the paternal Maglia. But Giuseppe's sincere, clumsy pampering left Marguerite vaguely discontented, and his ardent but tender embraces merely increased an indefinable yearning she had hoped would be stilled in marriage. Two years of unbearable conjugal serenity brought her to the breaking point. After an emotional upheaval that bewildered her doting husband, she disappeared one night and left no trace behind her.

Marguerite boarded a bus at random and landed at a metropolis several hundred miles away. Destitute and at a loss for anything else to do, she entered training in the nursing school of the municipal hospital under the name of Margaret Maclin—apparently to signify a compromise between paternal affiliation and Americanized emancipation. She found that the long hours, hard work, and unremitting responsibility afforded her relief and forgetfulness; she considered no duty too arduous, and soon won high favor. After graduation Marguerite was offered, and accepted, a desirable position on the hospital's nursing staff. This sinecure, however, proved a misfortune in disguise, for with the return of comparative leisure her vague restless, yearnings returned. Within a year, Marguerite was considering a second flight; she knew neither why nor whither. And then, Marguerite's inarticulate prayers seemed suddenly answered.

Burke first saw Marguerite at a nurses' dance, and promptly singled out the slim brunette as being eminently desirable. Waiting for no introduction, he swept Marguerite away from her friends and crushed her to him dance after dance. A crude, lumbering giant, Burke resembled Marguerite's physical image of her father only in his frank overbearing ruthlessness, but almost instantly she felt the same attraction to him that had drawn her irresistably, if only temporarily, to Giuseppe. Moving in a sort of trance, Marguerite followed Burke to a saloon, and then to his room. Here, however, she remembered that she was still a faithful Sicilian matron, and momentarily resisted. Burke, drunk and furious, beat her. Marguerite submitted, and found a transcending ecstasy of fulfillment she had thought never again to experience. Marguerite cried from pain and joy.

At Marguerite's suggestion, they lived together during the intervals Burke was in town from his interurban truck route. Marguerite seemed to have found her happiness, and, for a few months, her paramour too remained satisfied with the arrangement. Then Burke, following his custom in such affairs, began to bring home other women. Marguerite objected. Burke tried persuasion by methods he had hitherto found infallible, only to make the surprising discovery that Marguerite's sexual demands seemed to increase in direct proportion to the perversity of his requirements and the severity of his beatings. Completely puzzled, Burke admitted defeat and left town.

It is impossible to estimate to what Marguerite's remorse and sorrow might have led her had not fate now played a gambit inadmissable in fiction, but disconcertingly frequent in life. Three days after Burke's departure, there came into the emergency ward of her hospital a pale, pathetic derelict whom Marguerite recognized as Helene. Listlessly, Marguerite's sister told her story: She had been deserted by her seducer, had drifted through drink and thievery to narcotic addiction and prostitution. What matter? A street brawl had brought her in.

Marguerite took Helene to the apartment Burke had left. Tenderly, patiently she nursed Helene until once again there showed in her sister's face the swarthy smoothness reminiscent of a father whose memory Marguerite cherished. With health Helene also recovered the paternal Maglia disposition and was soon repaying Marguerite's solicitude with abuse and taking Marguerite's consequently redoubled loyalty for granted. At this point Burke, broke and out of a job, returned.

For a few weeks, Marguerite slaved for the two persons in all the world who most nearly filled her secret needs. Marguerite was happy and blind to the growing attraction between her charges. Fate, however, played no more tricks: When Burke and Helene eloped, the months of physical and mental overstrain finally told, and after an attempt at suicide, Marguerite was returned to her husband in Baltimore.

I was called into consultation and from various sources, pieced together Marguerite's history. I then spoke to her still devoted and bewildered spouse to the following effect:

"Mr. Chiappi, I know you love your wife, but to understand her you must know about her childhood. Her father was what most of us would consider a violent and some would call a perverted man, but he was all she had, and so she got used to his ways and even grew to like them so much that they seemed to her a necessary part of love. So, you must change your ways of treating her. You must learn to be more direct, more firm, more energetic. As you say in music, more *forte* and occasionally *sforzando.* Do you understand?"

Mr. Chiappi, a gentle soul at heart, had some difficulty understanding but finally in portentous silence, took Marguerite home. For a while, Mrs. Vanzetti objected to his newly energetic uxorial methods, but their results soon spoke for themselves. At latest reports, the Chiappi family is increasing, and Marguerite and her two swarthy sons seem relatively content.

With Adolf Meyer at Hopkins

It was under the tutelage of Adolf Meyer at the Phipps Psychiatric Clinic at Johns Hopkins University, that my vistas of psychiatry were opened. I knew that as the patriarchal dean of American psychiatry Meyer had attracted and trained Stanley Cobb, Franklin Ebaugh, Edward Strecker, Leo Bartemeier,

Lawrence Kubie, Robert Knight, Edward Billings, Spurgeon English, Maurice Levine and many others who were already leaders in the field, yet in personal appearance and manner Professor Meyer hardly appeared to be so charismatic a figure. Short, slight, spitz-bearded, painfully reserved, he spoke with a Swiss-German accent in long, orotund sentences sprinkled with obscure words and recondite allusions. When he talked of "anergasias," "dysergasias," "pathergasias," "holergasias," "neregasias," "oligergasias," "parergasias," and "thymergasias"—terms that could not be found in any dictionary—no student could know what this peculiar terminology meant; fortunately, some eventually learned (many never did) that Meyer was trying to replace the sterile pseudo-Linnaean stereotypes of "mental diseases" listed by Kahlbaum, Mayer-Gross, Kraepelin, et al., with a better understanding of how psychiatric patients, differentially but always "pluralistically," channelled their *ergs* or "behavioral energies." *Ergo, an*-ergasias connoted states of exhaustion; *dys*-ergasias were toxic reactions; *path*-ergasias, organic defects; and the rest in order were roughly translatable into psychoses, neuroses, intellectual defiencies, schizophrenias and affective disorders. Every human being, then, was seen to be capable of every possible form of reaction, simultaneously or in succession, and became "a patient" only when one or more of these modes of behavior became so deviant or excessive as to elicit cultural concern and require social readjustment.

Despite the inroads of psychoanalysis, avid disciples were still gathering about Dr. Meyer, certain that he would promote their careers to university chairmanships as he had done for their illustrious predecessors. Many close contemporaries, among them Oscar Diethelm, Wendell Muncie, Thomas Rennie and Theodore Lidz, were inclined to be a bit patronizing to those they considered less enlightened or in lower academic echelons, but were on the whole scholarly, dignified and dedicated men who later fulfilled much of their promise to American psychiatry. But there were a few who hardly seemed to fit The Hopkins. One such was Jerry Conn, shrewd, articulate and competitive; he became an advocate of authoritative hypnosis, which he used with predictable success in private practice.

Another was Norman Cameron, brilliant and literate, who, after his analysis became remote and retiring to the point of inaccessibility. But the most puzzling member of the coterie was Esther Richards, a stridently assertive dowager whose principle pedagogic pleasure seemed to be to hold "clinical conferences" in the Childrens' Outpatient Department to "demonstrate," in the presence of its distressed family as well as before her increasingly disbelieving and indignant students, that some deprived and mistreated child was a "hopelessly constitutional inferior who would always be a hopeless burden to society." Fortunately, my concurrent instruction in developmental psychiatry at the Bobs Roberts Children's Hospital under the benign direction of the gently avuncular Leo Kanner and his dedicated associates salvaged my conceptions as to what should constitute the rationale and practice of this subspeciality.

The most intriguing and instructive experiences at Phipps, however, were provided by Professor Meyer himself in his weekly Seminars in Psychobiology. Here literally anything from the metabolism of mice to Hegelian heuristics was discussed. In the former category, I recall a presentation by Curt Richter, director of the Phipps Animal Research Laboratory, in which he reported that when he made rats diabetic by removing their pancreases, and then offered the animals various foods, they spontaneously chose ratios of proteins, fats and sugars then considered the ideal diet for diabetic humans. Since the notion of a proper diabetic diet has changed considerably, I wonder what those of Richter's rats which had kept up with later medical reports would choose now.

More broadly stimulating were Meyer's excursions into the cerulean regions of philosophy. In one of these, devoted to the clarification of the epistemologic roots of consensual validation, he illustrated his points by holding out a blank card and expounding as follows:

> "Zis, ve agree, iss a vight card. But vhy do ve agree it iss a vight card? Because you see a mutually neutralized spectrum of colors und call it vight, and I see a neutralized spectrum and I call it vight, so ve

> agree vot is vight, und also vot is rectangular! Zen you touch it, und I touch it, und ve both know vot iss smooth, und cool, und so on, und so on. Und so if ve add the dimension of time do ve alzo haf common knowledge pluralistically about human actions and ergasias, und den ve can agree vot could be the best to do in psychobiological therapy."

The circle of disciples, arranged as always by hierarchic order alternately right then left from his chair, agreed in properly respectful turn with this logical excursion, quoting Aristotle, Aquinas, Spinoza, or anyone else they could think of to support it. However, when it got down to the outer tier where I sat, I recalled my more current readings in Whitehead, Calkins, Langer, Carnap, et al., and essayed the following comment:

> "But, Dr. Meyer, there seems to be a difficulty with that countersolipsistic position about which I would greatly appreciate your thought. You may see the card as green, and I might sense it as yellow, but if you called your green 'white' and I politely agreed to call my yellow 'white,' we could never really be certain we were perceiving or describing the same 'reality.' So also, you would call 'rectangular' what I might see as oval, and I would call 'rectangular' what you might see as round; or our 'smooth' might be your hot and my soft, and so on. Again we would 'agree,' but our 'consensual validation' would be merely verbal. How, then, can we really know and communicate a 'common reality'?"

There was a moment of awkward silence in the group after my brashness, but Professor Meyer, as always, was equal to the occasion. With a repressed twinkle, but with intellectual appreciation rather than pedagogic censure, he replied:

> "Dr. Masserman, I respect your ruminative thinking, but there is an old Sviss saying that perhaps you should remember: 'Vhere it does not itch, there is no need to scratch!' "

Although the itch, present then, has never quite abated, it took a number of years for me to realize the manifold wisdoms in Dr. Meyer's remarks. Among them: One can live and relate pragmatically in a world that is never completely tangible; questions about ultimates are not necessarily as searching as they might sound; and sometimes a bit of whimsey is the best coda to a futile dialogue.

Dr. Meyer's penchant for pertinent wit became evident on other quotable occasions. Once, after being introduced with somewhat embarrassing fulsomeness as speaker of the evening, he rose to the podium, gazed at the ceiling for a few seconds, stroked his beard reflectively and remarked to no one in general: "Praise, I suppose, iss like smoking—warm, soothing und satisfying. Und it may do little harm—if von does not inhale." But a much more impressive display of his talent for incisive parody occurred on a far different occasion. In 1950, Dr. Meyer was invited to attend an APA seminar on the topic, "What Are the Essential Qualifications of a Psychoanalyst?" Stanley Cobb of Harvard presided, and assorted analysts with assorted dialects had already spoken lengthily and sometimes not a little pompously to the effect that a psychoanalyst must possess one virtue above all, namely, integrity. Dr. Meyer had sat through all of this discussion apparently lost in his own thoughts. When invited to comment on the proceedings he at first demurred, but at the chairman's polite insistence he eventually got up, stroked his beard, and proceeded in his customary deliberate, imperturable manner.

In view of the fact, he said, that the Hippocratic Oath pledged *all* physicians to integrity, the speeches that evening had seemed a little redundant unless the psychoanalysts wished to differentiate themselves from the rest of the medical profession. That subtle point made, Dr. Meyer went on to develop what he thought *truly* characterized the analysts of the day—though, as will be seen, he did it in a manner few understood at the time. Stroking his Van Dyke and again lost in thought, he began (here I shall make no attempt to indicate his Swiss accent or *andante* tempo): "When I was a child [this was in itself a startling opening because few in the audience could conceive of Adolf Meyer's ever having been a child] . . . I had a profound belief in a Calvinist God. And when I wanted to do something different from what I had been taught, I would look up at God, and God would say, 'No!' [Here Dr. Meyer illustrated God's gesture by solemnly shaking his beard] . . . and so of course I wouldn't do it . . ." At this point Dr. Meyer had already taken about ten minutes, during which time many of his hearers had begun to wonder whether the aging dean of American psychiatry had gotten a little too old and tired to think clearly so late at night. But Dr. Meyer went on completely unperturbed: "As I got a little older . . . I gradually lost my faith in my childhood God. I finally knew this because now, when I would want to do something different and would look up at God and God would say, 'No,' I would go ahead and do it anyhow. . . ." This took another ten minutes, and by now more of the audience was really a little sorry for the aging patriarch who really should not have been invited to indulge in such public rambling. But Dr. Meyer went on: "Eventually I got to be a young man and I had to make a major decision. The decision was this: Was I going to be a religionist or was I going to be a scientist? I thought and I thought and I decided that if I were going to be a religious man I would be a Catholic, and if I were going to be a Catholic I would be a Jesuit. . . . But after thinking it over even more carefully I decided I was not going to be a religious man—either Catholic or Jesuit; instead, I was going to be a physician and a psychiatrist!" Here Adolf Meyer sat down. He was completely untroubled by the predominantly strained, puzzled, commisserative silence. But those of us who had spent three years learning to interpret the cryptic savant's wisdom thoroughly enjoyed yet another virtuoso performance.

He had implied, of course, that what really characterized the psychoanalysts of that day was not their vaunted "integrity," but the fact that many retained a childlike faith in self-imposed authority and therefore never deviated from official Freudian dogma. But this was hardly all: Not only did analysts constitute a quasi-religious cult, but, like Jesuits, they felt it their divine mission to spread their revelations lest the souls of the heathen unanalysed be forever lost. True, Dr. Meyer, as usual, had either overestimated or not been sufficiently concerned with the perceptiveness of his audience, but was there a better way to express a sage analogy?

My last contact with Professor Emeritus Meyer was much sadder, and occurred when I visited Baltimore some years after his retirement. As was my custom, I had called enroute through the city to pay my respects via the telephone, but unexpectedly, Mrs. Meyer, who answered, relayed a request from him to please come to their home. I did so, and after talking briefly with Mrs. Meyer, I sensed the situation. As noted, Dr. Meyer had been the center of a quite influential circle in American psychiatry, but after he retired from Phipps he had lost a great part of his national academic influence. Most of the people who had previously congregated around him had since become self-important in positions he had secured for them, somewhat forgetful of how much they owed to him. There were, indeed, few of us left who, contrary to the new fashion, still paid open respect to this retired scholar, and he recognized that I, though not among the major luminaries, was one of those few. He was lonely, and he wanted to reconstitute pedagogic associations that had once meant a very great deal to him.

Another aspect of this appeared when I was admitted to his presence. He was lying in an isolated upstairs bedroom, surrounded by his books and by various mementos of his public life—plaques, awards, and academic honors. He had obviously suffered an occlusion of the left middle temporal cerebral artery, and was partially aphasic and hemiplegic. However, he was sufficiently articulate to inform me that he had had an adverse neurologic diagnosis from someone who had not been trained at Hopkins and in whom he could not, therefore, "repose complete confidence." Then, still in his shy, courtly fashion he said (and I shall not attempt to convey his failing speech), "Dr. Masserman, I may hope to presume that you yourself were fairly well trained in neurology at Phipps as well as in psychobiology. May I ask you to please examine me to see whether or not this leg of mine, which had become slightly paralyzed after my mild stroke, is getting better fast enough?" It was obvious what he was seeking: a friend to reassure him and to welcome him back to physical and social recovery. I therefore did a careful examination and interpreted my findings as euphemistically as I could—or to put it more bluntly, I cheerfully equivocated about what was obviously a poor prognosis. Thus comforted, he began talking more freely to me, and as he spoke, he himself showed the failing powers of a truly remarkable mind. Among other examples of wishfully colored amnestic substitutions, he said, "I have just seen a review of your book in the *American Journal of Insanity.* It is an interesting book . . . but I do not believe it covered sufficiently . . . all the subjects it should have." (He was referring to my *Principles of Dynamic Psychiatry,* published in 1946, whereas the *American Journal of Insanity,* which he had edited, had actually ceased publication decades before.) "I think you did not stress sufficiently the many viewpoints of psychobiology. . . . In your future writings you will, of course, expand more on individuation and the ergasias? . . . It is my *Verdacht das heute oder morgen. . . .*" And his voice trailed off into the soft, then unintelligible Schweitzer Deutsch of his happier days.

Epitomized here were his fading efforts to perpetuate his intellectual heritage and to live vicariously in the minds and writings of loyal disciples. The last memories I have of Dr. Meyer are poignantly symbolic; his bed was placed against a west window. It was sunset. I had paid what proved to be my last respects to him and Mrs. Meyer; a few weeks later he died.

3. PSYCHOANALYTIC FANTASIES

"Americans are Jung and easily Freudened," wrote James Joyce.

When, at the invitation of Roy Grinker, I came to the University of Chicago from Hopkins in 1936, I was thirty years old and convinced—along with nearly every other restless and relatively young man in the field—that if I were to improve my future as a clinician, teacher, and investigator, I had to be "psychoanalyzed." With the tacit though hardly enthusiastic approval of Dr. Grinker (who had recently returned from six months of occasional sessions with Freud, and whose twelve-bed psychiatric ward I was now assigned to supervise), I applied for and miraculously was granted a Rockefeller Fellowship at the Chicago Psychoanalytic Institute. The grant furnished the Institute fifteen dollars per week for three of my analytic hours, provided I could pay the remaining three dollars per hour out of my $1800 annual salary. Even more incredibly, Dr. Franz Alexander, director of the Institute, who was also continuing Grinker's analysis, chose to be my analyst also (a bit of serendipity which Hugh Carmichael, a senior colleague who was assigned as analysand to the newly arrived Therese Benedek, apparently never accepted).

Franz Alexander proved to be a continually fascinating

and intriguing enigma. Robustly handsome, energetic, zestfully and wittily Hungarian, he was constantly torn between professional loyalties and intellectual probity. On the one hand he tried to maintain his position as a leading proponent of the Freudian School—then in its heyday—a role which had secured for him an historic appointment as the first Professor of Psychoanalysis at the University of Chicago and which had, despite his one-year academic debacle there, borne him to international fame. On the other hand, his keen, inquiring and charismatic mind could not really rest content with much of the dogma and procedural stereotypy of the "classical" school, so that he was ever proposing new formulations to be "tested" (he meant proved) by elaborately uncontrollable programs of "psychosomatic research," such as the administration of atropine "to counter vagal id-inhibition" and thus restore "instinctual sympathetic zest." Unsatiably avid of "dialogue" and "clarification" (read missionary zeal), he was forever traveling to meetings to converse with brilliant ambivalence (and with predictably little effect) with his more orthodox and eventually outraged colleagues, and writing books on his "theories as to" (he really believed them to be "demonstrations of") the "specific psychologic causes" of various physical illnesses or on the transcendent revelations contributed by psychoanalysis to the "dynamic understanding" of history, art, politics, war, etc. He was a man of such peripatetic and kaleidoscopic interests that my meetings with him—however irregular—invariably stimulated an evocative reexamination of my previously superficial assumptions as to my own knowledge, my academic, interpersonal and social motivations, and my resulting patterns of conduct.

My analysis began in late 1936, at a time when Alexander, as one of his many passing interests, was trying to "objectify" the analysis of dreams by having analysands recall the "manifest content" (M.C.) of any dreams they remembered since the last hour, "free associate" (Ass.) to the dream "elements" and then (with some prompting from Alexander) arrive at an "interpretation" (Int.). The analysand was then required to write this all down in duplicate and bring one copy to Alexander as data for his "dream studies." However, this research was never published because unlike Thomas French, Alexander eventually had to admit that there were too many interpersonal and other contingent variables involved. Fortunately or not, one feature made this chapter possible: the analysand was required to keep copies of his dream reports to review at the termination of his analysis. This I did for the year the project lasted, never consulted them again, and discovered the secreted manuscripts in an old file thirty years later. For what they are worth as whimsey and to indicate the reciprocal naïveté of my early analysis, I reproduce some of them here.

Dream Oct. 23, 1936

Manifest content: It is afternoon and I am in an unknown city in a strange hotel. My apartment, however, resembles my present one, except that the furniture is in disarray. I feel that H, who stayed with me the previous night, had left that morning to return to her parents in a distant city. I have an impulse to call her but, in order to save money, postpone the call. I began to write notes on a case history, but feel an urge to defecate. In order to do both, I take the history with me and sit on the toilet bowl, when the dream ends.

Associations: Strange hotel: places in which H and I have slept on our trips together. Disarray of furniture: disorganization of my personality structure during analysis. Loss of H: Diminution of guilt feelings as to my affair with H. Economy: My tendency to give my women presents and entertainment as a compensatory mechanism (however unsatisfactory) for withholding affection. Notes on Case History: My recent unadmitted deficiencies in presenting a case for Dr. Thomas French's seminar. Lavatory authorship: The worthlessness of some of my history notes.

Interpretation: I am becoming aware of the anal emotional miserliness which has heretofore resulted in lack of true devotion both to women and to my work. [I added later: "Am I not a good analysand?"]

Dream Nov. 12, 1936

Manifest content: I am living in an apartment which combines the features of my present one and the home my paternal grandparents had when I was eight to thirteen years old. I feel the threat of impending danger, after which smoke and flames begin to issue from the floor and walls. I think: "I must save what is most precious to me," and rush from the apartment carrying my violin.

Associations: Grandmother: The stories I had heard from my mother as to how my paternal grandmother had pampered me in my infancy. Fire: Danger. Violins: My narcissistic pride in my precocious violin virtuosity during adolescence—an ability I owed to my mother's encouragement and sacrifices.

Possible interpretation: Under the fire of the analysis which threatens to destroy my haven of refuge in the admiration and protection of my grandmother (equated with my mother), I attempt to rescue my somewhat regressive narcissism.

Dream Nov. 16, 1936

Manifest content: I see a piece of "halvah" (a Russian confection made of almond seeds and honey) covered and being made by "maggots of spiders."

Associations: Halvah: my favorite candy in childhood, and frequently bought with money my grandmother gave me. I still like it. My spontaneous interpretation of the dream as possibly denoting disgust with oral passive receptive tendencies uncovered during analysis. Spider: Black widow—Alexander's virago wife Anne (who once stalked into his office to upbraid him loudly over some domestic issue during my analytic hour). Maggots: Nonexistence of "spider maggots" (an intellectually appreciated connection between maggots and siblings).

Possible interpretation: Anticipatory insight into oral aggressive tendencies toward my brother as also revealed by recent associated disappointments in mother-images, such as Esther Richards.

Dream Dec. 14, 1936

Manifest content: I am driving toward the Baltimore City Hospitals on a road from Johns Hopkins University and have reached an underpass about six blocks away from my destination. In the car beside me are F.C. and a dog a resident had operated upon experimentally and killed at the Baltimore Hospital and had then taken to Hopkins for expert consultation on post-mortem findings. F.C. points out to me, however, that the dog is again showing signs of life and seems to be suffering. In alarm, I begin to pound the dog's head with a heavy object in order to kill it, but its eyes assume an expression so pitiable and appealing that I feel deep self-reproach and the dream ends.

Associations: The locus of the dream: a place I frequently stopped to buy milk to bring to my room at the Baltimore City Hospital. The car: a symbol of my narcissism, possibly also of my liaison with F.C. Baltimore City Hospital: a protective, sheltering institution which supported me, as contrasted to Hopkins, which represented intellectual competition and academic prestige. The Dog: symbol of that portion of my ego primarily interested in institutional security and physiologic research as opposed to the more abstract, difficult and individualistic pursuit of psychoanalysis.

Interpretation: A call to overcome the reemergence of oral receptive tendencies (equated with institutional research and the reviving, appealing dog) in order that I may attain adult independence and possibly marry F.C. This might settle my conflict between masculine protest and residual oral longings.

Dream March 27, 1937

Manifest content: There is a committee meeting (no date or place) to decide whether I am to be fired from a clinical job paying $1800 a year. I am waiting in great anxiety outside a transparent door leading into the committee room when a woman (unidentified) comes through the door; I wring my hands in supplication for her help.

Associations: The committee meeting: a similar meeting in Baltimore called to request the resignation of my chief Dr. Goldsmith. My lack of anxiety at the time, since I had already secured the University of Chicago residency and had a government appointment available in addition. The woman: Esther Richards, my mentor at Johns Hopkins, and Dr. Margaret Gerard, Grinker's assistant, who is similarly objectionable.

Interpretation: Disappointment in later mother images.

Dream April 27, 1937

Manifest content: I have killed a bull amid general disapproval.

Association: The bull: father; Grinker (bull in a china shop); Dr. Slight's failings ("Grinker's successor throws the bull"); Alexander ("he lets his seminar get full of bull").

Interpretation: Expression of unjustified hostilities toward all father-figures.

Dream Jan. 12, 1938

Manifest content: I observe a factory flying about above me while I lie on a couch. A small furry animal comes up to me, and I remember that it sprang from a cockroach I had crushed. Alexander and another man are playing chess in a corner of the room. I shout to Alexander, "I am hallucinating," and I am reassured by him.

Associations: Crushing the cockroach: childhood dream of a threatening snake that sprang from an earthworm I had crushed. Flying factory: recent refusal of an offer of marriage to a wealthy manufacturer's daughter. Chess: my father's game.

Interpretation: After rejecting a protective mother, I appeal for reassurance and security from my father, yet still feel threatened by his indestructible potency.

As my more-than-verbal insights progressed sporadically but profitably during the next three years, Alexander and I both saw with increasing clarity that these "dream analyses," like those submitted by other Institute candidates, generally included a not always personally or scientifically constructive desire to comply with intercurrent analytic theories and procedures. Dreams in general, then, were far from "a royal road to the Unconscious," whereas a searching scrutiny of one's overt and covert behavior in or out of the analysis revealed much more about the undesirable effects of concepts, relationships, values and goals set early in life and incompletely discarded or corrected.

In 1937, Grinker censured me because I would not resign my University appointment when he did and accompany him to a new Psychosomatic Institute at the Michael Reese Hospital—a decision which Alexander helped me reach and which I have never regretted. He was also wise in his counsels when my second marriage—which he had cautioned me against—ended in divorce three years later, and again in 1946 during my turmoil about choosing between Northwestern and New York University after Henry Brosin accepted the chairmanship at Chicago in 1946. My respect for Franz Alexander thus deepened over the years although, as indicated in the introduction I wrote to his and Selesnick's *History of Psychiatry,* it was never stultified by blind scientific discipleship. My last image of him at the age of sixty-seven is embodied in my preface to Volume VIII of *Science and Psychoanalysis:*

In Memoriam: Franz Alexander

On a sunlit first Sunday in March, 1964, I paid my respects to an inspiring teacher and warm friend at his mountain home in Palm Springs, and listened with the unique admiration that only Franz Alexander can evoke to the news that he had just been appointed to a specially endowed Franz Alexander Chair of Psychosomatic Medicine at the University of Southern California, that he would expand his discovery of a "new human typology based on differential somato-psychic reactions to anxious anticipations," that he planned to issue a new volume on Freud's correspondence, one on his own personal memoirs, and others already sketched—in short, that he would continue to be the ever youthful, energetic, eruditc, creative and progressive leader of American psychoanalysis. Exactly one week later, on a grey day in Chicago, our mutual friend Hardin Branch sorrowfully informed me by telephone from Salt Lake City that Franz Alexander, after a brief respiratory illness, had expired that morning.

To dedicate this volume as a memorial to Franz Alexander, Past President of the Academy of Psychoanalysis, may seem trifling in view of the fact that much of the literature of modern dynamic psychiatry and psychotherapy has been either directly enriched by his intrepid originality, clarity of thought, restless research, and charm of expression, or has flowed from the students he enthused, prepared for high places—and then liberated. Nor can this necessarily brief tribute review the zestful, colorful, ever-changing, and yet often troubled life of this scientific adventurer, endowed as he was with the spirit of the sixteenth, the intellect of the twentieth and the vision of the twenty-first century. The measure of his passing, however, is as great as this: those who knew Franz Alexander best will feel most keenly that an erudite scholar, a thoughtful observer and a wise leader has departed, leaving us all and forever a little poorer, a little sadder, and a little lonelier.

4. THE WRITING OF TEXTBOOKS

Behavior and Neuroses, my first monograph, received favorable reviews which encouraged me to essay more psychiatric writing. Published by the University of Chicago Press, the modest volume had been essentially a review of the literature on animal behavior seen in the context of my own experiments on how to influence "normal" and "neurotic" human conduct.* The ensuing *Principles of Dynamic Psychiatry,* however, was a psychiatric text radically different from others in the field in being based on the "principles" of (1) biologic motivation, (2) experiential individuation, (3) versatility of "normal" response, and (4) failures of adaptation under environmental unpredictability. Moreover, I had acquired the partial confidence to submit the manuscript not again to the dilatory University of Chicago Press, but to one of the most prestigious of medical publishers, W. B. Saunders Company of Philadelphia. To my surprise and delight, the manuscript was read and accepted within three weeks of receipt, leading to a flurry of correspondence totaling no less than fourscore and seven letters and replies over the first year, and tapering off only gradually during the succeeding seven. I immediately anticipated a second volume:

*For a review of this work and its later elaboration, see Chapter 21.

March 23, 1945

Mr. Lloyd G. Potter
Vice President and Editor
W. B. Saunders Company

Dear Mr. Potter:

Thank you for your generous comments on my manuscript; I know of no publisher with whom I would rather place the book. Since receiving your call I have therefore definitely refused another offer, recalled two other submissions and signed the enclosed contracts.

As I indicated over the phone, I thought it advisable to continue the exposition in another volume entitled *The Practice of Dynamic Psychiatry* so that students of psychiatry or graduate psychologists, social workers, sociologists, anthropologists and others interested in the fundamental principles of normal and abnormal behavior would not be frightened away by a formidably large and expensive book, half of which also dealt with the technical details of psychiatric diagnoses and therapy. Incidentally, I have had advance promises of adoption of Volume I from various schools—notably Hunter College, Cornell and Columbia.

Volume II is completely outlined, is about half written and will make a book about equal to the present one in length. It is based on the principles presented in Volume I, uses the same eclectic and integative approach, is richly illustrated with experimental and clinical material and will also, I hope, make a useful text for medical practitioners and younger specialists in neuropsychiatry. I plan to have it ready for you in about ten months.*

Whereupon I proceeded to enlist the aid of my friends:

*In this and all letters following, my signature and the complimentary close are omitted unless their function is more than conventional.

March 25, 1945

Dr. John Romano
Chairman, Dept. of Psychiatry
Cincinnati General Hospital

Dear John:

A couple of weeks ago I completed the manuscript of a new book entitled *Principles of Dynamic Psychiatry* and sent it to three separate publishers. A few minutes ago, I got a long-distance call from W. B. Saunders, who seemed enthusiastic about the book and is sending me a publication contract. He suggested, however, that it would improve the appearance of the book if I were to include a few illustrations.

The reason for this letter is now obvious: I would appreciate permission from you to use your series of three photographs illustrating regression in a schizophrenic girl. It is understood, of course, that the eyes of the patient will be blotted out to conceal her identity, that no identifying history will be furnished and that you will be given due credit and appreciation for furnishing the material. Moreover, if you have similar photographs or other illustrative material that you would care to have published under the same arrangements, I shall be very grateful for its use.

Dr. Romano sent me a triptych of photographs of a schizophrenic girl that so vividly showed her resumption of the childish dress and appearance preserved in a picture of her taken eighteen years earlier that the illustrations, now with his and my own permissions, has since been reproduced in eight other psychiatric and psychologic texts.

I notified the administration of the Division of Biological Sciences of the University of Chicago which, under the peonage "academic full time" contracts enforced at the time, might well claim all royalties:

March 24, 1945

To: Dr. Harrison
Dean of Biological Sciences
From: Dr. Masserman, Psychiatry

I enclose a copy of a letter from the W. B. Saunders Co. about the publication of my new book. I cleared with Chairman David Slight, the Dean's Office (Dr. Park, designated by Dr. Harrison), and the University of Chicago Press before accepting the offer, and trust that Saunders, as an eminent firm of medical publishers, will give the book a dignified promotion and distribution satisfactory to the University. The title page of the first volume will read: *Principles of Dynamic Psychiatry,* by Jules H. Masserman, M.D. From the Division of Psychiatry, Department of Medicine, and the Otho S. A. Sprague Memorial Institute, University of Chicago.

I received the following reply, credible only to those familiar with the quasi-paranoid administrative policies of the Division of Biological Sciences at the time: "Returned herewith is your letter which I have taken the liberty of copying for University files. As you realize, we are collecting such letters for possible future use in defense against unwarranted charges made against us."

While the manuscript was still subject to alteration, I submitted a copy to a respected friend and colleague, who praised it in general but pointed out that some passages were "too contentious . . . polysyllabic . . . recondite" or so "challenging" to accepted ways of thought that they "might confuse . . . or alienate instructors as well as students." I replied:

May 16, 1945

Dr. Maurice Levine
Chairman, Dept. of Psychiatry
University of Cincinnati

Dear Maurice:

Many thanks for your prompt preliminary criticism; I am sincerely grateful for them. In one sense, I have no defensive comments whatever, since if you have read all of Part I of my book and it does not answer your objections, then your criticisms are thoroughly valid and require appropriate revisions of the text. However, if you have not had sufficient time as yet to read through the book, I might explain further as follows:

First, the preface is intended for instructors in psychiatry rather than students, and perhaps had better be so titled—possibly as a means of assuring that the students themselves will read it. In the preface I attempted to refer to the problems all of us meet in training the students rather than professional personnel in the various fields. I think it undeniable that many of these students do come with such distorted ideas as to the nature of psychiatry, that the initial task of the teacher is to start considerably back from scratch for corrective reorientation. The problems referred to in the preface are, then, those of the many students who fall into this category through previously misdirected reading or through outmoded teaching in accordance with the usual texts of "abnormal psychology."

In this connection, too, the "abstruse" terms you criticize are definitely nontechnical and, I believe, are either already in the vocabulary of our students or would stimulate them toward differential thinking; in any case, they are defined, along with some 500 others in a simply worded, dynamically arranged glossary which I have just completed for the book. On this topic, however, I have another, perhaps wishful conviction: that our students—or those up to the recent war years—are really more intelligent and cultured, more amenable to rapid teaching and less demanding of simple spoon-feeding with non-nutritious pap than we usually give them credit for. All of this does not mean, however, that I shall not modify some of my terminology throughout the book in accordance with your excellent suggestions.

A second and more important point is this: I did not intend this to be an elementary textbook on psychiatry, and I do not anticipate that it will have any great success along that line. What I intended was considerably more idealistic and impractical; namely, an initial attempt at a housecleaning of our science—perhaps the one modern discipline most in need of thorough airing, disposal of trash, and installation of communications with its neighbors.

I am looking forward to your further readings in the book and I sincerely hope that you will continue to criticize its weaknesses as frankly as only one's friends can.

Gratefully,
Jules

The correspondence continued for weeks during which Dr. Levine, in a highly literate style and with a spirit of deeply concerned friendship, averred that the "task of housecleaning a discipline cannot be combined with instructing students," and that my book had a "lone-wolf feeling." More specifically, he was discerningly critical of my having subdivided "character defenses" (a term which I have since abandoned) into "normal" *vs* "abnormal," my having summarily rejected the concept of "masochism" and the "death instinct," etc. He also suggested that I should be "more gentle . . . in dealing with psychoanalysis" since it provided a "90% solid foundation . . . for the house of psychiatry," only the "superstructure of which needed 10% . . . of additions, strengthening . . . or rebuilding." I answered seriatim:

May 21, 1945

Dear Maurice:

I am really delighted with your comments, since they represent perhaps the most intelligent criticism of an attitude in psychiatry which I hope my book will help correct. To be very direct about it:

1. The present confusion in psychiatry is only increased by attempts to deny it and is something the student will not only find for himself, but will inevitably participate in unless his readings and experiences are broadly enough guided and integrated in advance. With such a preparation, he can then be referred to current advances in the literature, as I do at the end of each chapter.

2. Clarifying discussions are essential in textbooks. One does not have to be apologetic in pointing out, for instance, that despite Gall's lasting contributions to cerebral anatomy his formulations about "mental faculties" are no longer part of scientific psychiatry. Equivocation on such topics, I have found, is sooner rather than later detected by students, and their respect for psychiatry as a science—its solid good as well as its persistent bad—takes still another drop, however earnestly they may try to conceal it from teachers they like. What I wish above all to avoid is yet another book in the Kraepelin-Ebaugh-Strecker-Kraines-Noyes tradition. Someone with courage must make a break so long overdue.

3. This does not mean that the real contributions from any field should suffer expressed or implied blanket indictments. As you read further, you will find Pavlov, Meyer, Freud, Kretschmer, Kraepelin and many others (even Korzybski and Moreno) given due and sincere credit, with extensive references to their works. So also will you find plain and pointed criticisms of certain of their concepts followed—and this is most important—by attempts at dynamic integrations. As you can see, right or wrong, I am not at all in favor of the types of terminologic and conceptual compromise that you both admit and deplore in your own preface to *Psychotherapy in Medical Practice.* We can't ignore a tangle of overgrowth—we've got to clear it before we can build on the solid foundation beneath.

4. Again, I feel neither wolfish nor "alone." There are quite a few biologists, physiologists, neurologists, analysts, etc. here with whom I can talk profitably about many things, although I occasionally disagree with what I consider the many illogicalities and mentalistic naivetes of orthodox theory. The University community is intellectually stimulating and broadening in many ways.

As to the pedagogic "success" of the book, I am little

concerned. Contrary to my expectations, the Saunders Company—top-notch medical, but also hard-headed business publishers—anticipates an unusual sale of the book not only among physicians, psychologists and psychiatrists, but also as an undergraduate text; in fact, the book has already been adopted for psychology courses in eight premedical colleges. What concerns me much more are the ambivalences and rationalized anxieties among some of my own colleagues, although the true leaders have never been thus affected. Adolf Meyer, despite his arcane scholasticism, did an immense service by undermining the self-complacent errors of the old Kraepelinian nosology. Freud was intensely "polemic" in perhaps the most arrogantly possible way—by ignoring almost every other branch of biologic and psychologic science—and thereby created an antagonism that has unnecessarily disrupted the field and retarded optimum progress. Moreover, Alexander, French, Rado, Kardiner, and many other psychoanalysts have had the scientific honesty to abandon outmoded trial concepts in their own discipline and broaden their thinking through contacts with other fields of social science. True, they don't have as large practices or as many palpitant devotees as those who are given to polite and vaguely erudite obscurities, but they can enjoy feelings of forthrightness and integrity, and they eventually win scientific standing and respect.

Incidentally, I especially deplore the easy propensity of some analysts to attribute such convictions and reorientations variously to "father-identifications," "father-aggressions," "narcissistic omniscience," "incomplete analysis," *ad amusiam;* I might with equal *hubris* contend that they thereby exhibit their own defensive and cyclic thinking. Too many men who otherwise might have made original and lasting contributions became subject to these complacent rationalizations.

Incidentally, you may like to know that you are the only authoritative person who has had a prepublication opportunity to examine the book, and that the entire manuscript was written in four months of odd hours taken from an extremely busy schedule—a fact I hadn't stated before to avoid any mitigation of your criticisms. I look forward to more of them.

To a request from the publisher's advertising director as to publicity for the *Principles,* then in press:

November 19, 1945

Dear Mr. Williams:

If you will permit the ungraceful (and, I suppose, impossible) gesture of casting modesty aside, I can answer your questions about *Principles of Dynamic Psychiatry* by saying that the book differs from the usual psychiatric texts in the following respects:

History: The history of psychiatry is presented not as a mere chronologic account, but as an analysis of the development of the modern science of behavior in relation to the evolution of other biologic and medical knowledge.

Scope: Nearly all of the leading systems of modern clinical psychology and psychiatry are presented, including behaviorism, semantics, psychobiology, psychosomatics and the various current schools of psychoanalysis and psychotherapy. Each is given a sympathetic but objective evaluation, their differences and similarities are analyzed, and finally, each is translated into biodynamic and medical terms and so assigned to its place in modern psychiatry.

Clinical Applications: Despite this basically scientific and integrative orientation, the book is predominantly gauged to the needs of those who must learn the rationale and practice the techniques of psychotherapy. For this reason the neuroses and character deviations are given extended consideration, and those aspects of the psychoses that are of especial relevance are emphasized. Similarly, the fundamentals of every mode of psychotherapy from environmental manipulation to formal psychoanalysis are clearly stated and then specifically evaluated.

For these reasons, the volume should be of value to prospective users as follows:

For students of psychology, medicine and the social sciences, the book will serve as a text which summarizes much of the current knowledge in clinical psychology and dynamic psychiatry. Students will find especially helpful the logical organization of the work, the use of simple experimental examples or clear-cut case histories to illustrate difficult points, the lists of recommended readings at the end of each chapter, the Bibliography of some twelve hundred titles, the detailed Index, and the complete Glossary containing explicit and meaningful definitions of over a thousand current technical terms in psychology, psychiatry and psychoanalysis. These and other features of the book are the outcome of the author's fifteen years of experience as a full-time teacher of medicine, neurology, psychiatry and psychoanalysis at three Universities in the country.

For the general physician the book will clarify many recent advances in psychiatry and present a scientific basis for the practice of psychosomatic medicine and effective psychotherapy for many of the behavior problems he meets daily in his patients.

For the psychiatrist and psychoanalyst the volume will prove interesting as a basically original reevaluation and reintergration of the various theories in their specialty (and perhaps a partial solution for some of their current controversies) by an author who has had intensive personal training in comparative psychology, psychobiology and psychoanalysis, and who has contributed much research in each of these fields. Psychiatrists faced with the task of presenting courses in these subjects will find the book useful as a text or as a convenient basis for special series of lectures.

Finally, anthropologists, sociologists, economists, linguists, personnel counsellors and others concerned with the dynamics of human behavior will find many sections of the book directly relevant to their special interest and a ready source of authoritative information.

All this has been difficult to write, since it very probably exaggerates the merits of the work. In any case, I am certain of your good judgment in keeping the publicity factual and restrained.

A subsequent letter from Robert Rowan, sales manager at Saunders:

June 15, 1945

Dear. Dr. Masserman:

Let me report that the book did a surprisingly healthy business at the American Medical Association meeting in Atlantic City last week. As a matter of fact, we sold very nearly as many copies at the AMA as we did at the APA, which is a nice compliment because, as you know, the only psychiatrists who frequent the AMA sessions are those who have run out of free samples of Gelusil or have been washed back up on the beach after a too lively session at the Devereaux School soiree.

Best,
Bob

Other comments on the *Principles* from colleagues—some of them leaders in psychiatry:

January 1, 1944

My dear Jules:

I was delighted to receive a copy of your new book, and I want to thank you from the bottom of my heart. I shall find it very helpful in teaching my students here at the Winter General Hospital. The organization of it intrigues me very much and I am sure that it is a step forward in the presentation of psychiatric material. It pleased me immensely and I am intrigued and interested and eager to read it.

Let me take this occasion also to extend to you and Christine the best wishes of myself and my wife for the best new year you have ever had.

Sincerely yours,
Karl A. Menninger, M.D.

January 7, 1945

Dear Dr. Masserman:

Some days ago I received the volume of your book *Principles of Dynamic Psychiatry* and found it extremely interesting. If you will not think this crass flattery, which it is not, may I say that I think it is the first thoroughly comprehensive and well written document dealing with modern psychiatry. I cannot praise it too highly—it is a real contribution and one you should be very proud of having written.

Sincerely yours,
Harry C. Solomon, M.D.
Chairman,
Dept. of Psychiatry
Harvard Medical School

December 27, 1945

Dear Dr. Masserman:

If you keep on this way, you will eventually get me educated. I am grateful for your earnest and generous efforts.

Sincerely yours,
Robert M. Hutchins,
Chancellor
University of Chicago

As their new editorial consultant, I was asked by the Saunders Publishing Company for advice as to a proposal by Dr. Levine that he edit for them a "definitive" *Compendium of Psychiatry by One Hundred Authors.* I counselled:

John L. Dusseau
Vice President and Editor
W. B. Saunders Company

Dear John:

As to Maurice Levine's project for a "definitive" multi-authored *Compedium of Psychiatry,* here are the "essential considerations," con and pro, you request with the inevitable treble overtones of "as I see them":

Con: (*a*) As you say, psychiatry is not as yet ready for definitive formulation by any one person or any hundred, and in the latter case the permutations of inconsistencies and contradictions would become almost infinite.

(*b*) The chapters thus loosely assembled would fill volumes, which might be bought by a few of each author's students as an external sign of interest, and even read by some.

(*c*) There already exists a plethora of compendia in psychiatry: *vide* the volumes edited by Alexander, Hoch, Zubin, et al. For eight years I've written the chapter on "The Neuroses" in Spiegel's annual *Progress of Neurology and Psychiatry;* Spiegel has an otherwise fine stable of perennial experts, but even so the work is used only as a reference.

And yet, Pro: (*a*) Maurey Levine is a good friend of mine, intelligent, hardworking, and considerably ahead of his successfully routine *Psychotherapy in Medical Practice* of 1943. He'd make a competent and careful editor.

(*b*) If Saunders doesn't help edit and publish the projected work, someone else less conscientious and capable will—and I'm for preventing all such public danger.

Ergo, on the whole, I'm inclined favorably, even though I have just included in the first draft of my *Practice of Dynamic Psychiatry* a review of most of the leading psychodynamic theories and techniques now in use, so that you may wish to glance through my manuscript to see if there would be any competition or duplication.

As to republishing a German book in English:

May 11, 1946

Victor Frankl's *Medical Psychotherapy,* according to the unsigned review you sent me, is concerned with the philosophy of existentialism, a school of thought dating from Nietzsche through Kierkegaard to its present expressions by Sartre in France and Jaspers in Germany. As applied to psychiatry by Frankl, this philosophy ostensibly discards abstractions and attempts to deal with "actual being"—although, in some respects, it is in itself essentially mystic. Frankl stresses each individual's "liberty of decision," "responsibility to fate," and a unique "sense of suffering" which gives life its "form" and endows each individual with a sense of human value. Therapeutically, this is applied by increasing the patient's capability for and acceptances of inevitable suffering.

In essence, Frankl is concerned with an introspective and fatalistic type of thinking now current among the intelligentsia of Europe who have withstood the harrowing experiences of war. The book will undoubtedly be of interest to philosophers and a limited number of sociologists and psychiatrists in this country, but I doubt whether it would have a wide appeal. Incidentally, the review also states that a French edition is already in press.

I regret that the facts at hand make it impossible for me to give you a more specific opinion, but if you can secure a copy of the book, I shall be glad to advise further.

Now John L. Dusseau, editor-in-chief at Saunders, elisively complained to me about the "possibly pretentious polysyllabic prolixity" he "sometimes found in the writings of *other* authors." He hoped he would not "shock me into stunned and depressive agitation" by implying that this might be relevant to my writing a second volume on the *Practice of Dynamic Psychiatry.* He ended his "Dear Jules" letter with the following story:

Under the joint sponsorship of the American Association for the Advancement of Science and the American Institute of

Textbook Publishers a la-de-la symposium was recently held on effective technical writing. The conference herded along under the tight rein of Rudolph Flesch and his disciples who espouse "the cause of clarity." After a suitable number of papers and corresponding debate and discussion, certain more or less obvious principles of writing and mechanical criteria for its evaluation were formulated. The delegates, happy in fulfillment and censure, were about to depart. Rose up then an elderly, distinguished, unknown man who spoke as follows:

> "Ladies" [for such indeed were present] "and gentlemen," he said. "After due deliberation we have enunciated certain methods, guides, and signposts for good technical writing. These have an apparent foundation in fact and a seeming validity. Unfortunately they are all overthrown, defied, and reduced to rubble by a single interesting example of technical writing. The tortured prose and elusive meaning of the book I have in mind makes mincemeat of everything we have formally concluded. Nevertheless, it is the finest piece of scientific writing I know of. Its hard reading will repay all effort, will stimulate the mind and encourage the spirit. It is the *Principles of Dynamic Psychiatry* by Dr. Jules Masserman."

A curious episode. How is Volume II coming? Have you concluded that therapy should be in and of it?"

Cordially,
John L. Dusseau
Managing Editor
W. B. Saunders Co.

January 8, 1954

Dear John Lorelei:

That story of yours is probably apochryphal, and therefore, all the more intriguing. But it may be compared to the comment of a friend of mine—I have many such—who introduced me to a large audience by commenting that my books were being translated into French, Japanese, etc., and then turned to me and somberly requested the right to translate them into English.

Your former letter (which, I repeat, I sincerely appreciated) did indeed throw me, as you hoped, into a depressive agitation. However, the depression was manifested mainly by a tendency to lounge in an easy chair with a wide arm for writing, and the agitation by motions of the right hand over virgin paper. Helos and Hippocrates willing, I hope thus to get the Vol. II hewn in the rough, then spend much of the summer aboard the good yawl Naiad joining, chipping, rounding, sanding, and polishing. Come keep the Naiad company; somebody should keep her happy sailing while I work.

The cover letter on my 2400-page manuscript of the *Practice of Dynamic Psychiatry* ready eight months later:

October 5, 1954

John L. Dusseau
Vice President and Editor
W. B. Saunders Company

Dear John:

I suppose you've had authors tell you that finishing a manuscript is like delivering a baby in that you don't feel like putting it back and doing it better, and you want all extrauterine operations done by somebody else. But, to discard that corny metaphor, my attitude toward your prospective editing is this: Poor ideas should be joyously eliminated; fair ideas should be stated once; exceptionally good ideas may occasionally be repeated, but only if really necessary in other contexts. I look forward to having this trimming done by you and Miss Dietz while I dispose of my end of the placenta.

In the *Practice* I reported an address I had presented to a medical audience—a bit of whimsey that has ever since elicited reactions ranging from Rabelaisian raillery to regretful reproaches. The account ran as follows:

The Psychosomatic Profile of an Ingrown Toenail

Let us consider what Bacon would have called one of our Idols of the Marketplace—the current adoration of a Janus-faced concept called Psychosomatic Medicine. The worship of this idol is, as we well know, conducted in dedicated meetings of the faithful and according to a somber litany composed chiefly of resounding and felicitous ambiguities. Please do not misinterpret my serious sentiments in this sphere; during 20 years of research I myself have been seeking to clarify the principles that simultaneously apply to both external and internal (*i.e.,* "psychosomatic") behavior, and my own first and still incompletely regretted contribution to psychoanalytic literature concerned an investigation of what might be called the bio-dynamics of anorexia nervosa. Yet during the past decade I have watched with increasing concern the development of what appeared to be quite another form of "psychosomatics," namely, the derivation of seemingly specific "profiles" and "psychodynamic formulae" for quite nonspecific and variable disorders of total function. In many such exercises it seemed to me that little more had been done than select some particular facet of everyone's experience, utilize an inexhaustibly free-wheeling but unprecise vocabulary of terms, and thus derive some "psychosomatic formula" or other whose acceptance depended on its superficial plausibility and the impossibility of determining its validity, its relevance, or even its meaning by any truly objective clinical or experimental test. Some time ago, when I was particularly bemused by this problem, I was, of all people, invited to lecture before a group of internists on the general topic of psychosomatic medicine. I accepted, in the hope that I could share my tribulations with my audience and that in this manner we might once again approach a clearer understanding. Let me here recount briefly the story of that lecture and its almost incredible denouement.

Consider, I said, the toenail. Anthropologists have pointed out that man's mind developed when his arms were freed of the task of locomotion so that he could walk about the earth in an upright position, manipulating its resources and thinking about the heavens. Moreover, osteologists tell us that all of this in turn depended upon the hallux and its toenail. But, libidinally speaking, the nail represents even more than this. Actually, it is the most protuberant part of the body, hard and rounded; in locomotion it describes a most suggestive to-and-fro movement—obviously, then, it is a basic phallic symbol displaced, for a change, downward. But let us also remember the anatomic origin of this important little penis, namely the *nail-bed*—also a most significant term. This in turn consists of an *invagination* of vascular tissue into a zone called, with intuitive propriety, the *stratum germinativum* or *matrix*—a region consummately feminine in its conformation, physiology, and import. Here, then, we have a psychosomatically significant microcosm; a womb-equivalent ever generating a masculine imago which goes forth to meet, explore, and conquer the external world.

But now consider what happens when this normal functioning is disrupted by frustration and conflict: when, specifically, the erect nail is stubbed and traumatized, or is too long opposed by unyielding reality in the form of a repressive shoe. Clinically and perhaps personally we know the effects all too well: the nail, particularly at the peripheral portions of its individuality (or more technically, its "ego boundaries") turns about and digs its way back into the flesh of its origin. To those properly indoctrinated with psychosomatic understanding, however, a much deeper significance can be discerned in this process. It will be obvious, indeed, that the counter-cathected ungual masculinity, blocked from its exteriorizing libidinal outlets, introverts upon itself and eventually even seeks final regression through the mechanism of re-encapsulation and vascularization—*i.e.,* a return to uterine existence. This formula, derived as it is by analogic thinking enlightened by metapsychologic insight, could of course stand on its merits alone about as well as others derived from similar research endeavors; fortunately, however, it can be further validated by objective clinical observation. Thus, it can be demonstrated that analysands of both sexes with ingrown toenails actually *do* have masculine aspirations and intra-uterine fastasies, and the mere fact that analysands *without* ingrown toenails have the same unconscious dynamisms serves merely to emphasize once again how the study of the abnormal can reveal profound truths about all mankind.

Here I ended my Lecture on Psychosomatics, rewarded by what I thought was an understanding gleam in the eye of some of my listeners and trusting that I might have aroused a healthy whimsey of doubt about some of the verbal gymnastics that pass for serious thinking and investigation in the field. Imagine my consternation, therefore, when on meeting some of the members of the audience days and weeks later I was actually congratulated on the clinical and analytic perspicacity with which I had derived the specific dynamic formulae for the etiology and possible therapy of that hitherto unexplored psychosomatic disorder—the ingrown toenail!

It was I, then, who had been naïve in so casting my discourse. I had not recognized how precious and ingrained was the power of the Word and the Formula; how avidly even trained and intelligent physicians will cling to the belief that, if only they can evolve and invoke the proper incantation, large or small diseases from onychocryptosis to alopecia can be magically exorcised and made to vanish on command.

After the *Practice* was published, I began work on a revised edition of the *Principles*. This was to be repeated periodically, sometimes less speedily than others:

March 22, 1960

Dear Jules:

I look forward with pure pleasure to talk and dinner with you and Christine on Wednesday, the 30th. I must confess, though, to the merest shade of a shadow of suspicion of your motives. I envision the evening like this.

I will stop by your office at 5:30. We shall then drive along the lake and you will discourse of the civic improvements lately visited upon Chicago and of future betterments to come. The Chicago drivers will courteously nudge over to the right to better expedite our sedate but swift progress on the left. A balmy breeze from the lake will bring nostalgic memories of ocean trips and oil tankers, and already a kind of subtle euphoria will have seized me.

We shall arrive. That big fat Irish doorman will somehow convey the impression that his day—perhaps even his week—has been made by our mere arrival.

We shall ascend with all the mechanical marvels of a scientific age at our disposal to this purpose. We shall then look out over the yacht basin and see the Naiad gleaming in the last rays of that sunset which is vouchsafed to rich and poor alike. This too will bring back tranquil recollections of past pleasure.

Then you and Christine will tell of your trip to Jugoslavia and of calm sailing off that beautiful coast and will speak too of your side excursions to Minsk and Pinsk. All the while we shall be sipping away at those behemoth-sized new-fashioned glasses for which you are distinguished. The soft warmth of the evening will bead the glasses with a gentle dew fragrant of fine whisky—the outward and visible sign, one might say, of an inward and spiritual beauty.

At this point I might well plunge into a detailed account of the chances of the White Sox to recapture the pennant and of Stevenson to recapture the nomination.

Dinner is announced. We sit down to elegant and exquisitely prepared food. Pauline will have outdone even Pauline. Hers are not perils but pearls.

I now light up a long, thin, green-tinted Havana cigar. Its fragrance lends added gravity to the weighty words I am about to pronounce.

They should be these: "Well, Dr. Masserman, what excuse can you offer for failure to conclude your revision on time?"

But all the foregoing will stick such words in my throat. Instead, I should not be surprised to find myself saying, "Well, Jules, I certainly can understand why the revision isn't finished. Perhaps by this time next year we may have the first two or three chapters."

Even the most seductive temptations should not lead an editor from the conviction that nothing—but nothing—is of sufficient importance to interrupt the steady progress of book writing. In short, I shall have failed in my duty.

Well, Dr. Masserman, what excuse can . . .

The anticipation alone is enough to stifle such hard thoughts.

Gratefully,
John

Six months later:

September 16, 1960

Dear John:

Herewith.

If you can control the immediate wild yen for Yucatan that a first glance at the manuscript might evoke, an intrepid second look will reveal that the book has been considerably lightened by tossing overboard two of its outdated chapters; flinging after them 32 Kgm or so of *neverthelesses* and *moreovers* (some seem to have fallen into your Suggestions for the Preparation of Manuscripts) plus a disconcerting number of redundant words, phrases, clauses, paragraphs, and overweighted ideas. The text is now comprehensible in places.

The waterline trim has been restored by a proper distribution of sections on communication theory, sensory deprivation, existentialism, phenomenology, drugs, and other topics of current and probably sustained interest; a new appendix on the contributions of modern ethology to behavior theory; a fairly unstultified chapter on an evolutionary and integrative appraisal of psychiatric therapy and a preface proclaiming these achievements with charming modesty. Selah.

Cum apologia,
Jules

John's commentary:

November 4, 1960

Dear Jules:

It was good of you to let me have the new section on [Office Therapy of Psychosomatic Disorders] and I thoroughly enjoyed reading it.

It happened at the time that I was reading part of a so-so manuscript on management of psychic disturbances by the general physician. The contrast between this dull presentation and your own chapter was startling. He too spoke of the harm the physician's words may do; but you said, "An overlong and seemingly over-concerned ophthalmoscopic examination may signify to our patient that we are gazing straight through the window of his brain at a cerebral tumor. A dolorous shake of the head as we fold the stethescope after listening to his chest —no matter what is said afterward—may mean to him that our all-perceptive ears have heard the footsteps of approaching death." He also spoke of the harm the physician's hands may do; but you said, "It is little excuse that many frightened, lonely people who employ hypochondria as their main mode of supplication for concern and help are willing to submit to— and may for a time feel relieved by—the most drastic forms of expiative sacrifice and suffering, or that patients who would rather have their abdomens than their eyes opened may actually welcome hospitalization, surgery, and protracted and certified invalidism. But we must control our *furor chirurgensis* and, as curators of our patients' ultimate welfare, beware of the futility of waving scalpels as though they were magic wands."

O well, I don't really think his was much of a manuscript anyway. . . . In case you are becoming anxious about progress on your next edition, you will want to know that Helen is hourly expected back from Europe primed to the manifold tasks ahead—manifoldest of all, your mansuscript.

Cordially yours,
John

The years passed, and as I became involved in other writings for other publishers, correspondence with John Dusseau and Bob Rowan became less frequent and finally ceased. Which was, and is, a pity.

5. AN ABANDONED MOORING, AND SQUALLS ON THE WAY TO A NORTHWESTERN HARBOR

In 1946, I decided to leave the University of Chicago, impelled not only by the niggardly salary and research stipends ($6,000 per year plus $3,000 research support while I was turning over to the university over four times that amount in patients' fees, book and film royalties, and honoraria from lectures elsewhere) but also by the objectionable maneuvers on the part of the administration that deposed Dr. David Slight, then Chairman of Psychiatry.

I had attempted to enter war service:

October 11, 1943

The Surgeon General
U.S. Public Health Service
Bethesda Station
Washington, D. C.

Sir:

I should like to accompany the enclosed application for a commission in the U. S. Military or Public Health Services with a fair statement as to my intentions.

During the past two years I have been devoting as much

of my time and effort as possible to the full-time teaching of clinical and military psychiatry to medical students and Army medical officers, in basic neuropsychiatric research, as consultant in psychiatry to the Selective Service System, and as chairman of the Morale Division of the Office of Civil Defense.

The National Office of Procurement and Assignment and the University of Chicago have declared these activities essential to the war effort, but I feel that should my training and qualifications make my presence elsewhere more valuable to my country, I shall be happy to be appointed to duty here or abroad, and for the duration or permanently as required. The only criterion for my acceptance of a commission, then, would be an assignment that would justify resigning my present duties and my responsibilities to the University.

Respectfully,
Jules H. Masserman, M.D.

N.B.: The report of my physical examination is being forwarded separately.

The denouement:

Chicago 37, Illinois
June 20, 1944

Colonel William C. Menninger, M.C.
War Department, Army Service Forces
Office of the Surgeon General
Washington 25, D. C.

Dear Colonel Menninger:

I regret that I have been unable to write you sooner and that I missed seeing you in Chicago. But perhaps in view of our recent correspondence, it would be fair to inform you of the latest developments at the University of Chicago with regard to my enlisting under your command.

During the past four years, four of the eight members of our psychiatric staff have left the University for various reasons. This year I, too, sent in my resignation three months ago in preparation to entering the military services. Since then, however, Dr. Charlotte Babcock and Dr. Jay McCormick, the only others remaining on the staff, have also resigned to enter private practice, leaving Dr. Slight to face the necessity of actually closing down the department with its teaching and clinical as well as research services should I, too, leave. You can therefore understand the pressure that has been put upon me by Dr. Slight—to whom I owe considerable loyalty—and by the administration to remain here until replacements can be found to maintain the teaching of medical students and the minimal clinical services necessary to the University.

As I wrote you, my personal inclinations have been to leave, but it now seems impossible for me to do so for the time being. I have therefore agreed to postpone my resignation for several months at which time, should you still need my services, I plan to be available. My best personal regards.

Respectfully,
Jules H. Masserman, M.D.

Copy of letter from the American Medical Association with reference to one activity of my Morale Division:

21 January 1946

Dean Wendall Harrison
Division of Psychiatry
University of Chicago
Chicago, Illinois

Dear Dr. Harrison:

In a series of electrical transcriptions about health problems of adults we scheduled Doctor Masserman for an interview on wartime mental hygiene. He took such great interest, and so liberally offered his cooperation in going further with the idea that we asked him to be interviewer on a series of dramatized mental hygiene transcriptions for radio use by our local medical societies. In the development of this series Doctor Masserman devoted a great deal of time to our script writer in the preparation of scripts. He procured the cooperation of eleven other psychiatrists, who furnished script material and were summarizing authorities for the program. He took so much of the work of procuring and organizing the medical cooperation that the whole program went off with extraordinary smoothness and a minimum of errors as far as this bureau is concerned.

The programs turned out excellent and are meeting with approval wherever they have been broadcast. We made twenty-five sets of electrical transcriptions of which sixteen have been loaned. Since we have an average of eighty outlets per week, it is a reasonable presumption that these programs will be broadcast from ninety times upwards over the entire United States.

Please accept this communication as an indication of our sincere appreciation for Doctor Masserman's contribution, without which we could hardly have accomplished what we did.

Sincerely,
W. W. Bauer, M.D.
Director of Public Education
American Medical Association

With reference to a later offer of a Professorship of Psychiatry at the University of Utah, Dr. Slight wrote the recommendation when my services were no longer essential to him:

Dr. M. M. Wintrobe
School of Medicine
Salt Lake City 5, Utah

Dear Doctor Wintrobe:

I am writing you on behalf of Dr. Masserman, with whom you have recently had some correspondence with reference to the possibility that he might come to Salt Lake City.

I need not tell you of Dr. Masserman's excellent training, which he will give you in detail, or of the fact that he is qualified in all respects as a psychiatrist of national standing. As to his two recent books, I can only add my voice to the reviews which they have received throughout the country as to their excellent worth and to the fact that they are both noteworthy contributions in the development of modern psychiatry.

I should like to speak more of Dr. Masserman from a personal standpoint, insofar as he has been associated with me since my coming to the University of Chicago in 1936. Dr. Masserman has proven himself an excellent teacher in both didactic and clinical presentations at all the levels of our teaching in the medical school program. His other colleagues, and especially the students, have attested many times to his excellence in this regard. He speaks very well in public and always makes an orderly and clear presentation of his subject, which is invariably stimulating and illuminating, and hence the appreciation of his efforts that I have mentioned.

Dr. Masserman has taught in other courses on the campus, as for example, to psychiatric social workers in training in the Social Service Administration, and he has conducted clinical conferences and discussion groups in the departments of sociology and human development, and in other departments which have been interested in the field of human relations. He has continued to be an active and stimulating agent to his colleagues in those other fields and has been of great service to them in an advisory capacity in their work, as well as a stimulating influence in those aspects of their work which called for guidance and elucidation from a psychiatric standpoint.

I should have indicated earlier that Dr. Masserman is an excellent clinician of great diagnostic skill. He has proven himself to be an excellent therapist and has much experience in all forms of psychotherapy and has achieved splendid therapeutic results in the practice of all these forms of psychotherapy. As a clinician, he has always been cognizant of the general medical aspects of the patient's problems, which is always a challenge to a psychiatrist in a general hospital, and I can safely say that he has always had the confidence and respect of his general medical colleagues in such matters.

In this Division, we have taken an active part in the various social agencies and medical societies directly connected with psychiatry and also those with interests in allied fields, such as sociology, criminology and the like. Dr. Masserman has taken an active role in various of these organizations and in connection with one of them, The Chicago Society for Personality Study, has, one might say, carried the whole organization for several years past.

I trust that there may be a favorable opportunity in psychiatry for Dr. Masserman with you in Salt Lake City and if so, I would highly commend him for your favorable consideration in any such post or opportunity.

Yours cordially,
David Slight, M.D.
Professor and Chairman of Psychiatry
University of Chicago

The position was offered, but the Mormon milieu seemed less than optimally favorable for free teaching and research. I therefore considered another offer in New York:

March 25, 1946

Dr. Florence Powdermaker,
Director of Personnel
Veterans Administration Headquarters
Washington, D. C.

Dear Dr. Powdermaker:

Thank you for your prompt and considerate letter. Dr. Howard Potter wired me that the faculty at Long Island has voted me an appointment as Professor of Clinical Psychiary, and in a covering letter he outlined the psychiatric facilities at the school (which sound very promising) and his desire that I undertake clinical, research and teaching duties there.

If I accept a full-time appointment at Northport, is it possible for me to spend enough time at the college to satisfy Dr. Potter's and my own obligations to the school in teaching and research? I am almost certain I could also get Foundation grants to help research at the College—something in which Dr. Potter is interested. Finally, a minor point, but important to one who has lived on an unsupplemented academic salary for lo! these many years; are there partial allowances to cover the expense—rather heavy these days—of moving to Brooklyn to Northport?

April 1, 1948

The General Superintendent
Department of Parks
New York, New York

Dear Sir:

I have been offered the post of Professor of Psychiatry at the Long Island College of Medicine and am planning to move to New York. Being an ardent yachtsman, I would greatly appreciate any information you could give me about the facilities for the mooring and storage of sailboats in or around Brooklyn and Queens. I should be glad to pay for charts, booklets or other material.

Eventually, however, Christine and I decided that we did not wish to leave our home and friends in Chicago, especially since Dr. Lewis Pollock, then Chairman of the Department of Neurology and Psychiatry at Northwestern University, offered me a most attractive academic appointment, and Dr. Clarence Neymann generously shared his private office and patient fees with me to tide us over the financial shoals. Concurrently, Dr. Frances Gerty, regional director of Veterans Administration Training, appointed me to initiate and develop a residency training program at the Downey V. A. Hospital.

This training program proved so rapidly successful that when Dr. Benjamin Boshes succeeded Dr. Pollock at Northwestern in 1948, he accepted the Downey program as a basis for building one at the university. Grants were applied for and received for research and training at my new post.

October 25, 1946

Dr. Robert H. Felix
U.S. Public Health Service
Bethesda, Md.

Dear Dr. Felix:

As you may know, I have left the University of Chicago to accept the following appointments: assistant professor in the Department of Nervous and Mental Diseases, Northwestern University School of Medicine; senior consultant, Veterans Administration, Chicago; research associate, Chicago Psychoanalytic Institute.

The first position affords excellent facilities, already arranged, for continuing my research in experimental neuroses in collaboration with Dr. Lewis Pollock, Professor of Neuropsychiatry, Dr. Wendell Krieg, Director of the Institute of Neurology, Dr. H. W. Magoun, Professor of Neuroanatomy, and Dr. William Hunt, Professor of Psychology, all of the Northwestern Faculty.

The second and third appointments make possible intensive clinical studies in collaboration with the personnel of the Veterans Administration (particularly at the Downey Hospital where I am in charge of postgraduate training and research) and with Dr. Franz Alexander and the staff of the Chicago Psychoanalytic Institute.

To develop these opportunities for research, I respectfully request a grant of funds to Northwestern University to support one or both of the projects herewith described.

Dear Dr. Masserman:

I am pleased to inform you that approval has been secured for the application entitled "Neurophysiology of Experimental Neuroses" in the amount of $11,600.

It is anticipated that Congress will make funds available for the purpose of carrying out the provisions of the National Mental Health Act in the near future. It is therefore expected that funds will be available around July 1, 1947, and voucher should be processed for transfer of funds soon thereafter.

Yours sincerely,
Lawrence C. Kolb, M. D.
Research Projects Director
Mental Hygiene Division
National Institute of Mental Health

The Downey-Northwestern University Residency Training Program soon attracted highly qualified young men, possibly because of the comprehensive doctrines and policies outlined in the introduction to the brochure I prepared for national distribution:

Residency Training Program: Principles and Objectives

As a medical specialty, psychiatry first requires a thorough understanding of the anatomy, physiology and pharmacology of the nervous system and other body structures, of their interrelated dysfunctions under stress, and of the modes of preventing, detecting and treating pathologic deviations in psychosomatic and behavior disorders.

Second, modern psychiatry is also a medico-social discipline which derives broad insights into human behavior and its vicissitudes from the fields of anthropology, history, philosophy, psychology, psychoanalysis, communication theory and sociology, and relevant contributions from other humanistic disciplines.

Finally, psychiatry as a progressive science requires the cultivation of accuracy in observation, logical sequence, and clarity of thought, versatility in clinical and research techniques, and methods of validating data and communicating results.

There are many fields of endeavor open to the trained psychiatrist: private, group, or hospital practice, community services, teaching, research, administration or any combination of these. It is evident, however, that whatever plans the candidate may have for a rounded, successful and creative career, a truly comprehensive training in psychiatry can best be provided by an intergrated Department of Psychiatry and Neurology in a university setting with many and varied facilities. These are offered at the Northwestern University Center for Graduate Training, as follows:

1. A large and well-organized Division of Psychiatry with outstanding instructors and excellent facilities for teaching the developmental, physiologic, individual and socio-cultural determinants of human behavior, its deviations under biologic or experiential stress, and current techniques of somatic, individual, group and social therapy.

2. An integral Division of Neurology similarly staffed and equipped to teach the anatomy, physiology, pharmacology and pathology of the nervous system, clinical neurology and modern metabolic, pharmacologic and surgical aspects of therapy.

3. Corresponding opportunities for instruction in the Divisions of Psychology and Social Work, supplemented by exchange teaching arrangements with the Departments of Anthropology, Sociology, Philosophy and Law at Northwestern University.

4. A wide range of hospital and clinical services to furnish the resident with supervised experience and personal tutoring in the diagnosis and treatment of every variety of psychiatric and neurologic patient: i.e., the behavior disturbances of childhood and adolescence, adult character problems, neurotic, psychosomatic and psychotic disorders, alcoholic and drug addictions and criminal court cases. The clinical material covers other spectra of problems, acute and chronic, long and short term, in young and old, and in hospital and outpatient practice.

5. A physically attractive University campus in which the resident is in constant contact with current developments in every field related to psychiatry and neurology, stimulated by an atmosphere of academic freedom and original thought, encouraged to participate in interdisciplinary studies and given

the means for original work in excellently equipped basic science and behavioral research laboratories.

Finally, if the trainee proves his ability, he will be given every opportunity to develop an investigative, clinical and teaching career on the faculty.

The Northwestern University Center for Graduate Training cordially invites into this program residents well qualified by motivation, intellect and personality who desire a broad and comprehensive training and who wish to dedicate themselves to advancing the knowledge, practice and teaching of psychiatry.

Each candidate's morale and loyalty were maintained by unremitting concern for his personal welfare. For example, the following notarized letter was sent in behalf of a physician threatened with being drafted into the army as a private because of his alleged "liberal tendencies"—a draft board euphemism for unsupportable suspicions that he was a "security risk."

August 25, 1955

Gentlemen:

This is to certify that Dr. Edward M. Wasserman, while serving as resident physician in Psychiatry at the Downey Veterans Administration Hospital, Downey, Illinois, from July 1, 1953, to July 4, 1954, rendered intelligent and effective medical service to the hospitalized veterans under his care and was conscientious in discharging his duties to the Veterans Administration. At no time did I see any evidence in his speech or conduct on which to question his adherence to democratic principles or his loyalty to the United States.

Respectfully submitted,
Jules H. Masserman, M.D.

The hoped-for result:

April 13, 1956

Dear Dr. Masserman:

Since you last heard from me I have had the good fortune to have received the rank of Captain in the Medical Corps. There is no need to tell you how thrilled and happy my wife and I are about this turn of events.

I want to thank you again as friend and teacher for having helped me with your support.

Sincerely,
Edward Wasserman, M.D.

Recruiting outstanding faculty members was another prime duty:

May 18, 1953

Dr. I. Arthur Mirsky
University of Pennsylvania

Dear Art:

A final series of direct and telephone conferences now makes it possible to inform you that the following opportunities are available for you in Chicago:

Appointments: As Professor of Clinical Psychiatry at Northwestern University and as Chief of Psychiatry at the newly-erected Northwestern University V. A. Research Hospital.

Clinical Facilities: A 32-bed inclosed Psychiatric Unit to be organized and conducted under your direction.

Research Facilities: The fully equipped laboratories (eight complete floors) of the Research Hospital and Northwestern University; liberal V. A. funds as requested, and full liaison with the Departments of Neurology, Surgery, Medicine, Pathology, and others as desired.

Income: The top level salary from the V.A., and additional

salary from the University, and consultation and practice privileges for at least $10,000 or more.

. . . And perhaps most important, you will be among good friends and, we hope, happy in your work here.

In line with the *Drang nach Vienna* of the times, some candidates desired concurrent training at the Chicago Psychoanalytic Institute. Although myself a graduate of this Institute in its scientific heyday under Franz Alexander, I usually felt constrained to advise the mentors of such applicants somewhat as follows:

August 15, 1957

George C. Sisler, M.D.
The University of Manitoba
Department of Psychiatry

Dear George:

Briefly and frankly, I believe there are now very few psychoanalytic institutes (Columbia, W. A. White, and possibly Washington) in this country where the training given is currently worth a fraction of the time and expense involved. If your candidate wants to come to Chicago, his best course would be to secure a psychiatric residency, undertake a personal analysis and control supervision with some progressive analyst (e.g., Grinker, Rapaport or perhaps myself) and participate actively in the many courses, seminars, meetings and other training opportunities available here. At the completion of this time he could take his American Board and thus secure his specialty status. True, he would still be "unacceptable" to the American Psychoanalytic Association, but (a) if he were a capable, conscientious, dedicated person he would be at least as competent a psychoanalyst as are most members of the APsaA and (b) their "approval" would by then be even of less public and academic importance than it is now. Unfortunately, some youngsters still don't believe this, but it is the most sincere advice I can give—and what my own residents successfully follow.

Best regards.

Conversely, when a "controversial" but potentially gifted candidate sincerely desired analytic training, I recommended him to the Institute as follows:

September 14, 1957

Joan Fleming, M.D.
Director of Training
Chicago Institute for Psychoanalysis

Dear Dr. Fleming:

Dr. I. R. has requested that I recommend him to the Psychoanalytic Institute as a training candidate. In this respect, permit me to call attention to the fact that, despite certain professional and personal crises which, as you know, Dr. R. experienced in the last two years, Dr. Benjamin Boshes and I agreed that his intelligence, scholarship and dedication to his work merited his appointment to an influential position on our faculty. We thus expressed our own confidence in his basic integrity and his potential value as a rounded scientist, clinician and teacher in our field—and we hope the Institute will find itself in accord with us.

Nominations for honorary awards in our field to be bestowed by Northwestern University and more on Psychoanalytic Institute training:

December 31, 1957

Benjamin Boshes, M.D.
Chairman
Department of Psychiatry
Northwestern University

Dear Ben:

Two names that occur immediately as eminently deserving of Honorary Awards from Northwestern University, though for quite different reasons, are David McK. Rioch and Robert Felix. And, again, for quite different reasons, granting them a degree would also be advantageous to the University.

I have talked to some of our residents who were refused psychoanalytic training explicitly because their "interests were too broadly psychiatric" and I believe they now see the Institute in better perspective. Joan Fleming's arbitrary letters bring up once again the whole scandal about so-called psychoanalytic training in general. Many of us here (Roy Grinker, for one) and throughout the country (Ken Appel, Sandor Rado, Bob Heath, Leo Bartemeir—and now even Franz Alexander) are becoming ever more firmly convinced that the best way to eliminate arbitrary discrimination, cultism, and narrow indoctrination from this field is to set up broadly integrated psychoanalytic training centers under university auspices, and thus improve the selection, preparation, and scientific dedication of neuropsychiatrists who wish to add to their knowledge and techniques what is valid and useful in psychoanalysis. Perhaps Northwestern might join with other universities in this in the not too distant future.

Suggestions as to how Northwestern could utilize the newly opened Illinois State Psychiatric Institute:

May 28, 1958

Dr. Benjamin Boshes
Chairman, Dept. of Psychiatry
Northwestern University

Dear Ben:

It is, of course, impossible to specify in final detail precisely how we can use the Illinois Institute until certain over-all policies for its administration have been formulated by all the schools concerned. These policies should be determined at a conference among Gerty, Madden, Garner, Aldrich (if he wants in), yourself, Bailey and the new Director of ISPI—probably Les Rudy, a graduate, I am proud to say, of our own psychiatric training program. Until this concordat is reached, Northwestern may plan independently as follows:

Facilities: Request our full 100 beds, since it will be much easier for us to relinquish excess beds, devote them to research or join them with others in a research pool than it would be to acquire them after they have been pre-empted for other purposes.

Postgraduate Teaching: I outlined a tentative plan for this in my letter of April 8th, a copy of which I attach.

Undergraduate Teaching: In view of Dean Young's understandable preferences, we can plan (a) to shift the senior classes from Downey to the Institute, and perhaps eventually also to use the Institute for (b) sophomore demonstrations and practice in mental examinations, (c) a few sessions for the juniors for actual clinical demonstrations of amytal, CO_2, EST, hypnosis and other ancillary techniques of therapy and (d) if possible, at least three weeks of externship for each student in our service for actual and continuous contact with hospitalized psychiatric patients sometime during his clinical years.

Staff: If State salaries are provided as they should be, we can help choose a Director of Education that would serve our own teaching needs, plus top-level consultants from our own staff at all undergraduate and resident levels. If we can have only a half-time man, Jewett Goldsmith or someone of equal calibre could be given the responsibility of daily teaching and administration and the rest of his salary provided from research grants, which I am sure we could get for him. Even with lesser resources, good men from our own staff (e.g., John Adams or Charles Schlageter) have indicated their willingness to take one or two mornings a week, and I certainly hope if possible to shift some of my own teaching at all levels to the Institute.

Qualified recommendations for a faculty member considering moving elsewhere:

June 20, 1958

Ian Stevenson, M.D.
Professor and Chairman
Dept. Neurology and Psychiatry
University of Virginia

Dear Ian:

I shall write you frankly about K.T., since I know that is what you want.

K. has many assets which, properly directed, may take him far: a keen intelligence) though as yet insufficiently disciplined and integrative), an incessant creativity and ambitious drive, and, oddly enough, sincere tendencies to be friendly and loyal. However, his impatient strivings for uniqueness and his unremitting hurry to achieve his goals have made his personal, social, and academic adaptations hectic and contentious, with occasionally disruptive crises. Though he has made undeniable progress since coming with us, he has not as yet learned to prevent or avert these episodes completely, and will need wise and continuous guidance for some time to come. We have tried our best to help him thus far and cannot and would not stand in his way toward advancement. Therefore, if you think he would fit at Virginia, by all means let your and his advantage be the sole consideration.

My note to Dr. Boshes could be more outspoken:

November 12, 1958

Dear Ben:

To keep you confidentially informed, K.T. asked for an interview, and after hearing his story—fairly familiar by now—I advised gently but unequivocally:

That I could not, on his present record, nominate him for appointment as consultant at the Illinois Psychiatric Institute.

That he must not involve the University or either of us, however indirectly, in any activities of his without explicit consent.

That he had best postpone all public activities, especially organizational ones, until he was under the personal care of a competent therapist.

That he should appreciate the effort which we had made to keep him on the salaried staff as a final opportunity to redeem his status.

Unfortunately, he regarded this advice as "well-intentioned but impossible to follow" because it was contrary to his "temperament." I think that our consciences can now be quite clear that we have done all we could, and he must take the consequences of his behavior without further special favor.

When administrative directives imposed from above miscarried, and a basic reintergration of our postgraduate teaching of psychiatry seemed essential:

December 11, 1958

Dear Ben:

This letter is written in the hope that it may lead to the solution of a problem important to all of us: namely, a well-coordinated and progressive VA resident program of postgraduate training under the auspices and direction of Northwestern University.

Background: The history of our program can be reviewed very briefly. In October, 1946, at the recommendation of Dr. Francis Gerty, then Regional VA Co-ordinator, I was appointed by Dean Miller and Dr. L. Pollock to be Chairman of the Dean's Committee on Psychiatry at Downey, and commissioned to organize three years of resident training and to establish liaison with the Institute for Juvenile Research, the Criminal Court and the Children's Memorial Hospital for supplementary instruction. During its first five years this program was highly successful: for example, in four years it graduated five residents who have since become Chairmen of Departments of Psychiatry, several (locally, Drs. Lester Rudy and Tom Tourlentes) who have become managers of important hospitals and many others who have attained high rank in our field. On the basis of this reputation our program was rated as among the three best in the country by George Raines, President of the American Board of Neurology and Psychiatry, in his 1956 address to the APA, and it has received other honors.

To maintain or improve this record soon after your own appointment as Chairman of our Department at Northwestern, I proposed to the Central Office that the second and third years of training should be moved to the Northwestern campus under our joint direction. This was made official in a conference we arranged with Harvey Tompkins (VA National Director of Psychiatric Services), and for some time the new program continued to be among the best in the country. However, during the last several years the arrangement has been less satisfactory for various reasons, among them these:

1. A period of nation-wide decline in the quality of resident candidates, from which other programs in this area are suffering more than we are.

2. Staff depletion at Downey, so that residents were occasionally overloaded at the cost of sufficient time for study and supervision.

3. Dr. Arpad Pauncz' recent illness, so that for a time he could neither carry his full administrative and teaching load at Downey with the success he had achieved previously, nor conduct the proper supervisory liaison between Downey and the campus which we had officially entrusted to him.

4. The arbitrary conduct of our first appointee to the VA Research Hospital, who also failed to carry out our commission to integrate and develop the campus program, with a resulting

loss of morale which none of us could completely counteract. I therefore proposed:

1. That there be but one integrated Northwestern-Downey-VA Research Postgraduate Training Program, for which all residents will be recruited.

2. That all resident candidates must be approved by all members of the Dean's Committee, which shall also assign them, in any order it considers best and in accordance with VA regulations, to training courses and rotating services at Downey, VA Research Hospital, the campus hospitals, the Illinois Psychiatric Institute, or elsewhere.

3. That the first year of training may be either at Downey or the VA Research Hospital, depending on the needs of the hospitals, the suitability of candidates and other factors considered important by the Dean's Committee. In the case of assignment for first year training at the VA Research Hospital, the program shall not be considered as a "pilot plan," but as an integral and permanent part of the total program, with later training and rotation as directed in individual cases by the Dean's Committee.

4. That the expense of the entire program, including resident's stipends, course material and staff and consultants' salaries, be jointly carried in the training budgets of the Downey and VA Research hospitals, thus conserving our Departmental funds.

5. That duplication of courses and expenses be kept to a minimum by the following steps: (a) My own time and duties, as to lectures, seminars, demonstrations, etc. shall be scheduled so as to integrate best with the conjoint programs. (b) Exchanges of other staff lecturers between campus and Downey shall be made more feasible. (c) All residents shall be released for at least one entire day every week for conjoint courses with their colleagues on the campus (actually, they are so released for a bimonthly afternoon and evening now) so as to inculcate an anticipatory orientation to the program as a whole. So also, campus residents may attend visiting or special staff lectures, my Great Lakes Naval Hospital seminars, or special scientific meetings at Downey whenever that does not interfere with necessary clinical duties on the campus. Our annual prepara-

tion of a chapter on neuroses for Spiegel's volumes in the *Progress* series now authored by only the Downey residents and myself, should include all the residents. (d) With these modes of closer communication, we shall schedule productive staff consultations at least monthly as to the progress and best future course of all residents in each of the three years, with referral of important questions of policy, promotion or suspension of undesirable candidates to the full Dean's Committee for conjoint action.

This general plan was adopted at an executive session of the department, coincident with a fortuitous increase in my own influence in the national VA:

December 28, 1958

Dear Ben:

You might like to know that, over my demurrers, last Friday I was elected Chairman of the National Advisory Research Council of the Veterans Administration.

To deal with the startling demands of certain Veterans Administration psychologists presented in accordance with what they called "an overdue professional reorientation":

February 16, 1959

Dear Ben:

With regard to the proposal of the VARH psychologists that they, in effect, take over clinical diagnosis and therapy (to be followed no doubt by the social workers, "personnel counsellors", et al), my sentiments are unequivocal, and counter to the naivete some of our own "leaders" showed until recently in insisting that we open wide our gates to their Trojan Horse. It was not until three years ago that the American Psychoanalytic ceased training self-styled psychologists as "lay analysts"; and only a year ago that the APA Committee reversed its stand on "State Certification of Clinical Psychologists." You will remember that when I was president of the Illinois Psychiatric seven years ago, I mobilized the Society to help defeat such legislations in Illinois, and at the time repeatedly warned Paul Huston, chairman of the APA committee on liasion with psychologists, that his advocacy of "certification" for psychologists, despite our best intentions, could end only in interprofessional conflict and public misunderstanding and confusion. My sentiments on this score cannot be ascribed to personal prejudices; as you know, my *Practice of Dynamic Psychiatry* is the only current psychiatric text with a full section on psychologic tests, several of which, including the Thematic Apperception Test, I had a hand in developing; moreover, I have personally worked long and cordially with many respected psychologic colleagues both in research (Sanders, Pechtel, Aarons, et al) and clinically (e.g., with Pathman, Yacorzynski, et al). And yet, while I advocate a collaborative approach, I teach our residents and staff that if they transfer their clinical and therapeutic responsibilities in psychiatry to any profession not trained in the biology as well as the psychology and sociology of behavior, they are as guilty of medical malfeasance as if they turned over the exclusive treatment of a diabetic to a urine tester, a fracture to an X-ray technician or a general paretic to a dance therapist.

More specifically as to the pending proposals of the VARH psychologists, what they advocate is that we not only relegate to them many of our clinical teaching and research functions, but even our intraprofessional relationships, e.g., our role as consultants to our medical colleagues as to the diagnosis and therapy of medical and surgical patients (*vide* their demands that they be given—and I quote from their letter—the rights for "exclusive diagnostic screening," "group therapy for ulcers," "hypnosis for asthma," etc.). I find these proposals almost incredibly uninformed and presumptive, and sufficiently indicative of disorientation in what should be our joint fields of endeavor as to make highly questionable (a) the wisdom of continuing to teach outmoded "analytic formulae" to psychologic trainees, (b) the validity of most of the "psychosomatic research" they conduct, and (c) their assignment to clinical responsibilities independent of the control of the medical staff in a medical hospital.

In effect, I advocate friendly collaboration without, however, any compromise on the now belatedly reaffirmed AMA and APA principles: namely, that the diagnosis and therapy of behavior disorders are primarily the responsibilities of the psychiatric profession as the only one broadly enough trained to assume them. If ncessary, this should be officially re-stated at Northwestern, after which the details of administration can be worked out at VA Research or, if necessary, with the VA Central Office.

But periods of misunderstanding and discouragement occasionally recur even in the best of academic and personal relationships:

February 24, 1963

Dear Ben:

I am writing this confidential note to you in all friendliness but also in all sincerity.

I have now devoted nearly seventeen years to securing monetary support for, and maintaining the operation and development of, our Conjoint Residency Training Program at Northwestern at considerable cost to me not only in income but in time away from my research, creative thinking and writing and even essential rest and recreation. There have, of course, been many appreciations and satisfactions, including grateful and highly successful trainees (eight are now chairmen of various Departments of Psychiatry) we can all be proud of: nevertheless, I have begun to feel that my personal sacrifices have for some time not been justified by the rewards. For one thing, I appreciate the kind comments in your last departmental note to me that "through research, publications, lectures and honorary offices" I am "nationally and internationally known to represent the most advanced theoretical and clinical intergrations of medicine, neurophysiology, psychiatry and psychoanalysis," and that thereby I have "helped attract and retain desirable students and staff"—yet I cannot reconcile this with your implications that I would compromise the academic standards of our Department one iota more than necessary to provide the essential personnel from available applicants for the clinical services we require and thereby make possible the continuation of our program—also my main motivation in proposing and securing our annual $50,000 grant from the Illinois State Research and Training Authority. Nor can I agree with your comment that "our program stands for no central theme"; I submit that, as made explicit in our training brochure, the avoidance of outmoded indoctrinations and the emphasis on original thought, basic research, breadth of scholarship and their comprehensive applications constitute the highest academic and medical standards. Therefore, to restore what I hope will be a more equable status, I now make the following requests:

1. That as soon as possible I be relieved of massive candidate correspondence, file keeping, residency assignments, lecture scheduling, brochure preparations, committee reports, and a multitude of other time-consuming tasks which, especially in the past decade, have demanded excessive amounts of time and effort.

2. That my teaching and supervision at Northwestern be concentrated on advanced theory and practice in neuropsychiatry and modern psychoanalysis. This should eventually entail reducing or discontinuing my physically demanding duties at Downey and concentrating more effort on higher levels of teaching on the campus, with a reasonable annual stipend which I have up to now declined—as, for that matter, I have also declined many well-paying offers of editorships, lectureships, professorships and chairmanships elsewhere in order to devote as much time as I could take from private practice to the interests of our department. You will remember I returned to this after instituting a highly successful program at the Illinois State Psychiatric Institute in only two years.

3. Finally, I would like assurance that I can look forward to more suitable modes for collaborative planning, research and publications with more appropriate academic responsibility and dignity. Failing this, a long-delayed sabbatical or resignation from most of my current commitments would be in order.

In view of my proved loyalty and friendship, I trust you will understand these sentiments and will reply in the same spirit.

Rapport and collaboration were reestablished, whereupon Dr. Boshes wrote the following letter to Dean Young:

March 12, 1963

Dear Dr. Young:

Pursuant to our discussion and in keeping with the policy that I am developing in organizing integral divisions in our Department of Neurology and Psychiatry, I should like to recommend the appointment of Dr. Jules H. Masserman to the position of co-chairman, Division of Psychiatry. This will initiate the establishment of a chain of command through this division so that we can build up a core of younger men, full-time, geographic full-time, and part-time, to become the future faculty of psychiatry at the medical school. Thus all three sections of our Department will be brought in parallel with Dr. Masserman co-chairman of the Division of Psychiatry, Dr. Yacorzynski chairman of Psychology, and myself chairman of Neurology. I shall keep the department integrated at the top from the administrative standpoint.

If this is agreeable to you, will you inform Dr. Masserman.

Sincerely,
Benjamin Boshes, M.D.
Chairman, Dept. of Neurology and Psychiatry

When a faculty member resigned and applied for an academic appointment elsewhere, in fairness to all concerned it was necessary to reply as follows to inquiries from other departmental chairmen:

December 30, 1964

Dear____:

I presume that S. D. has described himself to you as an intelligent, serious, highly trained and sophisticated young clinician dedicated to teaching and research—and within limits, he is. Unfortunately, he also tends to be a little martinet whose patronizing and dictatorial manner toward "inferiors" often discourages applicants and alienates residents and staff. Nor are his dealings with whomever he regards either as his "peers" or "superiors" much better: envious, competitive, and ambitious, he has been ambivalently subservient when seeking favors (and I have given him many) or overtly hostile even to Ben Boshes and me whenever he believed it to his advantage. For such reasons, some months ago Ben and I considered it necessary to confront him with the alternatives of mending his ways, ("personal analysis" or no) or facing withdrawal of confidence and support. To be completely fair, he is generally an effective, though dogmatic teacher, and his overt behavior has been more carefully controlled since our series of interviews with him some six months ago; moreover, I really believe that he is capable of further improvement under directively dynamic rather than classical analytic therapy, supplemented by kind but firm guidance by you and your staff. Since you asked for a frank appraisal, and as a personal and academic friend, here it is. For further background data you may wish to check with Knight Aldrich, Roy Grinker and Percy Bailey.

Best of New Years.

Only one other dissonance needed to be resolved into the keynote before my departure to the Center for the Advanced Study of Behavioral Sciences:

April 29, 1968

Dear Ben:

Letters from Drs. Valerija Raulinaitis, Lowell Wigdahl, Gilbert Bogen, and Frederick Webber concern me very deeply. In effect, we are reminded correctly that about thirty months ago Drs. Wigdahl, Bogen, and Webber—three of the best residents we have ever had enrolled in good faith in what you and I then affirmed was a Conjoint Downey—Northwestern University Residency Training Program, and that they have since served our department in various assignments in an exemplary manner. Yet now, in my name but without my consent or even knowledge, they have, without preparation or explanation, been summarily informed by the Dean's office that they will receive only a one-year university certificate. Had they known this in advance, they could easily have transferred to any other university of their choice—and, as an invited visiting professor to many universities throughout the country, I know that any of them would have been glad to enroll and graduate men of the caliber of Wigdahl, Bogen and Webber. In contrast, while our Department would advantageously welcome each of these residents to our own faculty, we deny them a fully earned Departmental certificate of which they and our university should be equally proud.

If the Residency Training Board so rules, we can in the future make explicit to Downey candidates that they can expect university credit for only their second year of training; this will then be fully understood by all concerned. Even so, out of our Department's deep indebtedness to Downey, we should continue to help their program maintain its high standards insofar as possible. Parenthetically, six other residency training brochures in Chicago, submitted to me as chairman of the Illinois Research and Training Authority, indicate that the scope, variety and quality of teaching of our combined program compares favorably with any other in Illinois, and that Downey has been, and may continue to be, a highly valuable asset.

You will recall that twenty years ago, in full consultation with you, I expanded and strengthened our dormant university program by transferring Downey stipends, residents, and personnel to the department, wrote our successive brochures, planned the curriculum and clinical services, and have since devoted every effort to recruitment of residents and staff, teaching and administration—and I trust I can continue to do so. However, if an injustice is done to Drs. Wigdahl, Bogen, and

Webber that may well handicap their careers, then as a teacher who cherishes his rapport and friendship with young psychiatrists not only in Chicago but throughout the country, I must regretfully ask to be relieved as chairman of the Residency Training Board and director of the Program.

The residents duly received their three-year university certificates.

At Palo Alto, I replied to a kindly note from Ben as follows:

September 17, 1968

Dear Ben:

This note of appreciation of your gracious letter is being written from a new office—luxuriously furnished and provided with a picture window over San Francisco Bay and its surrounding verdant mountains. Even more gratifying are the people who have been appointed to the Center this year with me: Meredith Wilson, a most thoughtful, courtly and effective administrator, and Fellows of the calibre of Dave Riesman and Lou Coser in sociology, John Crook in ecology, Richard Falk in political science, T. C. Koopmans in economics, Norman Malcolm in philosophy, Robert Sears in psychology, George Schultz, who will soon depart for Nixon's cabinet as Secretary of Labor, and many others of equal calibre. As the only neuropsychiatrist selected this year, I shall try to do my utmost to preserve our status among our fellow scientists at their level.

My best to Virginia, Nelson Borelli, and our other faculty (I regret missing our first board meeting in over a decade) and especially our residents. If you would like to post a copy of this to serve as greetings to all, please do so and add that I shall be happy to see as many of them as possible when I return to Chicago for my monthly seminars preparatory to flying to Australia for a month as Roche Visiting Professor to the Australia-New Zealand Academy of Psychiatry.

Cordially
Jules

6. A WORLD OF TRAVEL

To one who periodically feels imprisoned by the protocols of patients and podium, and persists in the belief that there is much to learn and enjoy beyond these parameters, travel becomes an almost undeniable urge. Whenever possible I had driven as far from home as I could during brief vacations, and every summer since residency had sailed some sort of boat to far waters where I could anchor, read, and write. What remained was to explore the further reaches of the world, and to expand my parochial horizons in the arts and humanities—as, indeed, what human endeavor is more relevant to psychiatry? This peripatetic urge (reinforced by Henry Brosin, newly appointed departmental chairman, who expedited my desire to leave the University of Chicago) led to an appeal to a British friend for help in arranging a visit to England and the continent in the autumn of 1946.

September 5, 1946

The Honorable Walter Maclay
British Minister of Mental Health

Dear Doctor Maclay:

After five years of intensive, vacationless, wartime work, I am hoping to devote a few sabbatical months some time next year to a European trip. In the manner of the occupational neurosis that affects our kind, I shall, of course, not be thoroughly happy unless I can exchange ideas, knowledge, and fantasies with my scientific colleagues in England, and in particular, learn from their clinical advances in the postwar era. I should therefore be very interested in an invitation from some department of the British Government or a British university to present a lecture or two in England—or a series of these if desired—in return for an opportunity to visit and learn. I do not intend the implied request to be presumptuous, but your own experience has doubtless indicated how greatly such an invitation would facilitate the mechanics and scientific progress of my trip.

Nothing came of that gambit; obviously, I had brashly overestimated what little research reputation I had then attained. However, as I gained academic status at Northwestern, invitations to lecture abroad accummulated and led to a series of foreign travels. I have reported some of these in previous writings,* but never the first such excursion, which was submitted, confidentially to our State Department and to the WHO Secretariat of the United Nations in the troubled days of 1952. That report, which can now be published, was as follows:

Report to the U.S. State Department

Itinerary: En Route to England

Detroit, Michigan: Stopped for talks with Dr. L. Bartemeier, President of American Psychoanalytic Association, re

*See travel titles in the bibliography.

psychiatric and international contacts and missions in Europe. *Washington, D. C.:* Made final passport arrangements at the Pan American Sanitary Office and secured a *laissez-passer* for the four reels of lecture films—a precaution that, in the case of the French and German customs, proved to have been essential. Lectured at the Army Medical Center at the Walter Reed Hospital; learned from the Research Director, Dr. David McK. Rioch that direct interchanges of knowledge among American and European military neuropsychiatrists had almost ceased since the last war.

Notes Aboard S. S. Queen Elizabeth: Psychologic: An interesting shipmate was E. H. Gombrich (of the Garburg Institute, South Kensington, London), a psycho-aesthologist who, through his researches into the internal meanings and symbolisms of art forms, had reached the quite tenable conclusion that each work of art invariably expresses the internal needs, longings, values and behavior patterns of its creator, and that its "universal" significance springs only from the fact that these symbols and forms are in some ways significant to all human beings—if not, indeed, to many higher organisms.

Economic: Of a somewhat different order was the strong impression gained that the majority of American physicians ostensibly traveling to international scientific meetings in Europe (including one who said he was going to England to hear my lectures there) have only a perfunctory interest in these meetings, and quite frankly intend to use their record of registration as a means of making their vacations income-tax deductible.

From conversations with small industrialists, engineers, teachers, economists and civil servants returning after a brief sojourn in America to their native European countries I gathered an almost unanimous gloom and discouragement as to the basic economic vitality of these countries or their ability adequately to support higher education and scientific research on their own (exceptions were Sweden, Switzerland, and possibly Belgium).

England

Oxford University: Perhaps most striking is the fact that at Oxford University there is no professor, department, lectureship or even readership in psychiatry; whatever instruction medical or other undergraduates receive in this field is furnished quite inadequately by a loose conglomeration of philosophy, physiology, and psychology in a subdivision of the school directed by a professor of philosophy.* A year or so ago the University had considered appointing a professor of psychiatry, but inasmuch as Drs. McInnis and Skottow, heads of the two local sanitaria, had expressed their unwillingness to furnish either private or teaching patients for any prospective professor, this would have necessitated building an institute of psychiatry in which students could receive clinical instruction. Since funds were not available for such an institute, tentative plans for a department of psychiatry were dropped, and clinical teaching was confined to neurological cases at the Radcliffe Infirmary. Student instruction in neurology under Drs. H. Cairns, C.W.M. Whitty and their associates seems to be excellent.

Research Activities: In the field of comparative and experimental psychology Dr. P. Glees and J. Cole are continuing their interesting work in demonstrating that lesions of the paleocortex of the monkey, particularly the cingulum (area 24), may induce passivity and tameness, and that precortical functions of memory depend on mass action rather than specific tract connections. Another study concerns the emergence of right or left-handedness in previously ambidextrous monkeys when they are trained in skilled acts, and the limited effects of even repeated lesions of the ipsilateral cortex on these unilateral skills. Prof. N. Tinbergen, justly famed with Lorenz for his ingenious observations of innate behavior patterns and their "social releasers" in all organisms, is now on a permanent teaching appointment at Oxford, but seems to have little opportunity to continue his field of research.

Lectures: My own presentations at Oxford, as elsewhere, were designed along the following lines: (1) demonstration of sufficient competence in the special field of the group I was addressing (e.g., psychiatrists, neurologists, psychologists, biologists, sociologists) to win their initial interest; (2) avoidance of treading on local prejudices and susceptibilities; (for example, psychoanalytic theory is an anathema at Oxford) so as to

*This was still essentially true in 1969.

avert futile polemics; (3) presentation of what I knew of the recent progress in thought and practice in the field, whether the contributions came from America or elsewhere, and finally and most important (4) an attempt to show the fundamental interrelationships of the several specialities and their possible intergration into a total holistic and scientific understanding of "normal" and "abnormal" behavior.

I shall refrain from commenting as to the supposed success or failure of any of my lectures, seminars, or demonstrations, since the relatively large attendance nearly everywhere may bespeak local curiosity rather than scientific interest, whereas kind comments from chairmen and discussants may but have been part of the gracious consideration with which I was everywhere met; in any case I am sure that you will receive more direct and objective reports than those I could furnish. However, it may be of interest to note, in general terms, the nature of the discussion in various places as reflecting local theoretical or clinical preoccupations, or, as I first found in the case of Oxford, those generally held throughout Europe. Among the latter were these:

Much concern about heredity and genetics, with corresponding interest in group statistics rather than individual variations and experiences.

A corresponding preoccupation with various systems of typology, some based on hoary but quite unscientific premises dating from Galen: for instance, I was more than once asked what percentages of my experimental animals or patients were of the choleric, melancholic, sanguine or phlegmatic "types." This is reflected clinically in an excessive concern with phenomenologic descriptions and minute diagnostic distinctions to the neglect of a dynamic and operational approach to symptom and therapy.

Whenever specific factors in etiology were considered, there was a tendency to resort to vague postulates of "constitutional susceptibilities," or premises of specific tissue failure or disease, even though these could not be demonstrated by any available means.

Outside the meetings of the psychoanalytic societies themselves, I encountered nearly everywhere a special dislike of Freudian metapsychology and analytic jargon—a semantic aversion with which, despite my own years of psychoanalytic training, I was quite in sympathy. However, whenever I translated basic dynamic principles into more operational and scientific language, I found them readily understood and accepted even by previously prejudiced audiences.

A characteristic at Oxford which I found again especially at the Sorbonne was a movement among some of the psychologists and sociologists to drift away from the objective and inductive methods in science altogether and revert to intuition and introspective revelation with "existentialist philosophic" connotations. However, men in clinical or research neuropsychiatry, with the exception of a few diletanttes, did not seem to be taking this reversion to scholastic mysticism seriously.

As elsewhere in England, there was a tendency to dwell somewhat idly on past glories: the founding of the University by Henry VIII and Cardinal Wolsey, the competition of Mary and Elizabeth for Queens' College, the doubtful beauty of Wren's Sheldonian Theatre vs. the unquestionable beauty of the ancient college gardens, the privilege the University Senate retains in passing criminal sentence (including the death penalty) on its own faculty, and so on—preoccupations which seem occasionally designed to mitigate the fact that Oxford is slipping from her former position as one of the great universities of the world.

Cambridge: Cantabrigians pride themselves on their technical and realistic orientations (as compared with the scholarly abstraction of Oxonians), and yet in one of the most important fields of medicine—neuropsychiatry—there is little difference between the two. True, here Dr. H. C. Harris and his staff are conducting interesting experiments on the effects of diencephalic stimulation and on corneal pituitary transplants, but since Professor Adrians' retirement, no fundamental contributions to neurology have been made, and the subject is taught in routine and uninspiring fashion. As at Oxford, there is no professor, department, or clinical facility for teaching psychiatry; Beresford Davies—an intelligent, fairly well trained and articulate young man—holds the only readership in the subject, but must tread lightly to keep his post and his referral practice in view of the prevailing academic and clinical antipathy to (really ignorance of) recent dynamic advances in the field.

The Problem of the Press: The evening of my arrival in London I was first subjected to what proved to be a minor problem repeated in every country; namely, requests for press interviews by reporters who had little real idea as to the purpose of my trip, who would generally not say how they had been informed I was coming, and who nevertheless wanted statements, preferably startling, about my work and opinions. In all cases, I hope, I was able to keep the so-called "news release" tactful and objective, but I was moderately concerned that, without at least a day or two in the country to learn at least a little of its current attitudes, I might be quoted as saying something that might embarrass my local colleagues. Dignified publicity for visiting WHO lecturers is, I believe, favorable for our purposes, but it might be well to suggest to the well-intentioned secretaries of societies that invite these lecturers to postpone sending reporters for personal interviews for at least a day or two after the lecturer's arrival.

Status of Psychiatry: In general, senior British psychiatrists, as exemplified by Strauss, McKenzie, Harrowe, Garmany, Clifford Scott, et al., seem to possess a broader general education and wider cultural interests than their American prototypes; nevertheless, within their specialty some men even of the calibre of Sargant and Curran currently retain various convenient prejudices. Among these were blind beliefs, contrary to the weight of experimental and clinical evidence, in the harmlessness and efficacy of various drugs or forms of electroshock for specific "types" of psychoses, the "constitutional" untreatability of cases in which these limited therapies fail, and a reliance on post-hoc reasoning to justify arbitrary diagnostic categories. As is true also in America, some of the men who cherish these convictions also believe it necessary, for the sake of consistency, to condemn the supposedly fanciful theories of social psychology and psychoanalysis; and such men usually misuse the argument, inherently valid but here misapplied, of the necessity for keeping psychiatry a specialty completely within the medical fold—as though medicine were not itself a social science.

Fortunately, in England as in America, this spurious dichotomy between biologic and dynamic concepts is being bridged in three ways: (1) by a growing number of respected specialists such as Gillespie, Stengel and Lewis who think and teach in both fields, (2) by the almost universal regard with which some nonmedical analysts and psychologists such as Anna Freud and J. C. Fluegel are held and (3) by the recognition that modern theory and research (including, I hope, some of my own) paves the way for a comprehensive organon of psychiatry in much the same way as the previously incompatible corpuscular (Newtonian) and wave (Huygens) theories of light are correlated mathematically in modern physics. This re-integration in psychiatry can be fostered in Britain by a non-cultist presentation of objective experimental and clinical research leading to tenable principles. As one bit of evidence, I received the following letter as an aftermath of the most august assignment in my entire schedule, the address before the Royal Society October 24, 1951.

Dear Professor Masserman:

This is to say how very much we all appreciated your most stimulating and fascinating address last night. I am sure you must have realized how deeply interested the audience were from the attention with which they listened, and I have heard nothing but praise on all sides and how stimulating everybody found it. So thank you very much indeed for coming and giving us such an excellent evening . . .

Yours sincerely,
Dr. Desmond Curran
Chairman
Section on Psychiatry
Royal Society of Medicine

Status of Psychoanalysis: Unfortunately, in this field, too, old schisms remain and in some respects seem to have deepened into personal animosities. Ernest Jones, the dean of British analysts, is retired, and his most illustrious colleague, Edward Glover, became so embittered over internecine strife that he resigned from the British Psychoanalytic Society to join the Swiss. Melanie Klein, who teaches that all behavior is determined by the infant's experiences during the first few weeks of life, peremptorily heads an entrenched wing of the society; Anna Freud, with more reasonable views, shares the leadership of another faction with Gillespie, Balint (president and secretary of the Society), Stengel and others. Both groups were present at the special meeting which I addressed, but I noticed that the ardent disciples of each took occasion for indirect attacks on the other during the discussion, and that the Kleinians were conspicuously absent from the reception given me in Anna Freud's home, where the memorabilia of Freud are lovingly but rather inadequately preserved in cardboard wrapping under a bridge table. I had the impression that my talks may have furnished some basis for a rapprochement of views, as well as modifications of some aspects of analytic theory to bring it into greater accord with biologic facts, but combinations of psychoanalytic circumlocutions and ambiguities with British politeness and reserve rendered this far from certain.

Maudsley Hospital: This institution, because of current sterling exchange and travel restrictions, continues to be the center of postgraduate training in neuropsychiatry within the British Commonwealth, and still draws students from places as far away as India, Malta, and Malaya; Canadians and Australians, however, now generally study in our country. Under the directorships of Aubrey Lewis, Maudsley is markedly progressive in various clinical fields, particularly in its well-organized provisions for outpatient care and in its diversity of therapeutic techniques for hospitalized patients, both child and adult. Research is well subsidized, but at present seems to lack both inspiration and direction. Teaching, in the tradition of the psychobiologic school of Adolf Meyer (with whom Lewis studied) is exceedingly eclectic; indeed, so much so that students not yet capable of selective and integrative thinking might become either confused or one-sidedly partisan. Thus, they may be dogmatically told in the morning by Eysenck, a psychologist who is a devout adherent of Kretschmer, that "not only manic-depressive and schizophrenic psychoses but probably, according to Holzinger's H^2 factor, eighty per cent of neuroses also are hereditary and invariant disease entities," whereas that same afternoon they may be required by other instructors to treat these states either as somatic accidents reversible only by drugs or surgery, or, more operationally, as partially alterable patterns of physiological and behavioral responses, each replete with individual symbols and meanings, derived from each person's unique interactions with his physical and social milieu. Finally, in an evening seminar at the Psychoanalytic Institute, the same aberrations of behavior might be attributed to the actions of a topographically distinct region of the "Psyche" called the "Unconscious," torn among conceptual boojums yclept "Id," "Ego," and "Superego," and treatable only by cathartic verbalisms emitted in a horizontal position an hour daily for several years. I met some students at Maudsley capable of reconciling such contradictory teachings without pedagogic guidance; I also met many who apparently could not.

Bristol: Burden Neurological Institute, subsidized by the estate of the wealthy wife of a former asylum chaplain, constitutes with Gloucester the two leading psychiatric hospitals which have remained outside the British system of socialized medicine. Unfortunately, the inflation and devaluation of the pound has rendered its endowment inadequate, but despite limitations of staff and funds Burden is still one of the brightest spots in British neuropsychiatry. Professor F. L. Golla, director of Burden, is an eminent neurologist who still supervises that branch of the work at the Institute, but it is to his even greater credit that since he assumed the directorship in 1937, he has also gathered about him a staff of well-trained and dynamically orientated psychiatrists and psychologists. The latter are directed by Dr. Hadden who, with Miss Stapleton and others is doing interesting research in studying the progress of psychotherapy as shown in projective drawings and other synesthetic self-expressions.

The two luminaries of the first order of magnitude at Burden, however, are W. Grey Walter and H.W. Shipton (Clement Atlee's son-in-law) who are not only cultured gentlemen, competent neurologists, and well-read psychologists, but who possess a rare combination of originality and technical skill in neuropsychiatric research. As examples of their current pursuits I was shown the following:

1. A multiple-channel electroencephalograph that furnished analyses in either graphic or mathematical form.

2. A closed-circuit apparatus that, by reinforcing a subject's cerebral rhythms through amplified photostimulation, could alter his physiologic and subjective state, induce hallucinatory experiences, precipitate epileptic equivalents and produce other effects of great psychiatric significance.

3. A twenty-nine channel recorder that, on a luminous screen depicting the outline of the subject's brain, could trace the spread of a visual impulse, its elaboration by the parietal, temporal, and frontal lobes and the subsequent interaction of various parts of the cortex as they might occur in the formation of ideas and actions.

4. An ingenious mechanical "tortoise" which, equipped only with two electron-tube "brain cells," sought out "satisfying" stimuli and fled "unsatisfying" ones, "learned" to avoid obstacles by trial and error and returned home to rest and recharge its batteries when "tired." Another toy, possessed of three cells, was capable of acquiring "conditioned reflexes," storing them in "memory," and becoming neurotically compulsive under the stress of conflict.

5. Dr. Ashby, who works at the Gloucester Institute, also demonstrated an electrical apparatus that, like the brain, preserved the essence of a perceived pattern despite random or even traumatic interferences with the internal connections.

Perhaps the most impressive feature of these demonstrations was not their life-like parallelisms, but their significance, well understood by Walter, Shipton and Ashby, as a basic biomathematical approach to understanding the dynamics not only of the central nervous system but of behavior in general. As our knowledge progresses, this work at Burden will receive greater appreciation.

It may be worth recording that Dr. Golla and his family live in a large but old and decrepit house, and that they and their staff, like nearly everyone of whatever social stratum in

England (including Dr. Maclay of the Health Ministry) suffer uncomplainingly post-war deprivations of food, clothing and other everyday necessities that would be counted unbearable by their colleagues in America.

Socialized Psychiatry: I could gather few determinative data as to the successes and failures of socialized medicine as it affected psychiatry in Britain. Laymen everywhere almost unanimously favored the former; but since the British public was far less preoccupied with matters psychiatric than their Hollywood-and-television-bemused American cousins, I could get few data as to British attitudes in this special field. On the other hand, psychiatrists themselves evaluated the system variously: thus, the staff of Burden, outside the scheme of socialized medicine condemned it as economically wasteful and scientifically stultifying; whereas the staff of Maudsley, a hospital supported by the system, praised it as a boon to public, profession and progress. Similarly, the opinions of other specialists in the field seemed highly correlated with the effect of current conditions on their personal incomes.

France

Paris: French psychiatry is rent by schism perhaps more deeply than is the case in any other country, and each school seems correspondingly more subject to isolationist dogmatisms. Aside from his aversion to Freudian analysis, Dr. Jean Delay, Professor of Psychiatry at the Sorbonne, is perhaps the most eclectic thinker, but he appears to exert little academic leadership over colleagues who range from existentialist mysticism to the most irrational clinical practices: e.g., decerebratingly extreme electroshock therapy even for neurotic symptoms (P. Michon) or the intravenous injection of alcohol as a cure for inebriety (Fouquet). Psychoanalysts are also split into openly hostile groups: a loosely organized but relatively progressive one which uses *Psyché* as its journal, and an exceedingly orthodox one headed by Madame Marie Buonaparte, now in control of the French Psychoanalytic Society. Dr. Por'cher has wide clinical interests and excellent intentions, but his effectiveness as an executive is handicapped by lack of funds for his work and by his advanced age. Moreover, scientific thinking sometimes gets mixed with political convictions both among faculty and students: as an example of the latter, I heard that prior to my lecture on "Neurosis and Alcohol" there had been a communist-flavored, pamphlet-distributing student demonstration at the Sorbonne against the Croix Bleu, a French anti-alcohol society and presumably myself, apparently on the ground that alcoholism is a sacred right of the downtrodden worker and no imperialist exploiter who might question that fact (which I did not) was welcome.

Since I had so little time in France, I thought that perhaps the best way to cultivate further communication with French psychiatry was to contribute two articles on American psychiatry to *Psyché,* and at Professor Delay's request, to publish a longer monograph, also in French, in *L'Encéphale,* the authoritative French journal of neuropsychiatry.

Denmark: Copenhagen

Status of Psychiatry: The specialty is well accepted at the university and apparently everywhere else, largely because of the common sense and personal qualities of its practitioners in Denmark.

Status of Psychoanalysis: The telephone directory in Copenhagen lists about a dozen "psychoanalysts." None of them, I learned on inquiry, has had either medical or analytic training, but all are permitted to practice under Danish laws dealing with the regulation of extramedical cults. On the other hand, there is a promising "study-group" of five young Danish doctors, two of whom are being analyzed and all of whom are being guided by Dr. Hjalmar Nielsen, a visiting analyst from Sweden. I was asked by Dr. Lindemann, their local leader, to address this group, and found them to be a promising nucleus for the future of analysis in Denmark, although none of the group has official or academic status at present.

It hardly needs comment that the Danes, before World War II, were among the most progressive people on earth with regard to their provisions for the care of children, mothers, the indigent, and the aged, and for their intelligent handling of sexual and social deviations, alcoholism, drug addiction, and criminality. This enlightenment, leavened by typical Danish empathy and humor, is maintained even though its applications are limited by the post-war poverty of the country and the stresses currently placed on its democratic and social institutions. Nevertheless, to take but two examples, the redemption and occupational rehabilitation of girl delinquents from Nyhavn and the medicolegal treatment of sex offenders by Dr. G. K. Sturbys at Herstedvester can still serve as models of their kind. As may be inferred, I liked almost everyone and everything Danish.

Finland: Helsinki

Status of Psychiatry: Dr. Polaheimo, who had had two years of training in psychiatry and psychoanalysis in Baltimore and Boston and who was now associate director of the Psychiatric Institute, immediately dedicated himself to being my personal Vergil in Suomi and very efficiently—but quite considerately—saw to it that I was continually occupied in lectures and meetings, where he acted as interpreter whenever necessary. Moreover, he stated his reasons for thus devoting three days of his time very frankly: since his return from America three years previously, he had been only minimally successful in inducing either his psychiatric colleagues or the university faculty to accept modern dynamic approaches in the field, and he hoped that if I talked to as many groups as possible, his campaign in this regard might be helped. Actually, my experiences in Finland subsequently indicated that Dr. Polaheimo had either exaggerated the resistance to dynamic concepts among Finnish physicians and psychologists or that he himself may have used Freudian or Meyerian language which evoked unnecessary misunderstanding or confusion; certainly, the response to my mission could mean only that the Finnish profession was deeply interested, or that, after their long isolation, the Finns would welcome any foreign visitors and be excessively avid of in their scientific contributions. In effect, nowhere else in Europe did I find larger and more varied audiences, or ones more receptive of or sympathetic to a holistic viewpoint, if the latter were presented in a manner such as to encompass rather than minimize or exclude the special interests of the various auditors. While this statement may reflect some wishful thinking, the following data are nevertheless significant:

Despite my heavy schedule and the necessity of some review of each lecture for the sake of newcomers, leading Finnish neuropsychiatrists kept reappearing at successive lectures until, at my final appearance before the Duodecem in the large Hall of Parliament, nearly everyone I had met in Finland was there, and the audience also included people who said they had come all the way from Lapland. I was gratified that nonmedical academicians likewise attended this meeting, and was particularly impressed with Professor Veli Verkko, a sociologist who had written a penetrating analysis of Finnish character.

In the session with Professor von Fieandt and the Department of Psychology at the university I found the faculty and students well acquainted with developmental, comparative, gestalt and other current concepts in the field.

Similarly, despite the century-old buildings, poor facilities, and inadequate numbers of professional personnel at the Suomi State Hospital, Dr. Donner's staff there seemed intelligently appreciative of presentations dealing respectively with comprehensive, medico-psychiatric, institutional and social-rehabilitative approaches to psychotherapy, as contrasted with more limited custodial or empirical ones.

At the Institute of Occupational Health in Helsinki I found these approaches planned or actually practiced in a manner as well integrated as at any institution of my acquaintance anywhere in the world. Within the past five years, under the initiative and guidance of Dr. Leo Noro, this Institute has grown from a small clinic for the treatment of carbon monoxide poisoning to a beautifully functional six-story building, now under the jointly representative directorship of the government, industry, trade-unions, insurance companies, and medical societies, and staffed by competent physicians, neuropsychiatrists, psychologists, economists, social workers, nurses, engineers, statisticians, and research technicians. All of these coordinate their efforts, both at the Institute and in mobile teams traveling throughout Finland, in the following activities: (a) preventive medicine and psychiatry through surveying and advising industries and government bodies as to workers' health and morale (b) guiding employers and trade unions in formulating cooperative policies and practices in this regard (c) providing job-placement testing and counseling (d) teaching physical and mental hygiene at all levels: the public, general practitioners, and specialists in fields ancillary to medicine and psychiatry (e) providing both inpatient and outpatient diagnostic and therapeutic services at the Institute, and (f) conducting research on specific problems of public health, with especial reference to industrial hazards to well-being and morale. True, on close examination it becomes apparent that the Institute has attained neither its ideal of organization nor all of its objectives but it is also evident that its activities have already proved so advantageous to the many aspects of Finnish life on which they impinge that they have received wide support from government, industry, professions, and public, and constitute an index of the modern viewpoints and promising potentials of "community psychiatry" we envisage in the United States, as already present in Finnish medicine and psychiatry.

In my meeting with Dean Pesonin and the faculty of the Medical School I was informed, discreetly but unmistakably, that whereas the Professor of Psychiatry (Dr. Kailla, currently absent in America) had been opposed to any changes in his Kraepelinian concepts or traditional methods of pedagogy, other departmental heads felt that a more coordinated and expanded program of undergraduate teaching, particularly with regard to psychological and psychosomatic medicine, was needed and overdue. They seemed definitely interested in my sketch of the range of medicopsychiatric teaching at various American schools and asked particularly for copies of the curriculum and our outlines of courses and teaching methods at Northwestern University to serve as a basis for their own projected revisions.

Incidental Impressions: Finland is, of course, perhaps the poorest and most deprived country in Western Europe, with the highest cost of even modest living standards for both native and visitor. A cup of coffee costs about sixty cents, and the one present I could offer my various hosts with certainty that it would be well received was the promise of a pound of soluble U.S. brew. Nearly all Finns, including many Finnish communists, traditionally dislike and mistrust the Russians, and even more deeply, their erstwhile German allies; they long instead to identify with the Scandinavian countries from whom, however, they are separated by an almost unbridgeable language barrier (recently heightened by a nationalistic recultivation of the unique Finnish tongue) or with Americans whose sympathies they fear they may have alienated in World War II. They would therefore be particularly grateful for expressions of regard and offers of aid from the Nordic countries and would especially welcome concurrent scientific and cultural interchanges.

Sweden

Stockholm: The physical facilities of inpatient psychiatric care at the Karolinska Institute were excellent, and because of Government aid, remarkably inexpensive for both private and public patients; nevertheless, under Professor Torsten Sjögren's influence both the clinical therapy and the research seemed to be under a pall of genetic fatalism. Thus, nearly all behavior disorders were regarded as hereditary-constitutional diseases, and patients with "schizophrenic family taints" were solemnly warned that their children had five times the "normal" probability of becoming "schizophrenic." Despite all this, no one at the Institute could quite define what a "schizophrenic taint" was, or explain how the adverse familial and social (as distinguished from hereditary) influences exerted by deviant parents on their children could be excluded from descriptive "genetic" studies. Nevertheless, it seemed neither necessary nor advisable to press my own scientific criticism of such preoccupations at the Institute, inasmuch as (a) much money and effort was currently being expended on them, and would continue to be until their relative sterility was unmistakable even to the most ardent local disciples of the concepts of constitutional typology; (b) the chance that this conclusion would be reached was heightened by the fact that some of the more elaborate projects had already proved unrewarding (as for instance, Dr. Hallgren's recently completed work on specific dyslexia); (c) certain more independently-minded investigators had published results healthily corrective of current beliefs (for instance, Dr. C. H. Alström, in a well-controlled and extensive study of epilepsy, had shown that the hereditary factor is almost negligible even in this disorder); and finally, (d) some of the leaders of Swedish psychiatry (Lundquist himself, Törngren, Frey, Bingley and others) had quietly tired of the futility and therapeutic nihilism implicit in a purely genetic approach and were becoming relatively eclectic in their theory and practice. In my own lectures, I was therefore always careful to acknowledge the undoubted role of hereditary and constitutional predispositions in behavior, but tried to put these in the proper perspective of a much broader etiologic configuration of experiential and social factors. As nearly as I could judge, I found rational expositions of this more comprehensive approach and its clinical and therapeutic implications quite acceptable to most psychiatrists and other professional groups in Sweden.

Status of Psychoanalysis. The attitudes of most Swedish psychiatrists toward this specialty vary from strained tolerance (as Frey and Wolfart put it: "Some of us had that disease and have gotten over it") to the militant antagonism of Törngren, who resigned (the analysts say was expelled) from the Analytic Society about five years ago, now classes all analysts with quacks, and wants a law passed to prohibit them from "misleading social workers and harming [*i.e.,* treating] defenseless children." Actually, in my special meeting with the local analytic group I found them somewhat addicted to precisely the forms of Freudian jargon most likely to antagonize those unacquainted with its approximate meanings, yet on the whole the men were individually earnest, intelligent and relatively levelheaded in their studies and in their work. The Swedish Analytic Society is the only one in Scandinavia given official recognition by the International Psychoanalytic Association; nevertheless, it needs considerable guidance as to the strategy and tactics required to gain better professional status and academic acceptance.

General Impressions: Swedes are perhaps the most prosperous people in Scandinavia (if not in all Europe), proud of their cultural traditions, of their current social accomplishments and of their unpublicized but very great aid to their democratic neighbors—(including Finland) during World War II and after—yet, despite their ready explanations, most Swedes feel covertly guilty about having stayed out of the two world struggles for freedom. This mixture of pride and defensiveness renders many Swedes somewhat stiff and formal in their initial contacts with official visitors, and yet I found that what I had been told about them was quite true: anyone who shows a proper knowledge of and respect for their traditions (not forgetting the militant Charles XII) and a sincere desire to conform to their etiquette and customs is soon accepted with real warmth and friendliness—attitudes which any foreign guest, if properly instructed and willing to try, can readily elicit, thoroughly enjoy and utilize as well for constructive scientific liaison.

Norway

Oslo: I found Professor Gabriel Langfeldt to be an intelligent and personally charming gentleman, liked by his colleagues and students, and well qualified for his post in every respect except possibly two: first, a thirty-year lag in some of his psychiatric concepts (such as that of the "hypersensitive constitution" or the hereditary nature of "introversion" and "projection"—notions which, unfortunately, he incorporated into his *Textbook of Psychiatry,* the only one published in Norwegian) and second, his misunderstandings of and prejudiced antagonisms toward psychoanalysis, partially attributable to his lack of acquaintance with its modern developments. This prejudice, indeed had become sufficiently intense to lead not only to intramural discords with Dr. Schjelderup, Professor of Psychology at the university, but also to rather undignified polemics in the public press and to appeals to Dr. Evang (of the Royal Norwegian Ministry of Social Affairs) and others for national laws to curb the practice of analysis in Norway. The first of Dr. Langfeldt's minor deficiencies probably will be corrected during a period of study in America under a Fulbright Fellowship which Dr. Langfeldt wants and which I shall try to help him secure. The other difficulty, which has spread in Dr.

Langfeldt's case to a regrettable distrust of all dynamic theory and practice, has a deeper and peculiarly indigenous background in the recent history of Norwegian medicine. Nearly two decades ago the then Professor of Psychiatry at Oslo University became interested in Freudian theory and invited Otto Fenichel, who had written much in the field, to come to Norway and teach this newer knowledge. During his stay in Norway, Dr. Fenichel also interested Professor Schelderup and other psychologists in analysis; and, although he converted few physicians to its doctrines he was fairly well respected for his personal probity and sincerity. Unfortunately, Dr. Fenichel then emigrated to America and was succeeded by Wilhelm Reich, a man who, though he had once been a brilliant student of Freud, had subsequently been expelled from the Vienna Psychoanalytic Society for his wild theorizing and unethical practices, and had later created so great a furor during a brief residence in Denmark that he had been requested to leave that ordinarily tolerant country. By the time he arrived in Norway he had already developed what many currently regard as definitely psychotic behavior: a strange mixture of garbled analytic theory with Communist political dogma, paranoid feelings of persecution, and bizarre beliefs in the universal presence of a substance called Orgone which could be concentrated by "analysts" of his school in Orgone Boxes that could be employed not only to restore orgiastic potency in their patients, but to cure all somatic diseases including cancer. Dr. Reich's activities in Norway, of course, evoked a storm of antagonism not only against him and his pupils but also against all sane and sincere workers in psychoanalysis proper. Regrettably Dr. Langfeldt, when he succeeded to the Chair of Psychiatry at the University, thought it advisable to continue these attacks even after Reich departed Norway, leaving only one lone disciple and only one Orgone Box, whereas Professor Schjelderup thought it necessary to champion psychoanalysis without sufficiently clarifying his stand about Reich; moreover, since Schjelderup continued to teach psychologists in his department the techniques of analytic therapy, he enraged many medical men all the more. At the time of my visit to Norway the antagonism between the groups was still intense and almost no avenues of communication existed. In my talks to each, as usual, I tried to remove semantic misunderstandings and indicate the spurious nature of most of the conflicts about theory and practice; moreover, I was particularly explicit in my talks to the psychologists about the importance of biologic factors in behavior. Whether or not I succeeded in enlarging comprehension on either side during my two days in Oslo is questionable; perhaps Dr. Evang can report on this later.

Bergen: I found that Dr. Finn Rud, a former assistant of Dr. Langfeldt (and still a subscriber to his teaching*) had, as the new Professor of Psychiatry at Bergen University, quickly won the confidence of his academic and professional colleagues and was doing excellent pioneer work in establishing the teaching of psychiatry and in improving the administration and therapy at the ancient and decrepit Bergen State Hospital. He desires and would benefit from more direct personal contact with modern concepts in the field, and he deserves all available support and encouragement; indeed, these statements could well be applied to nearly every Norwegian psychiatrist.

Despite their current restlessness and intensity I found the Norwegians, too, a very likable people struggling simultaneously to resuscitate their devastated economy, to re-establish themselves scientifically in their universities, and to express themselves aesthetically in works of national pride such as the Vigeland sculptures and the Oslo Stadthus. Significantly, in the magnificent Stadthus murals depicting the evolution of various aspects of Norwegian culture in successive panels painted with supreme artistry, the Nazi invasion is almost always symbolized by the appearance of loathsome beasts or insects rather than men—only one expression among many others of the deep hatreds left in Scandinavia by the last war.

Germany

The Psychosomatic Institute at Heidelberg is actually the only school in Germany for postgraduate training in analysis, and apparently functions as such, partly because its name

*The epitome of such research is Dr. Rud's monograph "The Eosinophile Count in Health and in Mental Disease," in which, after 445 exhaustive and exhausting pages and threescore each of charts and tables, Dr. Rud comes to the predictable conclusion that the eosinophile count is of no particular significance in psychiatry.

averts the general prejudice among German academicians to psychoanalysis and partly because it actually maintains an outpatient service that accepts therapeutic referrals from other medical clinics at the university; even so, its activities and interests are divorced from (and largely ignored by) the regular Department of Psychiatry. Dr. A. Mitscherlich conducts the training of his residents (currently eight in number) along standard lines: a personal analysis of a year or more, seminars on psychoanalytic literature and dream interpretation, and long-term supervision of "control" cases in therapy; however, all these forms of analytic training at the Institute are at present handicapped by the circumstance that there are only two officially accredited training analysts and that one of these, according to Mitscherlich, taints his teaching with the philosophic mysticism that pervades much of German psychiatry. The Institute also conducts research on psychogenic factors in tuberculosis and investigates other "psychosomatic correlations," but most of this work seems lacking in medical controls and is subject to the same pitfalls of metapsychological speculation that Mitscherlich deplores in others. Despite all this, the Institute at Heidelberg still represents the broadest and most dynamic medical-psychiatric teaching and practice currently available in Germany, and may well serve as a nidus for future development in that country.

Berlin: My impressions were necessarily hurried and somewhat contradictory. Dr. Misgeld, one of the psychiatric group that six months previously had been most active in arranging my visit, was himself confined to a hosptial for what, I was told freely, was drug addiction. In his place Dr. Shober, an official of the Medical Society, spent almost an entire day out of what he described as an exceedingly busy medical and surgical practice taking me on a tour of Berlin. During this tour Dr. Shober placed particular emphasis on the destruction allegedly caused by American bombers, on the inflation occasioned by the flow of American dollars, on questions about what he obviously hoped was corresponding poverty and destruction in England, and on complaints that West German medicine was being "ruined" by an influx of refugees (implicitly Jewish) from the East Zone and from Austria—sentiments echoed more or less frankly by a number of his medical colleagues we met during the day. Even more revealing of certain aspects of German thought was a two-hour address by Professor Nonne of Hamburg, ostensibly as an introduction to my formal lecture before the joint Medical and Psychiatric Societies. This venerable gentleman traced the scientific development of neurology and psychiatry during his sixty years of professional experience in accord with a simple theme, to wit: that all lasting contributions to the field had been made only by Germans, whereas men of other nationalities (such as Charcot, Janet, Bernheim, Freud, Meyer, Hughlings Jackson, et. al.) had served only to vitiate, mislead, or degrade neuropsychiatry; moreover, although it was true that the world was temporarily forgetful of German greatness in this field, Professor Nonne assured all his hearers that here, too, they need but remember that Germany had always risen thrice as strong from her ashes to reassert the eternal watchwords "Deutschland über alles!" This ringing peroration, delivered in most polished High German, brought the large audience to its feet in what was obviously a resounding ovation to both the speaker and itself. Naturally, the demonstration also left me exceedingly doubtful as to whether it would be possible to follow Professor Nonne with a soberly scientific discussion of advances in psychiatric thought outside Germany since World War I—the time when Professor Nonne's own researches, as presented at the meeting, had ended. Moreover it was obviously necessary, by implication if not directly, to contradict Nonne in many ways, and thus very possibly offend his enthusiastic partisans. Accordingly, I spoke as tactfully as possible and suited the content and manner to the changing temper of my listeners—whereupon I experienced one of the many paradoxes of German thought and behavior referred to previously. The audience, despite the lateness of the hour and my undoubted lack of eloquence in German, seemed to follow my talk closely and sympathetically, registered approval of nearly all the points I made, discussed them intelligently, and closed the evening with another standing ovation followed by many personal expressions of appreciation; moreover, I was accorded similar treatment at an exclusive banquet with some of the officers of both Societies after the lecture. I mention the incident merely as an illustration of how the German temperament invades and sometimes pervades German science: high intellectual resources and technical skill combined with a capacity to perceive, evaluate, and integrate (if not preempt) the work of others—and yet all of this occasionally clouded and vitiated by aggressive chauvinism that not infrequently repels and alienates potential friends in scientific as well as other fields.

I had an opportunity to talk confidentially with only one psychiatrist from the East Zone, a Dr. Georg Destunis, who informed me in all seriousness that *whereas* Pavlov was now a scientific saint in Russian hagiolatry and *whereas* I had dared to differ with St. Pavlov's conceptual system in some of my own writings, *therefore* the Russian authorities had *resolved* that the favorable reviews that Destunis had written for the German literature of my work were scientific errors not to be published or read in Communist spheres of influence. Dr. Destinus, who may have a penchant for the dramatic, also informed me that, although he is allowed to attend scientific meetings anywhere, the Russians never permit the entire family to travel: instead his wife or one of his two children must stay at home as hostage.

Switzerland

Zurich: Dr. Eugen Frey of the Department of Neuroanatomy, University of Zurich, explained that his research is designed to confirm Freudian dream theory. His methods consist of hypnotizing subjects, directing them to dream, playing various types of music, waking the subjects, and finally securing from them colored sketches of successive scenes in their dreams. As might be expected, the *traumerei* so "reproduced" as paintings (generally watercolors) are supposedly replete with phallic, mammary, and vaginal forms, Medusa heads, waterfilled uterine caves, representations of Frey in various transference guises, and other vivid Freudian symbols; some of Frey's subjects also experienced a sudden burst of color in their dreams when the music penetrated their hypnotic fugue. Unfortunately, Dr. Frey, who has had no formal psychoanalytic training and does not work in collaboration with the Department of Psychiatry, did not investigate the life histories of his subjects minutely nor attempt to confirm the individual semantics of the dream and synesthetic symbolisms, ergo his studies remain original, intriguing—and inscrutable.

Burgholzi under the younger Bleuler retains its traditional prestige as the most advanced and best-organized neuropsychiatric hospital in Europe, but must nevertheless contend with certain handicaps, among them a lack of quarters and services for inpatients adequate for present needs, and a serious limitation of funds and facilities for psychiatric research. The day I was there Professor Bleuler had appealed to the government for a new hospital and sufficient funds to correct both deficiencies, but was far from certain that he would be granted either request. It was also somewhat surprising to learn that in this center of continental teaching undergraduates received only one course each of lectures in psychiatry and psychoanalysis during their entire medical curriculum, and that only about one student in eight has an opportunity for individual work with psychiatric patients. Another problem described by Professor Bleuler seemed easiest of all to solve: namely, an influx of second-rate students from various countries who had failed to gain admission to medical colleges at home or in America and who had then come to Zurich because of the policy of that University, in conformity with its cherished democratic and tolerant traditions, to admit everyone who applies with a record of having passed his premedical courses. Many of these students, once enrolled, did unsatisfactory work and some even refused to learn German, with the result that the morale and efficiency of undergraduate teaching at Zurich had sometimes been seriously impaired. Dr. Bleuler seemed genuinely grateful for the information that American medical colleges used standardized psychologic and personality tests and direct personal interviews as well as scholastic records as criteria for the admission or exclusion of medical students, and that Zurich would in no way be considered "undemocratic" if its faculty, under the guidance of the Department of Psychiatry, adapted similar means for selecting its medical freshmen. In this connection, I arranged to send Dr. Bleuler samples of the tests and procedures employed at Northwestern.

Italy

Rome: The most impressive person I have met here was the venerable Professor Ugo Cerletti, a scholar who had sacrificed academic posts at the University of Rome and his livelihood rather than subscribe to fascist doctrines, who had attained fame as the codiscoverer of electroshock therapy (and who now deplores the world-wide misuse of his discovery), and who, currently restored to status but not to an adequate income, continues to teach and practice a sane, eclectic, socially orientated psychiatry. Dr. Gozanno, the new director of the Neuropsychiatric Clinic at the university, is rapidly improving its facilities and services so that the teaching of psychiatry here, now quite inadequate at the undergraduate level, should improve materially.

That report was written nearly a generation ago. As Heraclitus would have it: no man steps into the same river twice—and yet, European psychiatry is still pretty much the same river.

Many hegiras followed to many far places: Latin America in 1957 and 1958; Czechoslovakia, Yugoslavia and again Italy in 1958; Greece in 1961; Japan, India, Israel, the Middle East, and Central Europe in 1963; Africa in 1964—each under unique circumstances and with special trials and lasting enlightenments. Each also led to opportunities for service to newly made friends. For example, after my return to the United States the late Dr. Iracy Doyle, director of the Institute of Psychological Medicine in Rio de Janeiro, appealed to me for help in getting her new Institute of Psychological Medicine officially recognized by the government of Brazil. Since the affair has long been settled fairly and favorably, I can reproduce her letter:

December 28, 1955

Dear Dr. Masserman:

It occurs to me that you, as a recognized international authority, might very handily get in a word to the Brazilian Ministry of Health in Rio de Janeiro to the effect that the William Alanson White Institute, where my staff and I were certified, is a training institute in good standing in the United States. It would probably be very impressive, too, if some mention could be made about the new Academy of Psychoanalysis, some of the better-known names that are making it up, and the fact that I am being invited as Associate Member.

This officialization would involve very real benefits, aside from the formality of recognition as an institute of post-graduate level, including the possibility of financial assistance and immunity from persecution.

Now to lighter matters! Under separate cover I am sending you some Brazilian records, and herewith some clippings *re* your visit, and snapshots. Also a letter from the University of Brazil, which might come in handy at income-tax time.

Cordially yours,
Iracy Doyle

January 5, 1956

Dear Iracy:

I have phrased the attached in the stilted professorese that seems to awe authorities, and I hope sincerely it will help "officialize" the Instituto. If need be, I'll put on my Lasker Award medal (and, if they can't read English, a more impressive one I got for playing chess), come down again, and try to act officious and imposing.

Meanwhile, our best hopes for your health. And our regards to Margarida, Henrique, Jorge, Horus, Carlos, et al. I really hope to see you again soon.

A letter commending the clinical, training, and research potentialities of Dr. Doyle's Psychoanalytic Institute was duly sent to the Brazilian authorities, and may have helped secure for it official certification as a facility for higher professional education. However, not long afterward, I had to write this sorrowful in memoriam letter for a volume to be dedicated to her:

April 25, 1957

Dr. Augusto D'Esaguy
Imprensa Medica
Lisbon, Portugal

Dear Dr. D'Esaguy:

It would indeed have been a treasured distinction to me to have been, as your letter implies, "one of Dr. Iracy Doyle's closest friends." Instead, it is my sorrow that I did not have the opportunity to be one for long. Mrs. Masserman and I met Dr. Doyle for the first time less than two years ago while on a mission to South America for the World Health Organization. We were both immediately impressed by her broad erudition and independent wisdom, and later even more entranced by her youthful initiative, modest gentility, personal warmth, and unfailing charm; we therefore spent as much time with her and her group as was possible. Unfortunately, we were obliged to leave Rio in only a few days, and though we corresponded thereafter, we never saw her again, and therefore experienced an even greater sense of sorrow and loss at the news of her death. Somehow, it did not seem that so vibrant and well-loved person could really have departed, and we shall prefer to regard her as eternally present.

I also undertook to help another friend arrange an American edition of his monograph under somewhat trying circumstances:

August 30, 1956

Dr. Angel Garma
Professor of Psychiatry
University of Buenos Aires

Dear Angel:

Your book *Peptic Ulcer and Psychoanalysis* arrived precisely at a time when it was most difficult for me to give it the careful attention I wished: I had just been simultaneously elected president of three national societies, each with its peculiar problems and duties, and had to meet a deadline on a book *Progress in Psychotherapy,* besides all my usual teaching, research, and clinical routines. However, I went over your manuscript as carefully as I could to correct typographical and stylistic errors, and shall now send it to Nolan Lewis for consideration as a "Psychosomatic Monograph," as you direct. The main difficulties which it may have in being accepted are:

1. Psychosomatic thinking in the United States is on the whole swinging away from the "specific unconscious formulae" concepts of Dunbar, Alexander, Szasz, etc. toward a more comprehensive bio-dynamic approach.

2. The theories of Melanie Klein which you advocate are here accepted by very few behavioral scientists.

3. Your manuscript, especially in its sections on etiology (such as "that a bad introjected mother [literally] eats the gastric tissues and causes ulcers") presents notions not taken seriously in this country.

4. Your style, whose Spanish grace I can sense, has unfortunately been rendered into rather awkward English by your translator. I reworded many paragraphs, but the manuscript needs further revision.

Despite the above, your writing is consistent and sincere and deserves consideration by our English-speaking colleagues. I shall recommend it to my friend Nolan Lewis, and hope that his editorial board will think as I do. As you suggest, please also send him your curriculum vitae; his address is New Jersey Psychiatric Institute, Princeton, New Jersey.

Christine and I ardently hope that you and Betty will come stay with us as soon and as long as possible. Please do.

Meanwhile, other prospective American travelers began inquiring, more or less directly, as to how they, too, might get invited to lecture through South America. A typical reply to one mentor:

November 6, 1956

F. C. Redlich, M.D.
Professor and Chairman
Department of Psychiatry
Yale University

Dear Fritz:

South Americans, although always receptive and cordial, invite people to their countries (a) because of their scientific status through publications and lectures and (b) because of previous personal friendships. Confidentially, I am not sure that the scholastic and pedantic "classical analytic" approach or your protege Dave Rapoport is what most of our southern cousins currently need or want; ergo, his best course would be to inquire through whatever contacts he might have with analysts in Montevideo (Baranger) or Buenos Aires (Garma, Rascovsky, et al.). If I were to initiate this, it might later be interpreted in their Latin American way as a rebuff to me if they did not invite him, but if he has a favorable reply I shall of course do all I can to help.

Thanks for your glowing comments on my last book. I still hope that the new Mrs. Redlich and you can visit with us soon.

I had occasion for more important services during a polio epidemic in Argentina:

August 31, 1956

Senor Hernando Pastrana
Consular Attache
Buenos Aires, Argentina

Dear Senor Pastrana:

Herewith enough Salk vaccine for the 18 children of our mutual friends, plus another vial to be used for Dr. Susana Lustig and the two Rascovskys.

This is but a small token of appreciation for your friendship and hospitality. Christine and I sincerely hope to see you and your charming wife again soon.

Con abrazos

Nevertheless, not all was sweetness and light. To a member of the faculty of the University of Sao Paulo who took exception to certain passages in my South American report that he thought reflected unfavorably on his city and University School of Psychiatry:

January 22, 1958

Dr. Publio Salles Silva
Clinica Psiquiatrica
Sao Paulo, Brazil

Dear Dr. Silva:

I regret that possible verbal misunderstandings seem to have led you to a partly prejudiced reading of my psychiatric travelogue on South America. I respectfully request that you reconsider the following passages, here precisely reproduced:

"*Psychiatry in Sao Paulo:* My schedule was arranged to reflect the pace of the city: in only three days I was to visit the University Psychiatric and Neurologic Clinics, lecture twice at the Assocoao Paulista de Medicine and at the University, attend various dinners and luncheons, and spend a day at the

Juquiri State Mental Hospital. My impressions—necessarily somewhat tachistoscopic—were these:

"Most influential as policy-maker, administrator, and representative of Brazilian academic psychiatry abroad is Professor A. C. Pachéco e Silva, who has the unusual distinction of holding the chair of psychiatry at both of the medical schools in Sao Paulo. A dignified, gracious gentleman, Professor Pacheco entertained us ducally in his magnificently furnished mansion, set in a small park about which, in patrician Portuguese tradition, he had built small homes for his son (also a psychiatrist), his daughters, and his sons-in-law. We were also shown proudly through his recently opened University Institute of Psychiatry, well constructed and excellently equipped for teaching and research, but containing many locked cells viewed through barred portholes and ceiling mirrors ingeniously arranged, so we were told, 'to prevent the patient hiding in a corner and then jumping on the doctor.' Only a section of this Institute is in operation, but Dr. Pacheco is employing every persuasion to obtain additional funds from the government. Even more important, he has gathered about him or sent for further training in the United States (e.g., Dr. Paul Vaz de Arruda who is studying electroencephalography with Dr. F. Gibbs in Chicago) an eager and alert faculty and staff. With their help, Dr. Pacheco hopes to make his institute, in association with the adjoining Institutes of Neurology and Neurosurgery, the acknowledged center of neuropsychiatric study and research in South America.

"However, despite Dr. Pacheco's prevailing influences, psychiatric thought and effort are not nearly as unified in Sao Paulo as we later saw exemplified in Santiago or Panama. The psychoanalytic group (Dr. Mario Yahn, Dr. Durval Marcondes, Dr. Anibo Silvera, et al.) do not feel accepted at either university, and have in turn isolated themselves from academic contacts and communication to a greater degree than possibly anywhere else in South America. Perhaps even more unfortunate is the position of several intelligent and sincere young psychiatrists eager to pursue eclectic and dynamic training either in Brazil or in the United States but, afraid that if they departed from local traditions and policies they would be barred from teaching or research position at the university. It was my privilege during my brief stay to be of help to some of the young men who, justifiably or not, considered themselves caught in such a situation."

As you will note, the first paragraph completely acknowledges my personal respect for Dr. Pacheco e Silva and his staff —a respect I also expressed later in the article for the psychiatrists at Juquiri who were commendably overcoming tremendous odds. The only possible objections must be to the second paragraph, but the information here can hardly be questioned on factual grounds. Neuropsychiatric opinions and loyalties of course differ in Sao Paulo as they do everywhere else on earth, but as a counter to those you express, permit me to quote but two passages from many letters I have received from Brazil since publication of my report:

From Dr. Oswaldo Camargo, Director of Mental Hygiene, Rio de Janiero:

> Let me present you the warmest congratulations for the paper. Everything you wrote about Brazil reveals a great sense of observation, an accuracy on details, a full justice in the analysis of the people, the country and the sceneries. I should say you have put on that fine piece of work a bit of talent and tons of heart. Remarkable the expression: "This country is in advance of most on the road to human brotherhood."

From Alberto Seguin, Professor of Psychiatry, University of San Marcos:

> Concerning your (report) I must confess that I am amazed by the sagacity and comprehension with which you were able to penetrate our affairs; from the reading of these travelers' impressions, I was able to draw conclusions of great usefulness.

——And many other similarly gratifying expressions.

As to your quite justifiable civic pride, please let me add that, of the many physicians in South America who expressed a desire (though perhaps only in courtesy to me) to train further or live in the United States, only one was from Sao Paulo. In any case, I greatly regret that you found anything troublesome—let alone "malicious"—in a report that repeatedly stressed my great respect for the scholarship, graciousness and hospitality of my South American colleagues.

Con abrazos

cc: Dr. Pacheco e Silva

January 12, 1958

Professor A. C. Pacheco e Silva
Clinica Psiquiatrica
Sao Paulo, Brazil

Dear Professor Pacheco e Silva:

I attach a copy of my reply to a recent letter from one of your colleagues. I regret that any member of your staff should have misunderstood my comments and felt as he indicates. Permit me to assure you once again of my sincere professional respects and my appreciation of your most gracious hospitality to Mrs. Masserman and myself during our visit to Sao Paulo. We hope that some day we shall have an opportunity to entertain you in like fashion in Chicago.

Most respectfully

Professor Pacheco e Silva replied with a most courtly apology in perfect Spanish and, I am afraid, implied disciplinary action against Dr. Salles Silva.

In May of 1963, as program chairman of the American Psychiatric Association, I also helped arrange a series of Round-the-World Conferences in Japan, India, Thailand, and Israel for some 300 American psychiatrists. My reports of these conferences were published in *Psychiatry: East and West.*

A follow-up letter from the late Walter Maclay, British Minister of Health, after this hegira:

June 10, 1963

Dear Christine and Jules:

I had a few delightful days of rehabilitation in Cyprus, sunbathing and swimming in Kyrenia and Famagusta and visiting the new archaelogical discoveries at Salamis. I just missed seeing Aphrodite rising from the sea at Paphos; she only does it when the moon is full, conditions perfect and the onlooker in the right frame of mind.

Jules must be feeling very gratified at the success of his part of the tour. Indeed the whole expedition seemed to me an immense success. I judge this first by my own constant enjoyment of it all and secondly by the apparent enjoyment of everyone else. Others can decide whether or not it served some great international function of world brotherhood, etc.

My main impression is of all the friendliness and kindness of my fellow travelers and more especially of Jules and yourself. The travel arrangements were so good that I began to fear that never again would I be able to accept responsibility for my own welfare.

It was grand to be able to see something of you both and I hope you will come to England soon.

Yours sincerely,
Walter

Another follow-up:

Department of State
Bureau of Educational
and Cultural Affairs
August 12, 1963

Dear Mr. Masserman:

It was nice to hear that you had such a successful trip. . . . We have had reports on your visit from Ankara and Budapest only. The references to you are very nice indeed.

I am sorry to say that the Department does not have funds

for the reimbursement of your expenses incurred through your generous donations of books, publications, gifts, etc. You are certainly to be commended, though, with respect to your efforts and your willingness to carry on.

We shall be most happy to see you in our offices when you come to Washington in October. Mr. Netherton asks that I send congratulations on so successful a trip and tell you how much he looks forward to seeing you in October.

Sincerely yours,
Virginia E. Orem
Program Officer
Division for Americans Abroad

Subsequent lecture tours to Africa, Australia, New Zealand, and elsewhere are described in the books and articles listed in the bibliography.

7. THE AMERICAN PSYCHIATRIC ASSOCIATION—PERSONS, PROGRAMS, AND POLITICS

I had qualified for membership in the American Psychiatric Association in 1942, and had presented a more or less "scientific" paper at each of its subsequent annual Scientific Sessions. But it was more than a decade before the APA assigned me even a minor role in its Establishment.

June 16, 1953

Kenneth E. Appel, M.D.
President, APA.

Dear Dr. Appel:

I shall be honored to represent the American Psychiatric Association at the Chicago convention of the World Federalists, and to report to you any transactions of interest to our Association.

Congratulations on an administration that already shows great promise, and best personal regards.

Respectfully,

My entry into organizational politics:

April 2, 1954

E. Thayer Gaston
President
National Association for Music Therapy

Dear Thayer:

The little brochure on Music Therapy you submitted to the APA is excellent; I would suggest only that under Psychology a course on Group Dynamics and Therapy be specifically recommended as very important in the use of music in therapy. I suggest that you now send a letter to Daniel Blain, medical director of the American Psychiatric Association, to the following effect:

> Dear Dr. Blain:
>
> At the instance of Dr. Jules Masserman, member of our Research Committee and Psychiatric Advisor to this Association, I am writing to you for counsel as to how we can best coordinate our special interests, training programs, and service to patients.
>
> The National Association for Music Therapy was formed about four years ago (mention meetings, activities, annual publications, etc., as you think best).
>
> May I respectfully suggest that your Association appoint a small committee of those specially interested in this field to meet with a parallel one of ours: The joint committees could then work out a program of training, service, and research that will be in the best interest of patients, and therefore also of both Associations.
>
> We would greatly appreciate your referring this letter at your discretion to the proper officers of the Association, and letting me know your recommendations.

I have also written to Dan—a sailing friend of mine—and will talk to him at the St. Louis meeting of the APA.

April 2, 1954

Daniel Blain, M.D.
Medical Director
American Psychiatric Association

Dear Dan:

Professor Thayer Gaston of the University of Kansas will be writing you soon to request the formation of a joint committee with the National Association for Music Therapy to set proper standards of personnel training, service, and psychiatric direction in this rapidily growing field. I have known Dr. Gaston and his associtess in the NAMT for several years and am glad to say that he and the other officers and, for that matter nearly everyone in this organization is sincerely interested in keeping the field scientific, and in cooperating sincerely and effectively under the direction of physicians and psychiatrists in the care of patients. An instance of my belief in this is the fact that I have devoted considerable time and effort to the NAMT and shall continue to do so. Now, however, may be the time for the APA to take official cognizance and leadership, in a manner best decided by the Council.

P.S.: Your room overlooking Chicago and the lake (you may overlook the former if you wish) is ready any time. The Naiad is, I hope, being launched this weekend, and wé shall be happy to have you aboard in June whenever you come.

The noncommital reply:

Dear Jules:

For some time I have been thinking of writing you for an autographed picture of yourself which I can frame and hang on the walls of my office.

Cordially yours,
Dan

April 20, 1956

Dear Dan:

Well, if you insist, I'll be hanged. Herewith.

In answer to a later inquiry as to just how peripatetic I was among APA membership:

February 26, 1957

Dear Dan:

You request a record of vagrancy nearly equal to yours. Reprehensible as it seems in review, in the last three weeks I have given the following lectures:

February 7–8	University of Oklahoma
February 9–13	University of Utah
February 12	Leonard Taboroff Memorial Address, Salt Lake City, Utah
February 15	Center for Advanced Behavioral Study, Palo Alto, California
February 18	Northern California Psychiatric Society, San Francisco, California
February 18–19	University of California, San Francisco, California
February 23	Invitational Address, American Psychopathological Society, New York, N.Y.

Over and above which, I am scheduled for:

March 2	American Association of Music Therapists, Jacksonville, Illinois
March 3	Galesburg State Research Hospital, Galesburg, Illinois
March 27	Association of Medical Psychoanalysts, New York, N.Y.
April 3–10	Marquette University, Milwaukee, Wisconsin
May 23	Post-Graduate Lecture, Marquette University, Milwaukee, Wisconsin

This, then, my contribution to confusing professional intercommunication for the trimester. Incidentally, I collect personal greetings for you everywhere.

Possibly on the basis of such evidence of grass roots contacts, in May, 1958, I was appointed to the program committee of the APA and assigned by John Donnelly, its chairman, to special mentorship over the Section on Psychoanalysis. The then chairman of the Section, Norman Reider, promptly informed me that he was planning to devote its May, 1959, meeting to a panel on research in perception; he proposed that the program committee invite the usual "panel of psychoanalysts" whose record (with one or two exceptions) in research had consisted of somewhat opaque public statements of their private fantasies. With a freshman's trusting innocence, I suggested to Dr. Reider that he might be introducing a bit of fresh air by opening his wooden panel as follows:

September 18, 1958

Dear Norman:

I appreciate your informing me of your choice of psychoanalytic research as the topic of your tentative roster of speakers. My own immediate suggestions would be based mainly on the now well-known hypothesis of Gödel: namely, that theory-building on research within a system cannot, of itself, validate its concepts, and that therefore partial closure must be secured from other fields. I agree that the Section on Psychoanalysis ought to remain primarily within that field, but would its program gain in general as well as scientific appeal if your projected symposium included "analytically oriented" speakers who have approached your topic of "Perception"—and hardly anyone now supports the doctrine of the Immaculate Perception—from a wide variety of other angles? For example: Harry F. Harlow of Wisconsin, who can make baby monkeys prefer warm towels to cold mothers; Jim Olds of Michigan, who, after "operational conditioning," can make rats prefer septal-stimulating levers to essential food or water; or my own associate Curtis Pechtel who, by perceptual manipulation, has developed highly symbolic "fetishistic" behavior in monkeys.

On the clinical side, Jay Haley of the Bateson group in Palo Alto has some interesting data on hypnotic percept-transactions, and Herbert Spiegel of New York has a series of drawings from his patients in "hypnotic regression" which may reflect the unconscious ideas of Herbert Spiegel. Then again, Jolyon West of Oklahoma has done some good work and clear thinking on the subject of "subliminal" perception and hallucinogenesis under drugs, and Hebb, Vernon, Lilly and others on the effects of sensory isolation; finally, Dave Rioch has some intriguing inferences on the subject.

These, I repeat, are merely off-the-cuff suggestions in immediate reply to your letter; if you are interested, I am sure I could expand or improve the list. In any case, we shall have time to correspond before the program committee meets on October 31st.

Dr. Reider rejected all of these suggestions and instead, deliberately or not, tried to schedule the panel as a "joint meeting," not of just the APA Section on Psychoanalysis, but of the entire APA with the American Psychoanalytic Association. Such maneuvers and the counteractions they elicited from the program committee eventually led to the abolition of the Section on Psychoanalysis, and eventually of all Sections, and a return of the scientific sessions of the APA to the sole control of the committee. My own part in this:

May 6, 1959

John Donnelly, M.D.
Chairman, Program Committee

Dear John:

Suggestions, as requested:

Adolf Meyer Lecture: If our other intended victims of last year don't accept (I would still like to see Leonard Bernstein and his orchestra in leotards or Maynard Hutchins heckled), E.

Strömgren of Oslo, who seems to be doing an excellent job in his current lecture tour of the United States, may serve. If you are interested, we can get him to serve as our academic lecturer in 1960.

Section on Psychoanalysis: This section, you will remember, turned down our suggestions, sent in its list of speakers too late for committee review, and listed itself in its own American Psychoanalytic Association program as holding a "joint session of the American Psychoanalytic Association and the American Psychiatric Association." Of the six authors selected, four were nonphysicians, and the papers they read on "preconscious perception" described work which had been presented many times previously. The audience dwindled from only about 300 in the vast main hall to about 75 for the last paper by Art Mirsky, and no discussion was permitted for any of the papers. Even more amusing was the "business meeting": Franz Alexander was nominated for chairman and, according to the tellers appointed by Reider himself, was elected on first ballot by 33 votes to 31 for Bob Morse. However, Reider apparently didn't like this result, called for a revote, and declared Morse elected by 38 to 35. After that, no one opposed the election of the secretary, or protested when Reider closed the meeting with no discussion of future plans or program. I shall be glad to continue as the program committee's liaison officer with this Section—in fact, my friend Bob Morse will be much more satisfactory to work with than was Reider—but perhaps the APA should reconsider the whole matter of Sections.

Section on Psychotherapy: This Section had an attendance of standing room only on Tuesday morning, a predictably worded but fairly lively program by four old APA stalwarts, and considerable discussion of each paper thereafter. Since its officers have a two-year term, there was no new election; instead, there was much discussion of future themes and plans and speakers. The topic selected for next year was "Reintegration of Psychoanalysis and Psychiatry," for which the Academy of Psychoanalysis was invited to a single joint meeting with the Section. When asked, I informed its officers that I shall recommend that all Sections, however cooperative, should eventually be abolished as troublesome anachronisms, and that in any case they would have to clear this with both yourself and the APA Council. They said they would do so.

When my term on the program committee expired, I wrote Dr. Donnelly:

October 20, 1959

Dear John:

As a departing Cato I submit the attached suggestions which your committee may or may not recommend to the council. Even if we act now, it will probably be years before these recommendations will be put into effect, but sooner or later something must be done to develop and improve what is one of the principle functions of the APA—our scientific sessions.

Numbers of submitted papers and other program arrangements: Since the number of proposed papers now exceeds 400 per year, and the annual lecturers, special sections, round tables, luncheons, discussants, etc. add up to hundreds of items more, the time the program committee can spend on each item of the annual program, even if it met for a total of twenty uninterrupted hours of executive session, must necessarily average less then two minutes. As a consequence, major policies sometimes receive only hurried consideration, whereas excessive time must often be accorded to special pleading by individuals and committees on relatively less important issues. The committee has thus inadvertently held itself open to criticisms implying "political influence" and careless or even prejudiced selections.

Deficient control of the program: The Committee currently delegates many of its selective and executive functions to officers of the various "scientific sections," to committees of other Societies who arrange joint meetings, to round-table and luncheon chairmen, and to other such functionaries, who compete with each other and encroach on other portions of the program more directly arranged by the committee. This has given rise and will continue to give rise to charges of hierarchic control by small groups, undemocratic practices, special favoritism for various societies, and doctrinaire section and round-table policies.

The above diffusion of program planning has indeed made some parts of our annual APA program seem so unorganized, repetitive, random, and uneven in quality that any member interested in the best papers in any single field must spend much time scuttling about from session to session, yet missing much he may want to hear—again giving rise to allegations of lack of interest or competence.

I recognize that the conditions that sometime occasion such criticisms can in no sense really be attributed to deficiencies of the program committee—I have worked long enough with the committee members to know better. Rather, the failure is in the outmoded routines and executive limitations under which the committee has labored. For these reasons, I submit the following proposals to expedite the committee's work in the future:

1. *Selection of Papers:* Deadline for all abstracts shall be October 1st, with nine copies distributed to the committee members as previously. These are to be graded by each member according to lucidity, originality, methodology, and import, and returned to the chairman about a week before the fall meeting. The chairman can then survey the grades and list the papers in order of their approval, saving a great deal of meeting time now devoted to this mechanical function. Copies of this list will be made available to each member in advance of the meeting so that objections or special pleas for changes in the order of selection can be seriously considered by the committee as a whole. The committee can then apportion the programs among twenty-two coded major subfields with equable topical assignment.

The total of thirty-two sessions would allow six of the more important subfields, (e.g., clinical psychiatry, social psychiatry, psychotherapy, psychoanalysis, hospital administration, and research) to have two sessions each (one early and one late in the week) and each of the twenty others to have one complete session. At six papers per session the program committee (with a total of about 192 papers) can then select twelve of the highest ranking papers in each of the six principal subfields, and six in each of the twenty others. Authors of papers ranking next in the average grades of the committee will qualify as discussants, thus converting each session into an informative seminar among the best qualified and interested contributors in that year.

Since there will be one or two such sessions in every subfield (and only four running simultaneously) fully planned and organized by the program committee, there would be no need for independent, competing, and sometimes contentious sections in the same field, and these can be gradually eliminated as judged best by the APA council.

2. *Round Tables, Motion Pictures, Exhibits, etc.:* These have established their value in past APA programs, but can be more carefully considered as to topic, personnel, and place by the committee.

3. *Future Committee Functions:* With these procedural policies, the program committee can be released from the mechanical and increasingly overwhelming routines of considering each item without apportioning time in accordance with its relative importance, and devote its efforts to major issues of program content and organization such as: (1) The academic and other annual lectures. (2) The relative allotment of time and importance to the various subfields and sessions. (3) The encouragement of research and clinical contributions from promising younger members of the APA. (4) The invitation to scientific participation in our meetings by authorities in ancillary fields. (5) Other fundamental policies and plans that should currently concern the committee and the APA.

Whereupon Walter Barton, new APA president, reappointed me for another three years, during which the committee took a much more active part not only in scheduling sessions but in enhancing their pertinence and interest. As one example:

June 8, 1961

B. Cullen Burris, M.D.
APA Divisional Meeting

Dear Dr. Burris:

Many thanks for your note requesting suggestions for your proposed panel on ethics in psychiatry. As to how to "organize the discussion," you might consider the following subtopics:

The Psychiatrist and the Patient: Apart from the usual considerations of personal confidentiality, safeguards against legal subpoena of information, iatrogenic traumata, subversive or seductive influences, etc.; you might also scrutinize more subtle questions:

1. In private practice, how far can we expect the psychiatrist to relinquish doctrinaire theories and dogmatic methods, no matter how great their current prestige, and remain eclectic, comprehensive, and flexible in the best interest of his patient?

2. In institutional practice, can the psychiatrist justifiably preserve his status through (a) The legal powers of commitment and the withholding or restitution of civil rights? and, (b) Hierarchic dominance over—and implicit downgrading of—essential therapeutic roles by social workers, nurses, activities therapists, occupational supervisors, and other (sic) "ancillary" personnel?

Ethics among Psychiatrists: You might consider *en passant* the not excessively rare instances of (a) Psychiatrists who, both publicly and in their private communications to patients, depreciate each other's specialized training (e.g., among psychoanalysts of differing schools or affiilations), theories, and techniques. (b) Psychiatrists who, without such overt action, nevertheless accept patients who impulsively have discontinued therapy with a colleague, without a conference about nor permission for such a transfer, often to the patient's detriment.

The Psychiatrist and the Social Order: Here the discussion might include (a) The regrettable image of the idiot savant, or at best, learned naïf, presented by some of our colleagues who, though obviously uninformed about history, anthropology, sociology, politics, economics, esthetics, theology, or even the elements of logic, clarity, and good taste in communication, nevertheless issue patronizing and pontifical pronouncements through the press and air on every subject from Art to Zen. (b) Or psychiatrists who, even when they stick to their own field, couch their knowledge in such obscure jargon, outmoded nosologies, and fanciful "interpretations" that once again our obligations to enlighten and clarify are unfulfilled.

Obviously, this is only a first purview of what you might consider; I shall hope for a much richer discussion.

October 4, 1961

John Donnelly, M.D.

Dear John:

I was greatly disappointed with the number of papers in the batch you sent me for grading that were trite, obvious, baseless, repetitious, doctrinaire, opinionated—shall I go on? I don't think we should grade our program submissions down to their level, and I marked them accordingly. Hope the subsequent batches will bring up the batching average.

As to the Theoretical Symposium, I am bone-weary of equating glibness with erudition, and obscurity with profundity. Let's not have K again; how about really rounded people such as Dave Rioch or Ray Waggoner as psychiatric discussants? Or, with a dash of bitters, Roy Grinker?

In 1961 Hardin Branch, APA president-elect, instead of accepting my plea for relief from program committee duties to attend to other pressing commitments, appointed me program chairman, inferring correctly that, because of my great personal esteem for him, I would assume perhaps the most trying and thankless post in the APA. My inaugural address to the program committee at the May, 1962, APA meeting:

Careful research having revealed no constitutional provisions for impeaching a new program committee chairman—even if the procedures were initiated by himself—the prospects are that I shall have to preside for at least a year over the efforts of our committee to maintain the golden age of John Donnelly. So we may as well get together the first day of the May meeting to take up the following matters as well as all others that the committee desires.

1. *Standards:* In view of the many papers of questionable quality submitted every year—over 350 of the 450 or so submitted—we must consider the feasibility of condensing the annual program even further by raising our criteria of acceptance to a level best for the scientific status of the APA. A copy of my last note to John on this subject is attached.

2. *Format:* We might accomplish this and yet save our collective scalps by designating more sessions as symposia on definitive topics. The four papers rated best on any subject would then be accepted for reading (total maximum one and one-fourth hours), the authors of the next four listed as discussants (total one-half hour), and the remaining half to three-fourths hour given over to audience participation and speakers' rebuttals. The secretary of each symposium could then prepare a written summary of the discussion and have it added to the seminar if and when accepted for publication in the APA journal. This would get everyone into the act, help solve the problem of finding suitable discussants, and provide greater opportunities for scientific communication on various subtopics of psychiatry.

3. *Fellowship Lecture:* It is the traditional privilege of the president to select the distinguished speaker for this event. Dr. Branch asked me to contact Justice William O. Douglas during a recent Ford Foundation meeting in Greece to which we were both invited, and I am happy to report that Mr. Douglas agreed to address the APA in 1963 if the Supreme Court were not in session at the time. However, if he is not available, and Dr. Branch has no other candidate, the committee might suggest such interesting departures from the ordinary as Danny Kaye on "The Healing Humor that Helped Hippocrates" with

discussion by Martin Grotjahn and Hardin Branch, or Leonard Bernstein, Thor Johnson, or Carrol Kearns on "Music Therapy for Psychiatrists—Illustrated." Or please think of others more intriguing. I propose that the committee petition the council for an annual appropriation of $1000 to cover the expenses and token honoraria of such invited lecturers.

4. *Invited Symposia* (theoretical or teaching sessions): Space may also be made on our program for truly authoritative discussions on currently important topics by *invited* speakers, for example: *The Psychology of Survival in Atomic War:* David Rioch, Harrison Brown, Herbert Muller, Herman Kahn, Albert Glass, David Riesman, et al. *The Future of Psychiatry in an Historic Context:* Arnold Toynbee, L. Gottschalk, Walter Bromberg, Ilse Vieth, et al. *Durham Decision, A Re-appraisal, 1963:* Judge David Bazelon, Henry Davidson, Manfred Guttmacher, Melitta Schmideberg (or a more reasonable facsimile), *et al. The Joint Commission Report, A Follow-up:* Jack Ewalt, Edison Duval, Ed Billings, Paul Hoch, Francis Gerty, Ted Ginsberg, Dan Blain. *How Educators Look at Psychiatric Education:* Robert Hutchins, Ralph Tyler, John Whitehorn, Burt Lewin, Bernard Dyer (director, AMA Joint Study on Continued Medical Education), et al.

5. *Great Debates:* Apropos of the above, last year Don Greaves proposed that we deliberately stage formal debates, complete with rebuttals among authorities known to differ on important human issues. The idea is replete with fascinating possibilities (e.g., Tom Szasz *vs* Howard Rome or Henry Davidson) that might be explored by the committee.

6. *Sections:* Most of these have become citadels of entrenched cliques and the refuge of only marginally scientific programs. Papers are now subject to committee approval, but we may wish to take further action as to the final abolition of all sections.

7. *Evening Seminars:* Too many (k)nights, too much pageantry, and not enough Camelots. These multiple sessions compete for the same small coterie of speakers, and need some system of regulation.

8. *Exhibits:* Justified complaints are received annually

that some of our exhibits are far from scientific, informative, or even dignified; the committee may wish to make recommendations to the council on this matter.

9. *Committee Organization:* Next to the council itself, the committee has perhaps the heaviest burden of responsibility and hard work of any group in the APA; and our obligations are constantly growing. I therefore propose, with your consent, to apportion the committee's tasks as follows: (a) By delegating particular responsibilities, such as seminars, special lectures, films, exhibits, discussants, round tables, etc. to individual committee members. (b) By requesting that a part-time secretary be designated at the Washington office of the APA, while I provide one (free) at Northwestern University. These secretaries will receive all abstracts submitted to the committee, send them to each member for appraisal by our code of grading, and arrange them by topic and rank. In this way, the committee can devote its own annual meeting time to considering only controversial, special, or marginal papers and assigned discussants, and then have an opportunity for constructive deliberations on program policies and format.

10. *Time Limitations:* Session Chairmen are to be instructed as to their duties and privileges in conducting their meetings. Mechanical means considered for controlling speakers ranged from trap doors, through silenced mikes to remote-control chloroform sprays; but it was left to the committee chairman to work out a system of lights (and/or electroshocks) with the arrangements committee in St. Louis. There will also be a page of Respectfully Insistent Suggestions to Speakers and Chairmen in the printed program.

11. *For the Fellowship Convocation:* Much of the ritual can be abolished and the rest be made more literate. For the newly instituted annual session on the arts and humanities we may invite Danny Kaye to illustrate and explain his skill in establishing immediate interpersonal empathy, and designate Charles Osgood, president of the American Psychological Association, and Jurgen Ruesch as discussants.

12. *The Book of Summaries:* Its title is to be changed to *Scientific Proceedings of the American Psychiatric Association in Summary Form* and its contents revised so that the abstracts

will be in topic groupings [with] cross indexing of the subjects, thus making it a permanent, readable, accessible, and logically organized record of our scientific meetings.

The APA Council authorized all the procedures recommended and appropriated a modest $2000 to cover the committee's expenses.

Nevertheless complications arose in arranging the first APA Session of the Arts and Humanities:

January 4, 1963

Dr. Charles Osgood, President
American Psychological Association

Dear Dr. Osgood:

The attached letter from Dr. Pumpian-Mindlin, my local Ambassador Extraordinary to Danny Kaye, is, I believe, a sufficient reason abandoning any certainty that that international worthy, despite his past promises, will appear in St. Louis on schedule next May 8th. I therefore tried to call you at your university today, but learned you were in California—a bit nearer to New Zealand where, perhaps all of us should be. But in the hope that you are still possessed of the seasonal good will toward all men—even psychiatrists—I shall now make the following request in the august name of the APA.

If I can get no completely affirmative commitment from D.K. (who gave us one last June) within the next few days, will you please accept the role of our Honorary Academic Lecturer at the 1963 meeting of the APA, and talk for about forty-five minutes—as seriously and/or as entertainingly as you like on any subject of your choice? The token honorarium ($150) and the expenses provided (travel, hotel, honorary dinner) will be far less a reward than the credit for cementing the professional and personal relationships between our two organizations by being one of our principal guest speakers, the other being Supreme Court Justice Douglas. If you wish to talk on communication, I can retain Dr. Jurgen Ruesch as one of the discussants, and perhaps appoint Ray Birdwhistell to present the anthropologic and mimetic aspects and/or Dr. Martin Grotjahn to talk about the psychoanalytic approaches to speech and gestural symbolisms. We shall all rest much easier if we can count on you.

To the editor of the official journal of the APA, troubled by the plethora of papers submitted to him from the annual meeting:

July 16, 1963

Dr. Clarence Farrar

Dear Clarence:

I can well appreciate that you might consider the 1963 APA papers a deluge and would send a dove from your editorial ark to me in the hope of a sign that the flood will abate next year. My olive branch:

1. With an APA membership of over 12,000 and about 600 papers submitted, the program committee had to place a minimum of a third on the program, else be given the choice between lynching and hara-kiri.

2. The average merit of the papers was, on an absolute scale, only so-so; on a relative scale, however, it was actually better than most previous years.

3. Since we wanted to schedule many outstanding invitational lectures and topical sessions (Justice Douglas, human communication, nuclear anxiety, population explosion, peace corps, military personnel evaluation, etc.), we could minimize the protest about worthy APA members being "displaced" by listing their contributions on the program as "resource papers."

4. This is all actually favorable to the quality of the journal's content: Your editorial board is certainly under no obligation to print more contributions; instead, it has a wider variety from which to choose only the best.

5. This selectivity will also improve the quality of the APA program, since members will learn that whereas it takes a good paper to be scheduled at the APA meeting, only the outstand-

ing ones will be published in the journal—ergo, the quality must be improved if both are desired.

I hope this explains the committee's currently unanimous thinking; however, I would be most happy to have you meet with us in Washington so that we can reach complete understanding and accord.

Sympathetically

Planning the annual APA Session on the Arts and Humanities always involved tactical problems:

September 27, 1963

May E. Romm, M.D.

Dear May:

The only arrangements I've made so far for the 1964 session is to have Dr. Nick Dallis, an APA member who authors that sterling serial-strip psychiatrist Rex Morgan (don't you read the funnies?), present the "Art and Message of the Cartoon, Illustrated"—all of which may fizzle. We'll all therefore greatly appreciate you and Jack Lomas, chairman of the arrangements committee, filling the other hour of the two-hour session by inducing or seducing Stanley Kramer to comment on his *Mad, Mad, Mad, Mad World*—and I know I can trust both your judgment and your feminine charms.

October 3, 1963

Mr. Stanley Kramer, Director
Universal Studios
Universal City, California

Dear Mr. Kramer:

I am in receipt of most welcome news from Dr. Jack Lomas and Dr. May Romm that you may consent to address the annual meeting of the American Psychiatric Association in Los Angeles next May pending arrangements with me. Permit me to tender this official invitation to do so and to acquaint you with some of the circumstances of your lecture.

A high point at each of our annual meetings is a Session on the Arts and Humanities, when most of the professional personnel (expected attendance four to five thousand) at the meeting gather to hear some deservedly renowned director, artist, or virtuoso endowed with a deep understanding of, and empathy with, human feelings and aspirations, communicate his insights and describe the skills he employs in his special field. The auditorium is equipped for any audio-visual demonstrations, including sound film projection, you may wish to employ. Most regrettably, as a scientific society, we cannot offer you a proper financial inducement, but sincerely hope that you may consider broadening the intellectual and esthetic horizons of an informed, influential, and deeply appreciative professional audience a sufficient reward. And, of course, we would be delighted to have you as our honored guest at any of the other scientific or social functions—including the President's Dinner—throughout our convention.

I shall look forward to luncheon with you on Friday, October 18th, as arranged by Dr. Lomas.

Mr. Kramer agreed to deliver the address, which, with excerpts from his films, was enthusiastically received at the 1964 meeting.

December 9, 1963

Jack B. Lomas, M.D.
Chairman, Arrangements Committee
Beverly Hills, California

Dear Jack:

With the program book due at the printers next month, we must get the following details settled as soon as possible:

Official Opening: I trust that you and Jack Ewalt have made certain that Father Sullivan will give the Invocation, but to assure our entry into whatever competing heavens there may be we must also invite a Protestant minister and a rabbi for the interim and closing Benedictions.

Governor Brown's office wrote me that he was "favorably inclined" to give the Official Greeting, but could not as yet "be certain" of appearing personally—which of course doesn't help much. Please exert as much local pressure as you can to get a more definite answer, or permission to put his name in the program with the understanding that if, at the last moment, he cannot come, he will send an acceptable representative—perhaps his new Director of Mental Health. Also, if you want the Mayor of Los Angeles or any other big brass to give Five Minutes of Hearty Welcome, please let me know right away so I can list Hizzoner.

The Session on Coordinated Action for Mental Health is to be an *In Memoriam for John Fitzgerald Kennedy.* I therefore think it would be appropriate to have a moderately sized portrait of our late President hung behind the speaker's table, appropriately draped in flags and with some flowers around it —no longer in mourning, but in respectful memory. I shall check with Jack Ewalt as to whether or not, under the circumstances, he would want HEW Director Celebrezze on the platform for another ten minute greeting at the first Scientific Session.

VIP Accommodations: As soon as possible I'll give you a list of invited Personages who should be specially met, registered, and made comfortable in rooms reserved for them at the Biltmore. Are you planning a VIP registration desk, pretty-girl welcoming committees, etc.? Let me know so we can coordinate correspondence.

In response to a public relations' inquiry: I could restate the issues:

June 2, 1964

Zigmond Lebensohn, M.D.
Chairman, APA Public Relations Committee

Dear Zig:

Not counting over 700 summaries and panels prepared each year, I annually receive about 200 letters concerning every May meeting. Nearly all the letters begin with high praise for the preceding meeting, and then proceed to offer a wide variety of suggestions to the effect that we should have more, fewer, or different topics, speakers, debates, discussants, panels, sections, free time, jam sessions, periods of prayer, "joint" or "open" meetings, etc. For research interest, last year I made a matricial analysis of this significant resonance from the officers and membership of the APA, and found that (a) there was a most gratifying consensus of approval for the many changes made during the past two years in our committee procedures, publications, and annual program, and (b) all other suggestions neatly cancelled each other out. Put as briefly as possible, the real issues that governed our committee deliberations have been these:

1. To have relatively few papers, with invited speakers on major topics. This would undoubtedly raise the average scientific level of the program, but might confine it to a recurrently favored few, and exclude many.

2. To select about a third of the very best summaries submitted annually, arrange them in a wide variety of topical seminars to cover nearly all the interests of the membership, and salt these liberally with topnotch contributors of known ability to ensure that nearly every session would be of some interest. This course might admit some relatively weak speakers who had submitted fine-sounding summaries, but would favor wider interest and participation of the APA membership, develop the potentialities of younger members, and furnish a richer, and more varied meeting from which everyone could make wider choices to suit his special interests.

3. To combine the best features of (1) and (2) and add memorable sessions on arts, history, humanities, etc., thus assembling a program most likely to meet the widest range of expectations and fulfillments.

Ordinarily, the committee has done its best to implement the third course. However, we are always open to suggestions and would welcome expert help with all aspects of the program.

The success of the 1963 and 1964 meetings led to a bit of tentative over-wishfulness at the highest levels:

November 27, 1964

The Honorable Dean Rusk
Secretary of State
Washington, D. C.

My dear Mr. Secretary:

The American Psychiatric Association, comprising 14,000 psychiatrists, with additional authorities in the behavioral sciences from around the world as guests, will hold its annual meeting at the Americana Hotel in New York from May third to May seventh, 1965. The high point of this meeting will be a Convocation Address on a topic of importance to all mankind —whether in statesmanship, law, philosophy, or any branch of the humanities—by an authority who has attained universal respect in any or all of these fields. You may be interested to know that Justice William Douglas was the honored speaker at our last convocation.

I most respectfully inquire whether it would be possible for you to be our convocation lecturer on any topic of your choice. A generous honorarium will, of course, be available, and every effort will be made to make your visit with us personally enjoyable.

I shall be in Washington on December 12 and 13th, and would greatly appreciate the privilege of calling you on this matter if you would like further details.

Most respectfully

Daniel Blain, the newly elected APA president, intimated (in retrospect, justifiably) that this invitation as well as other arrangements for a joint APA meeting with the Royal Medical Psychological Society of Britian which I had been commissioned to explore, should have been initiated by him, and elicited what I now consider a bit of overreactive pique on my part:

July 27, 1964

Dear Dan:

Your telegram to me in London that "I make no final decisions" as to our Edinburgh meeting and your more recent note, awaiting me on my return, on the copy of the invitation to Dean Rusk I sent you seem to require this reply:

As to the former: in the next mail you and all members of the Ad Hoc Committee will receive a full report on my meeting —on my "vacation" time and at no expense to the APA—with our opposite numbers of the Royal-Medico-Psychologic Association—a report that will, I hope, make clear that though our deliberations were most cordial and productive, we all wanted them to be exploratory, and our recommendations only preliminary to the full meeting in August. I certainly never planned to make "final" arrangements about anything. In fact I attended this meeting at all only because your medical director, Walter Barton, asked me to do so, and because I hoped you, he, and Harvey Tompkins might also be there. You will recall that I have always referred important issues first to my committee and then to the APA president and council, and have invariably abided by their advice and decisions.

As to the second matter, you were personally present at our program committee meeting in Los Angeles last May when we reviewed and approved the list of important personages to be invited for 1965, including President Johnson, Dean Rusk, U Thant, Adlai Stevenson, *et al.* In my eight years of participation in program committee procedure, such preliminary invitations (which, incidentally, are never seen by the personage invited but always handled by his secretariat), have customarily been written by the program chairman for many good reasons: centralization of preliminary correspondence, coordination of possible program dates, avoidance of the indignity of a direct refusal to the president of the APA, etc. On the other hand, whenever the invitee's secretariat indicates interest, since I have been chairman I have always brought the APA president immediately into the picture for the final formalities, arranged for him to preside at the actual APA session, and had the program committee fade out of the picture. This was the procedure in the case of Justice Douglas in 1963, the late President Kennedy (tentative acceptance), and Governor Brown (who declined at the last moment) in 1964, and will be in the case of Dean Rusk, U Thant, Adlai Stevenson, *et al.*, if these prove available in 1965.

Now, regrettably, I must add a personal note. To serve the APA adequately, during the past two years I have had to sacrifice thousands of dollars of income and neglect many academic, research, university, editorial, and even familial interests in order to give nearly half my time throughout the year to the increasingly complex and manifold demands of the program chairmanship. I have done this cheerfully and, I hope, efficiently, my only reward being the promotion of the prestige and scientific status of the APA and the appreciation of my friends, including the successive presidents of the APA. Unfortunately, your telegram and note indicate either a desire to change all these customary procedures without explanation, or insufficient confidence in my conduct of the chairmanship. In the latter case, you are most welcome to my resignation without further prejudice.

The resignation was declined in a most courtly manner. I replied:

August 13, 1964

Dear Dan:

All clear; sorry I got grumpy, but that's a privilege among old friends.

Herewith the letter from Rusk's third assistant social secretary. This leaves U Thant and Adlai Stevenson as interested. So herewith also copies of my letters to them and their replies. Also, I got Dr. Sadusk of the Federal Drug Administration corralled for a straight talk on government policy on drugs. Want to carry on from here? I'll wait to hear from you.

Services were now requested by other departments of the APA:

28 August, 1964

Dear Dr. Masserman:

So—you've done it again? I refer, this time, to your "The Contributions of Experimental Psychiatry to the Art of Healing" (*Psycho-Anal. Rev.* 50:633-662, Winter 1963), which I stumbled across during one of my episodic quaffings at the National Library of Medicine. My pleasure and profit in reading it were marred only by pangs of regrettable envy.

Which brings me to my point: May we have your permission to buy reprints or to get the journal's permission to reproduce copies to make available in our packet and to readers of the *APA Bulletin*? You may recall that we have done this with others of your articles and that we make no charge for these reprints.

William F. Sheeley, M.D., Chief
APA-GP Education Project

September 1, 1964

Dear Bill:

Since I am a modest man who, in Churchillian language, has every reason to be so, I am far less sure than you are that my writings do much more than marginally amuse and minimally instruct. However, you are most welcome to use any of them for your good purposes.

A note of approbation from a colleague on the program committee:

November 11, 1964

Dear Jules:

While I'm at it, my friend, let me reiterate the sentiments I spoke at our last session. You have been a magnificant chairman of the program committee, and there is absolutely no doubt that the quality and interest-value of the programs have increased immeasurably under your leadership. I hope that you will continue at the helm of this crucial committee, or (if moving onward and upward) will keep your eagle eye on it. It was an honor, a pleasure, and an education to help you. I'll never forget it and I thank you deeply for it.

As always,
Jolly
L. Jolyon West, M.D.

I kept a personal check on motion picture films submitted for showing at the annual meetings, and ran across an old friend (see Chapter 11).

October 14, 1964

Dr. Jacob Moreno
Institute of Psychodrama
New York, N. Y.

Dear Dr. Moreno:

I reviewed your film on psychodrama at the earliest opportunity, shall return it to you shortly, and present it for consideration to the program committee as you requested. However, I must inform you that in order to meet APA standards of merit and ethics, the committee may well decide that the following changes will have to be made before it can be presented under the sponsorship of the APA:

1. Since your sound film identifies several hospitalized pa-

tients (by name, visage, speech, and even home address) to unknown audiences, you must obtain their written or officially authorized consent for such uncontrolled exhibition.

2. You must delete all injurious allegations, such as your principal subject identifying his fiancee by name and then stating publicly that "she was not a virgin." This is not only a regrettable breach of ethics, but would be legally actionable by her against the APA if the film were shown under its sponsorship.

3. Your closing soliloquy about "psychodrama making possible mass psychotherapy to cure [all] mental illness in the nation" might well be modified to less sweeping and more modest statements.

I shall be glad to convey your reactions to these suggestions to the committee before they make their final decision.

Dr. Moreno made no reply, but to avoid any allegation of past personal bias, I extended the deadline to the last possible day:

February 1, 1965

Dear Dr. Moreno:

The program committee was in complete agreement with the critique of your film that I sent you on October 14, 1964. Unfortunately, I have not heard from you in the ensuing four months, so the program had to go to press without listing your film. Nevertheless, if you can send me an acceptable version of the film within the next two weeks, I may still be able to enter it on the page proofs.

Dr. Moreno now wrote that he had made the changes requested and would send his film again for a final inspection. I reviewed the "edited" version and replied:

February 17, 1965

Dear Dr. Moreno:

In my letter of October 14th I outlined a number of serious scientific and ethical objections, fully endorsed by the program committee, to the showing of your film on psychodrama. You replied that you would revise the film accordingly and, relying on your good faith and pending a second review, I listed it for showing on Wednesday afternoon, May 5th, as the APA program was going to press.

I have now viewed the revised version you send me and find that among other uncorrected defects (e.g., poor picture and sound, questionable procedures such as directing physical contacts between patients, ordering one subject to pray publicly, lie on the floor, to hallucinate, etc.), the following violations of confidentiality as well as good taste remain:

1. Several patients at the Camarillo State Hospital are identified not only by closeups, but specifically by name and address.

2. The principal subject is similarly identified, and his past and current actions are revealed in a way that may seriously handicap his future occupational and social relations with possible viewers of the film.

3. Even more unethically, he was still permitted to give the name and address of his parents, his fiancee, and others, and to describe their actions in a manner that, true or not, may be seriously objectionable to them.

I have been legally advised that even should you obtain written permission from all the parties so adversely identified, their hospitalization as incompetents and the unprovable allegations recorded would render you liable to suit for violation of confidence and defamation of character; further, were the APA to show this film at its annual meeting, the Association would not only be open to public criticism but could be made a party to such a suit.

Since the program committee is entrusted with the responsibility of protecting the APA against such eventualities, I must regretfully remove your film from the program. It is being returned to you express prepaid.

After my nomination to the august serenity of the APA Council, I resigned as program committee chairman and presented my final oral report to the APA Membership, May 3, 1965:

President Blain, Ladies and Gentlemen:

On all previous such occasions I had asserted that my appearance here, though demanded by protocol, was completely unnecessary, since each of you had at hand the full report of the Program Committee in the form of a program brochure of some 200 pages rather fully packed with the organized details of our annual meeting. But since this is my third and last appearance as your Program Chairman, I hope you will grant me a few moments to review what the aspirations and objectives of the Program Committee have been, however asymptotic our performance. In essence, we wished to encourage an ever larger proportion of our membership to participate in the scientific and humanitarian activities of this Association in as many ways as possible, among them these:

First, by scheduling as many discerning and diverse papers as reasonable and practicable for the time and facilities available. You may like to know that each of the contributions to our annual meeting is read in summary form by every member of the Program Committee, and culled by careful consensus from thrice the number of submissions for originality, validity, clarity and other specific criteria—our only partial bias being that deserving contributions by our younger members should be particularly encouraged.

Second, by assembling the fifteen score papers finally selected into 50 topical sessions, each arranged as a logically progressive seminar on its special subject, with chairman, co-chairman, and discussants assigned with equal care for their competence in the field and subtopic.

Third, by so distributing the various sessions throughout the week as to occasion as little conflict of interest and attendance as possible.

Fourth, by seeding each day of the program with prearranged Symposia to which world-renowned experts in anthropology, sociology, law, politics, and others allied to psychiatry are invited for illuminating dialogues with our own authorities and leaders.

Fifth, by arranging what we hoped were esthetically as well as scientifically intriguing seminars on the arts and humanities including this year a showing of *David and Lisa* and a new professional film on the history of psychiatry.

But despite all efforts to the contrary, such scientific sessions and sections retain a formal, predominantly unidirectional flow of communication, and need to be supplemented by opportunities for a freer interchange of experience and opinion among our members. For this purpose the program committee further developed two other features of the annual meetings, to wit: (1) Eight "Questions the Experts Sessions'" at which our youthfully avid members could meet and interrogate, and stimulate and challenge, their professional elders in various fields of research, teaching and practice; and (2) Forty-five "Evening Panels"—filling every room available—on topics ranging from alcoholism to zoophobia, at which long dissertations were explicitly discouraged in favor of free and frank, friendly or ferocious discussions throughout the evening—and sometimes into the night and morning.

Two editorial duties also deeply engaged us: (1) to cooperate with the committee on information in replanning and revising the format and title of what is now our yearly volume of *Scientific Proceedings* so that readers throughout the world can have an organized permanent record of our annual meetings in summary form; and (2) to contemplate deeply and to formulate clearly further improvements in our annual and regional meetings.

Clearly, no one man—and certainly not I—could have done any of this unaided. Fortunately, I was blessed with eight tireless IBM computers who programmed themselves to sort incredible masses of data into useful categories and came up almost invariably with the right answers. I refer to my eight colleagues and personal friends on the program committee, in whose case the initials IBM could well stand for trios of qualities ranging from intrepid, burdened and masochistic to doubly insightful and intelligent, brave and broadminded and magnificent managers. It is to the work of John Ewing, Sherv Frazier, Don Greaves, Ed Harper, Will Peltz, Don Ross, Jolly West, and Larry Wolberg, and to the cooperation of Walter Barton, Bart Hogan, Robbie Robinson, Austin Davies, Phyllis Woodward and Liz Crossette in the Central Office, and not least to my own enslaved secretaries Miss Laird and Mrs. Schore that the organization and success of these programs were largely due—as I hope the current one will be also. But I am certain of this: you will be consummately well served by your new Program Committee and its able Co-Chairmen, Sherv Frazier and Jolly West.

My program notes for the 1965 Session on the Arts and Humanities:

Psychiatry, Art, and Ballet

In some moment of reflection on C. P. Snow's categorization of all men as either "scientific" or "humanistic," someone must have objected that *if* there are two types of human beings, one must be the type that sets up such untenable dichotomies. Are all "scientists" really cold, remote, and ruthlessly calculating, in contrast to all "artists" who are subjective, empathic and integratively visionary? Does science merely "codify" man's images of the cosmos, whereas art "creates" them? Alfred North Whitehead put it both scientifically and poetically: "Nature gets credit which ... should be reserved for ourselves: the rose for its scent, the nightingale for its song, and the sun for its radiance, whereas in truth . . . nature is a dull affair, soundless, scentless, colorless, merely the hurrying of material, endlessly, meaninglessly." Freud, too, commented to the Vienna Psychoanalytic Society: "Our understanding of science reaches only as far as our anthropomorphism"; thus, as had Locke, Berkeley, Kant, and Hegel before him, Freud emphasized that all man's arts and sciences equally reflect uniquely individualized forms of perception, imagery, and evaluation. Finally, since the *Oxford Dictionary*—that repository of the wisdom of aeons of philologic evolution—defines Art itself (from L. *ars*, to join) simply as "skill derived from knowledge and experience," can we as psychiatrists presume to distinguish our "art" from our "science"?

How, then, does art illumine (not differ from) science? Perhaps by contributing the ideal of grace (from L. *gratus*): pleasing, harmonious, elegant, excellent. Inevitably, in the comprehensive semantics of our language this root has become generalized to all of man's ultimate (*Ur-*) aspirations: first, for physical and mental perfection (Apollo, handsome and wise was the fitting deity of both art and medicine); second, for human dignity and gratitude ("your Grace," "*muchos gracias*"), and finally, for communion with the Divine ("the Grace of God").

Ballet epitomizes all of these, whether its five technically "scientific" positions are expressed in the classic Italian style of Cechetti, or in the flowing French school, or in the Slavic vigor of Diaghilev. All idealize beautiful bodies in perfect motion, strive for the harmony and counterpoint of the ensemble, and yearn for the transcendent and ethereal. Tonight, with a virtuosity ranging from the limpid classicism of "Swan Lake" to the stark earthiness of "Phoebe Snow," our world-famous principals—Marcia Haydee, the German prima ballerina making her debut in this country, and Edward Villela star of the New York Ballet—supported by the talented Boston Ballet Company, will convey not only the rhapsodies of gentle love but the poignancies of human frustrations and the tragedies of insensate passions. In this way the fifth annual session on the Arts and Humanities can well grace the one hundred and twenty-fourth scientific meeting of the American Psychiatric Association.

On my national election to the APA Council:

Bart Hogan, M.D.
Associate Medical Director
APA

April 26, 1965

Dear Jules

Congratulations. You did better than LBJ—swept *every* state.

Sincerely,
Bart

And from my publisher:

May 24, 1965

Dear Jules:

It is with great joy that I congratulate you on your election to the Council of the APA. The fact that you were elected by the largest vote in the APA history confirms again how highly your services to the Association are appreciated. I may add to it that although I attended the meeting for only two days, I enjoyed every minute of it. The program was excellently selected and prepared as uaual. The credit, of course, goes to you. To whomever I spoke had nothing but praise for your untiring efforts.

As ever yours,
Dr. Henry M. Stratton
Grune & Stratton

After being again commissioned by the program committee to arrange the arts and humanities session for the APA meeting in Miami, in 1969, I proceeded, as always, to secure the cooperation of the central office and the local arrangements committee. However, this time plans soon began to go awry, apparently due to the same administrative turmoil during the presidency of Larry Kolb that also resulted in the suspension of the transcultural conferences (see Chapter 20). Dr. Alan Lipton, a personable and popular Miami psychiatrist, was assigned to collaborate with me, and wrote that he was investigating what the Miami Symphony and the Music Department of Miami University could offer. I replied:

June 11, 1968

Alan A. Lipton, M.D.
Miami Psychiatric Associates

Dear Alan:

I am delighted by your letter and, as is my wont (or want?), responded with action by calling Mrs. Geraldine Freund, generous doyenne of the Fairview Hospital Foundation and getting a promise from her of another subsidy for the Arts and Humanities Session in Miami; the amount was unspecified, but last year's Ballet cost them about $16,000. The only catch is that, although Sherv Frazier, chairman of the program committee, and the council have cleared the matter, we would all want to cooperate fully with Walter Barton of the central office and with Bruce Alspach and Sam Hibbs of the arrangements committee so that everything can run smoothly.

If they agree, I shall be most happy to enlist you as local co-secretary of the 1969 Arts and Humanities Session so that you can begin to explore the following: (1) The availability of the Miami Symphony. (2) The best and most entertaining musicologist and/or artist to act as interpretive master of ceremonies, provided Conductor Alain Lombard won't do it himself *à la* Leonard Bernstein. I promise I won't ask anyone to play any of my own compositions or ask to sit in the violin or viola sections, but nearly every symphony has a voluntary swing, rock or other far-out combo who secretely play together for fun. If we can't bring them out in the open, perhaps a local "Jefferson Airplane" group can give us a coda to the classics. (3) The loan of ancient, medieval, Renaissance, Romantic, Victorian, baroque, and up to modern and psychedelic paintings (or archietectural photographs) to project on a screen in synesthesia with concurrent musical illustrations. (I presume we can't reproduce the differing smells of each period.) (4) Etc., as genius directs.

Dr. Lipton voted for the Miami Symphony. Ergo:

June 15, 1968

Bruce W. Alspach, M.D.
Chairman, Arrangements Committee

Dear Bruce:

Since Alan favors the Miami Symphony, I asked him to check with you if perhaps we could use some of the symphony players—many of whom must also be swingers—as a basis for an exploration of synesthetic history starting with excerpts from the classical with concomittantly projected illustrations of art and architecture at various periods and ending with Calypso and psychedelic music and posters. Duke Ellington would be great fun, but hard to get; I have an in with Isaac Stern and David Oistrakh, but not with the Duke; do you know anyone who does? Since you wish it, I'll be glad to welcome Herman Selinsky as collaborator; please write and we'll keep things going.

Dr. Selinsky at first seemed perceptive and cooperative:

June 19, 1968

Herman Selinsky, M.D.
Miami Committee on Arrangements

Dear Herman:

As you know, Al has proposed using the Miami Symphony to illustrate the evolution of musical idioms from "classical" to modern 12-tone sequential, possibly combining the expositions with illustrations of all sculpture and architecture from ancient to psychedelic during the corresponding eras for synesthetic vividness. In response, I wrote him, with a copy to Bruce Alspach which I trust you saw, that the proposal sounded most promising but that I would want to coordinate my efforts and choices with the advice and consensus of Bruce and any other members of the Arrangements Committee who would know best what Miami had to offer. Your own suggestions sound equally exciting, so that it now becomes a question of what is (a) most practical from the standpoint of availability, cost, relative predictability of performance, etc., and (b) esthetic, entertaining, and—since this is an APA Session—instructive as to deeper insights into the effects of nonverbal affective (i.e., "artistic") communications on human behavior.

As to costs, I believe that Dr. and Mrs. Freund of the Fairview Hospital Foundation may again subsidize the Session, hopefully to the tune of up to $8,000. Considering the fact that the first four Arts and Humanities Sessions I arranged including the first one on Music and Emotions four years ago, cost the APA less than $400 each, this is fairly generous, and we really should not strain the Freunds' generosity further. Within this budget, would it be possible, within the 3-hour morning or 2¼-hour evening allowed for the Session, to combine selected members of the Symphony to illustrate the evolution of Western music, and then, after a brief intermission, continue with combos to show how African idioms (including Cuban and American Negro) have infiltrated and enlivened our own in recent times? This might make a rich, unique, and memorable sequence, utilizing both the symphonic and Dr. Lee's supplementary resources—or, possibly it might make for conflicts of interest, clashes of temperament, and confusions. At this distance, I cannot know, and I shall rely on the combined good judgment of Bruce, Al, and yourself as to how to proceed to ensure the best Arts and Humanities Session ever.

To further clarify the purposes of the APA Arts and Humanities Sessions with their financial sponsor:

June 27, 1968

Mrs. Geraldine Freund
Fairview Hospital Foundation

Dear Gerry:

The famous philosopher of the comic strip, Pogo, once remarked that human communication occasionally follows the principle: "I don't understand a word you say, but I will fight to your death for my right to deny it!" Since this may have applied to some of our recent communications, let me clarify the issues in as clear and friendly a manner as possible:

As I have tried to explain on numerous occasions, the APA Arts and Humanities Sessions are not intended to be merely shows or exhibitions, although they should also be as artistically satisfying as possible. It is true that such excellence is promoted by high-priced professional talent, and that our last session on ballet was the esthetic high point in APA history—yet each session must be more than a "concert." In addition, it should explore some significant aspect of human behavior of scientific interest to the APA—how painting, drama, sculpture, architecture, music, dance, etc., can convey anger, awe, depression, love, rage, and other emotions, or illustrate neurotic and psychotic deviations of conduct and their alleviation through expression and catharsis. Incidentally, these combinations of art and psychiatry have in past highly successful Sessions been better portrayed by experts in human behavior who are only casually versed in some art, than by professional performers relatively ignorant of human dynamics. Of course, if both are available, so much the better—and we should seek such happy combinations.

As I have also tried to explain, in planning these sessions I must not only follow my own tastes and those of the financial donors, but necessarily satisfy the wishes of the officers and council of the APA, Dr. Barton and his staff at the central office, the program committee, the arrangements committee, and the general consensus of 16,000 members of the APA. In this connection, the council requested that I devote the next Arts and Humanities Session to two themes: (a) *Synesthesia*—which is a technical term meaning that various sensory modalities such as sound, vision, olfaction, and kinetics can be combined to make the total experience vivid and unforgettable. (b) *Musical development*—meaning not only twelve-tone and progressive, but the infiltration of Eastern, African, Haitian, and other "foreign" modes of music.

I hope you will now understand better what I tried to convey over the phone and in the letters I sent to the program arrangements committee, as always, with copies to you. The suggestions I made are entirely tentative and preliminary, and while I remain in nominal charge of the session, it cannot succeed unless we enlist the complete cooperation of these committees and the APA Council—and we must, without compromising either art or science, respect their preferences.

As illustration as to how such problems can be worked out with tact and judgment, please refer to my last letter to Dr. Selinsky (again with copy to you) and to the letter from Dr. Lipton (copy enclosed) which states that the Miami Symphony alone would cost $11,000—a sum I would expect you or no other donor to spend. This leaves Dr. Lee, the Miami University School of Music, Duke Ellington (whom we would hope to get), the famous Stan Kenton, and the excellent local professional or semi-professional talent to present the evolution of modern music—a very promising set of resources we can develop, and which we can correlate with modern evolutionary and revolutionary trends in all human conduct.

As to whether you wish to subsidize the next session, please consider these facts: (a) I did everything possible to have the APA and all others acknowledge and extend every tangible appreciation of your 1968 generosity—including having the council pass a special resolution and, for the first time in APA history, design a special plaque which is being prepared to hang in your office. From a purely practical standpoint —and there is no reason for not being realistic as well as idealistic—this will greatly increase your and Dennis' prestige in the APA, and may help his career in important ways; (b) As my letter to Dr. Selinksy indicates, I have no intention of having you or any other donor spend excessive amounts on any Arts and Humanities Session. I mentioned the sum of $8000 as maximum, but we can try to expend even less.

As always, my best to Dennis and yourself.

Meanwhile, Dr. and Mrs. Freund now requested that I arrange Arts and Humanities Sessions four or five times annually for the psychiatric community in Chicago. My initial introduction at one such intercurrent session, presented after an invitational dinner to about 150 psychiatrists and their wives at the Chicago Arts Club:

Ladies and Gentlemen: Some months ago, your genial host Dennis Freund, and your gracious hostess Geraldine Freund and I had a solemn conference—as solemn as we ever get—to see what we could plan that might most please you. We readily agreed that we were *not* going to have yet another lecture series, usually consisting of a procession of pompous and pretentious pedants pontificating about what you already knew and didn't want to hear more about. Instead, we were going to share with you an exploration of the Arts and Humanities in their psychiatric context. Of these, we chose dance, music, opera, sculpture, and theatre. I agreed to be moderator, but only on condition that I be immoderately brief in my remarks.

This promise I recently kept on a related occasion: some weeks ago I was privileged to give a succession of lectures at the Centennial celebration of the Alaska Medical Society. Its officers proved gentlemanly and tolerant, and with sly humor invited me back, not for some meeting in the immediate future, but for their next *centennial.* Came the inevitable banquet at which I was scheduled to give a final talk on "Sex and the Singular Psychiatrist." The master of ceremonies gave me a long and complimentary introduction ending with the suggestive "And now Dr. Masserman will give us his considered conclusions from his research and clinical studies of sexual relationships." The temptation was too great, and I succumbed: I got up and said: "Ladies and Gentlemen, I still rather enjoy them"—and sat down.

This is what I shall do now. The Arts are a supremely esthetic joy in themselves, and what little interpretation they need should be conveyed by the artist himself. Tonight we shall be privileged to witness one of the most ancient forms of artistic expression—namely, the varieties and depths of human emotion expressed in the eloquence and grace of human motion. As one of its most charming choreographers, ballet masters and interpreters we shall have with us that delightful doyenne of the dance—the picaresque, pixyish Miss Ruth Page, Directress of her own Chicago Ballet Company. To introduce her further would be like explaining to music lovers what a combination of Arturo Toscanini and David Oistrakh might be like. Ruth, would you please take over, and, in Biblical parlance, wherever thou goest, we shall go?

Prologue to a Chicago Presentation of "The Art of the Cinema"

As psychiatrists or psychiatrists-in-law, nearly all of us here are proud of being able, in an hour's interview with another human being to survey his character, assay his weaknesses and strengths, search for their origins in his past life, and discern his vicissitudes, the recent stresses that precipitated them, his current ways of dealing with reality, his patterns of transaction with his fellow men and, indeed, his probable fate. Incidentally, we also like to think that his future is deplorable if he doesn't change as we imply he should. But we have competition in this field of artistry—art being defined, as it is in *Webster's Dictionary,* as skill derived from training and experience. I refer to the art of directing a motion picture: Let me illustrate:

Five years ago, as some of you may recall, I induced Stanley Kramer, the producer and director of such classics as *The Treasure of Sierre Madre* (with John Huston), *The Bridge on the River Kwai* and *Mad, Mad, Mad, Mad World* to address the Arts and Humanities Session of the APA. With superb communicative skill illustrated by film clips, Kramer showed how, in a fleeting scene lasting not more than sixty seconds, a director with genius could delineate a whole personality, his background, his current transactions with reality and his fellow men, and his probable role in the rest of the story. Stanley Kramer could do this because a movie director has every modality at his command: the composite frame of setting, the choice of colors, the background of sound or music, the pace of the motion and the thrust of the drama itself. And he can add an infinity of animate and inanimate symbolisms: for example, he may, with a background of Beethoven's "Pastoral Symphony," dwell on the bucolic beauty of a springtime brook running crystal-clear to its destiny in the infinite ocean—and suddenly have a rill of raw blood appear on it to indicate that the beauties of nature cannot hide the cruelties of life. He can show a human face gazing at this shearing incongruity, and that face can express bewilderment, or awe, or fear, or horror, or be sated with evil revenge. Indeed, a movie director such as Bergman can for a brief moment create men and women in his image—and thereby relate himself once again to certain aspects of being a psychiatrist.

Like all others, the art of the cinema has both an esthetic and technical background. Moving pictures—in both senses of the word "moving"—originated in the middle Pleistocene age when Acheulian or Mousterian man, on the walls of his stone-age caves near Altamira in Spain or Lascaux in France, drew silhouettes of bands of men hunting the bison and sabre-toothed tiger; significantly, in these masterpieces of ancient imagery the animals were depicted in harmonic rhythmic movement, whereas the men themselves were symbolized as mere branched sticks. Forty thousand or so years later Peter Roget, in 1826, presented to the Royal Society of London his discovery of the persistence of visual images, and thus laid the physiologic groundwork for the illusion of the fluidity of motion in the sixteen-frame per second "motion" picture.

Interestingly, it was Jules Morey, a physician, who in 1882 first recorded movement by taking a rapid series of pictures of the flight of birds through a non-lethal camera he called a photographic gun. And it took twelve years more, until 1894, for Edison to market his Kinetoscope, a simple picture-exposure device which, in effect, provided only a fifteen-second peep-show. It then took another fifteen years for the first movie with a plot to appear: Edwin Porter's "The Great Train Robbery," and yet another decade passed before D.W. Griffith thought of moving the camera along with the action. I can still remember hearing the first sound film produced by the De Forest process, *The Jazz Singer,* in 1927, and it was only about fifteen years ago that Cinerama introduced the wide screen. I myself made my first movies of animal neuroses almost thirty years ago, and it was then considered a novel and expensive innovation in research or pedagogic techniques.

As to pedagogy, John Stuart Mill, Rousseau, John Locke, Pestalozzi, and many others long ago pointed out the supreme advantages of consensual reinforcement of learning through sight, sound and motion, and since then motion pictures, especially as disseminated by television, have become perhaps the most influential of all media for transmitting not only information (or propaganda) but also esthetics and culture throughout the world. They keep not only actors, but also writers (e.g., Truman Capote) and dramatists (e.g., Edward Albee) alive: Vaughn Williams and Prokofiev compose movie scores, and painters such as Ivan Albright are immortalized in *Portrait of Dorian Gray.*

Fortunately, we have with us tonight someone who not only knows all this, but has an advantage over Stanley Kramer in being a fellow psychiatrist as well as a movie producer. I always hesitate to introduce my associates in a way they really deserve, because I remember one occasion when one of my good friends, after such an introduction, turned to me and said: "Jules, now I know how a pancake feels when it's had syrup poured on it."

But we all know Jerry Schulman as one of the most productive and renowned child psychiatrists in the country, and some of us have already appreciated not only the pedagogic effectiveness, but the artistry as well as the clinical poignancy of some of his films on child behavior and therapy. He has most generously agreed to present the "Art of the Motion Picture" this evening.

To return to the APA: Since there was no reply from Dr. Selinsky about the Miami Session, I continued my effort to secure his collaboration, sensing that he was somehow concerned about his status:

December 2, 1968

Herman Selinsky, M.D.
Miami Committee on Arrangements

Dear Herman:

I trust that by now you have checked with Sherv Frazier and Don Greaves as to our mutual roles in planning and arranging the next APA Arts and Humanities Session. In essence, although I was specifically commissioned by the program committee last May again to present and chair the session, and although it has been customary for the current APA president-elect and arrangements chairman to be the co-chairman and secretary, if it is agreeable to President Waggoner and Drs. Alspach or Lipton, I shall be happy, in view of what I hope will be your very valuable local help, to have you act as co-chairman or as secretary, as you choose.

Incidentally, you will recall that last June I responded in detail and very favorably to your good suggestions about a program on the evolution of music, to be presented by the University of Miami, but unfortunately last July you unaccountably notified me that because of excess work you wished to withdraw from the project. Had you not done so, no other program would have been considered, and an excellent Arts Session might have been well set by now.

Alan Lipton, Miami Arrangements co-chairman, wrote that local help for the Arts and Humanities Session was temporarily in abeyance "because Dr. Selinsky was now ill," but wanted advice as to whether APA officers and guests should be given special tickets for the best seats, etc.:

December 4, 1968

Dear Alan:

Our letters again crossed, and again I appreciate your cooperation. As to tickets: we have usually set aside about 300 of the best seats for APA officers, council chairmen, the members of the program and arrangements committees, and visiting emperors, kings, dukes, barons, knights, and assorted ladies in waiting, recognizing that some members and guests of the APA are more equal than others. Ergo, to avoid any odious comparisons, it might be well to print tickets all one color and simply try to rope off a front center section of the auditorium (tactfully protected by ushers) for our "foreign guests," and allow APA churls who express righteous indignation to slip in anyhow. However, I suggest this only from five years of experience; it's the arrangements committee that should have the final say.

One other item is the usual four-page artsy-craftsy program brochure, handed out at the performance. To save time, money, stamps, and nerves, we could, under direct supervision, print it in Chicago—but that again is *sub judice.*

Again, my thanks and regards.

Retiring Program Chairman Frazier, apparently sensing the miasma in Miami, again telephoned that he wanted me to arrange and conduct the session, and would so notify Selinsky. However, since there were still no replies from the Miami group, I wrote Don Greaves, the newly appointed program chairman, asking to be relieved of responsibility for the contents of the 1969 Arts and Humanities session and requesting his counsel and that of APA President Ray Waggoner as to whether I should accept an invitation from Dr. Alex Simon, arrangement chairman for the 1970 meeting in San Francisco, to plan for the Arts and Humanities there.

January 23, 1969

Dear Don:

In a telephone conversation with Sherv Frazier about the 1969 Arts and Humanities Session about a month ago, he confirmed the fact that, since the program committee had commissioned me to arrange it as long ago as last May, he again wanted me to prepare the literature, plan and supervise the session in collaboration with the arrangements committee, and act as chairman. I promised to do my best as usual, and also offered to relinquish the chairmanship of the session to anyone else if it would help to secure local cooperation. Unfortunately, I have yet to hear of any. The situation is now this:

Ever since I initiated the Arts and Humanities Session in 1965, at practically no expense to the APA but with considerable expenditure of my own time and money, I have arranged annual presentations of music, sculpture, painting, drama, dance, etc., which most APA members thought of high esthetic quality and professional interest; indeed, the only even minimally controversial occasion was the 1967 theater of the absurd, a modality which the program committee itself selected. This year I had intended to maintain that tradition and had again, with official permission, secured a financial grant from the same source that the council honored with thanks and a plaque last year. However, I have since received so many conflicting communications that, unless I hear definitely to the contrary, I shall presume that the grant is not required and that other arrangements for the 1969 Arts and Humanities Session are being made.

My present inquiry is, then, whether as program chairman for the 1970 annual meeting in San Francisco, you wish me to take advantage of my current residence as a fellow at the Center for Advanced Study in the Behavioral Sciences in Palo Alto to explore the following possibilities for the session there: The American Repertory Company, one of the best theatre groups anywhere; Mobile Art, a specialty of the San Francisco Museum; or Architecture as Music Frozen in Stone and Steel, by the Stanford or Berkeley faculties.

With best regards.

Don's response was indirect but characteristically adroit and effective:

March 8, 1969

Raymond Waggoner, M.D.
President-Elect
American Psychiatric Association

Dear Ray:

Since the Arts and Humanities Session is considered a part of the program, since it is the wish of APA council, and since the committee on conventions have complete control over all matters relevant to the program, I must assume this responsibility for the San Francisco meeting in 1970.

Obviously, part of the responsibility must be delegated to others, even if they only advise the program committee chairman and the members of the program committee. You will be consulted since you will be president during this meeting. Alex Simon must be consulted because he is chairman of the local arrangements committee, and the local arrangements committee usually has a significant role to play. Walter Barton must be consulted because of his role as medical director, and his immediate knowledge of funds and budgetary matters. Jules Masserman certainly should be consulted because of his many contacts, his rather considerable talent,and his excellent judgment in the general area of the arts and humanities. I would propose a committee consisting of the above, plus Bob Garber, and with me as chairman to handle the planning, budgeting, content and arrangements . . .

It is unfortunate that this year there has been more than the *usual* amount of communication failure, budgetary misunderstandings, personal conflicts, and territorial struggles. I think a clearly defined structure should enable us to avoid most of these problems.

Don

March 13, 1969

Mrs. Geraldine Freund

Dear Gerry:

You will be interested in the attached copy of a letter from Don Greaves, the new APA program chairman, to Ray Waggoner, the new president. In effect, it apologizes for this year's mishandling of the Arts and Humanities Session—not by us, but by the Miami group—and promises much better coordination with me—and of course with you—for 1970. This confirms our wisdom in not getting involved either administratively or financially in Miami; however, at President Ray Waggoner's request, I agreed to be co-chairman with Selinsky to salvage whatever was possible.

At the Miami meeting musicians from Miami University performed, Stan Kenton ad libbed from a prepared script, and the evening passed into relatively forgettable history.

8. THE ACADEMY OF PSYCHOANALYSIS

At the annual meeting of the American Psychiatric Association (APA) in Chicago in May, 1956, a group of psychoanalysts—most of whom were members of the American Psychoanalytic Association (APsaA) and all of whom were weary of that body's reactionary policies, isolationism from the mainstreams of psychiatry and medicine, and arbitrary presumptions that it was the sole arbiter of psychoanalytic training, certification and practice—met to organize an American Academy of Psychoanalysis. The group included many influential figures: Kenneth Appel, past president of the APA, Don Jackson, Donald Bloch, Judd Marmor, Alex Martin, Janet Rioch, Leon Salzman, Leon Saul, Natalie Shainess, William Silverberg, Edith Weigert, myself, and twenty-two others.* After about an hour of discussion we found ourselves in such nearly complete agreement that Henry Davidson, Parliamentarian of the APA and I were immediately commissioned to write a Constitution, and completed a draft in an hour. With only minor changes, the Constitution, as adopted at the same meeting, emerged with the following principal features:

*Invaluable preliminary work had also been contributed by Henry Laughlin of Washington, D. C.

Article I. The aims of this Academy are:

(a) To develop communication among psychoanalysts and their colleagues in other disciplines in science and in the humanities;

(b) To constitute a forum for inquiry into the phenomena of individual motivation and social behavior;

(c) To encourage and support research in psychoanalysis;

(d) To foster the acceptance of psychoanalysis and its integration in universities; and

(e) To advance the interests of psychoanalysis in all other respects. . . .

Article II: Officers (omitted here).

Article III. Fellowship and Membership. Only a physician who is psychoanalytically trained is eligible for Fellowship. Criteria of such training will be defined in the Bylaws. *This Academy will not license, supervise, certify, or accredit any training program or institute.*

Article IV. Scientific Associates. This category includes scientists in fields allied to psychoanalysis who may be able to make valuable contributions to the scientific discussions of the Academy, but who are not engaged in [analytic] practice. Scientific Associates shall be (*a*) psychiatrists who are versed in the dynamics of behavior; and/or (*b*) scientists who are active in psychiatric research and in fields allied to psychoanalysis; and/or (*c*) experts in other branches of the behavioral sciences who meet the requirements of academic status of this Academy; and/or (*d*) full-time teachers and heads of departments of psychiatry in recognized medical schools.

Dr. Janet Rioch, leader of the New York group, on my nomination was elected the Academy's first president, I its vice-president, Dr. Frances Arkin, secretary, and Leon Salzman, treasurer. For the first Scientific Session of the Academy, I secured as speakers Franz Alexander, Sandor Rado, Roy Grinker, Jurgen Reusch, Percival Bailey, Paul Hoch, Robert

Heath, David Rioch, the historian D. Walcher, and others of similar stature. Their assembled contributions proved to be of such high caliber that Dr. Henry Stratton, of Grune & Stratton, agreed to publish our proceedings annually under the title *Science and Psychoanalysis* if I remained as editor and the quality could be maintained anywhere near the first issue.

Progressive analysts, particularly younger ones, flocked to the new Academy. Of the eighty chairmen of departments of psychiatry, and distinguished anthropologists, sociologists, linguists, and other behavioral scientists whom I invited during my term as President to join as Scientific Associates, fifty-eight accepted, and the Academy rapidly achieved stability, solvency, and influence. Paradoxically, this troubled some Academy Fellows about its "image" and "status" vis-à-vis other organizations in the field. One such concern was legitimate: since the American Psychoanalytic Association had been having an exclusive "joint session" with the Section of Psychoanalysis of the APA at the latter's annual meeting, the impression remained widespread among APA members that the APsaA was the only psychoanalytic society "officially recognized." Therefore when in 1959 I was appointed a member of the APA program committee, I did what I could to make this arrangement more equable by writing Dr. Hardin Branch, then president of the APA, as follows:

> Dear Hardin:
> The American Academy of Psychoanalysis. . . , now comprised of over 250 fully qualified psychoanalysts, and over eighty Scientific Associates, all of whom hold high academic and research positions, respectfully requests equal participation in the Section on Psychoanalysis either by (*a*) proportionate participation of its members in the annual sessions of the Section on Psychoanalysis, or (*b*) "joint meetings" with the Section on alternate years if the Council of the APA prefers that policy. This request has as its only objective the reintegration of truly progressive and scientific psychoanalysis into its parent discipline of neuropsychiatry through the annual meetings of the American Psychiatric Association.

Dr. Branch's reply was personal and sympathetic, but with characteristic fairness he pointed out that the seven Sections of the APA were then semi-autonomous and could choose to meet with whatever society they wished, that this caused perennial program problems, and that the best course for the Academy was to have its own APA members register in the Section and vote for a joint meeting with the Academy. Since many of the Academy Fellows had already tried this democratic approach and had had their votes—obviously in the majority—flagrantly ignored at business meetings of the section, I replied:

> Dear Hardin:
> Thanks for your letter, which was certainly clear. Apart from both our personal preferences, the facts seem to me now about so:
> (1) The Section on Psychoanalysis will remain under the control of the American Psychoanalytic Association, since
> (*a*) That Association has made it a public, explicit and permanent policy to stock and control the "business" meetings of the Section and ignore all opposition even if outvoted. Therefore, the Section on Psychoanalysis will never forward to the APA Executive Council, the Program Committee or anyone else any request from the Academy for a joint meeting.
> (*b*) In contrast, the Academy of Psychoanalysis is not a power-politics, electioneering organization and has no intention of becoming so unless its policy changes markedly in this regard.
> (2) Ergo, the Academy will petition the Program Committee directly for program collaboration.

The following year when I was made APA program chairman, the program committee voted to invite the Academy to a joint meeting and to recommend to the APA Council that the specialty sections themselves be abolished, including traditional "joint meetings." The Council agreed. But to mitigate this blow to the APsaA the Program Committee, at my recommendation, continued to schedule joint meetings of the entire APA with *both* the Academy and the APsaA during my tenure, after which these were discontinued except by special Council provision.

My Presidential Prologue to the 1957 Scientific Program of the Academy of Psychoanalysis

Ladies and Gentlemen: Permit me to welcome you to the third annual scientific meeting of the Academy of Psychoanalysis. Parenthetically the salutation "Ladies and Gentlemen," trite as it may sound at first, was chosen only after the thoughtful rejection of other alternatives. For example, to have addressed you as "Colleagues and Friends" would have been redundant: in this Academy, colleagues *are* friends. Or, to have greeted you as "Fellows, Associates, and Guests" might again have implied gradations of scientific or other status that none of us feels. There remained only the simple, Ladies and Gentlemen!—acknowledging the only distinction that *is* valid—and delightful.

Our program today epitomizes the highest purposes of our Academy: To join with our fellow scientists in a reexamination, elaboration, and integration of our knowledge of human behavior, so that we may better serve ourselves and humanity. To sincere adherents of the young discipline of psychoanalysis, a self-critical humility and receptivity is more appropriate than oracular dogmatism, and in line with search and research we have invited distinguished authorities in the other humanistic sciences to join with us today in transcending the artificial boundaries within our common field and extending and clarifying our understandings, our investigative methods, and our therapeutic techniques. A contrary approach would deny the epistemologic roots of psychoanalysis in history, philosophy, biology or sociology and would wrench it out of its proper context in the organon of behavioral sciences. Indeed, the latter approach would place analysis on the plane of medieval medicine that, in a defensive arrogance born of ignorance, disdained embryology, physiology, pathology—let alone logic—and instead based its supposed rationale and practices at best on empiricism, and at worst on mythology and superstition.

We are, therefore, happy to welcome to this symposium many fellow scientists—all thoroughly versed not only in psychoanalytic theory but respectively also in the sister fields of history, biology, philosophy, sociology, and systems theory. Now that my introduction is over, we may all begin to enjoy the meeting.

New applicants for fellowship had to be carefully screened:

March 12, 1959

Joseph H. Merin, M.D.
Secretary, Academy of Psychoanalysis

Dear Dr. Merrin:

I believe Dr. G. qualifies under the intent of our "grandfather clause" and is therefore eligible for consideration. Confidentially, however, though possessed of dynamic initiative, a constructive imagination, and much ability, he is so stormy a petrel in his interpersonal and organizational relationships that I do not wish to be put in the position of an urgent advocate of his election. Indeed, I would like to leave that to the judgment of the New York members of the membership committee, who may be better acquainted than I with his current status and activities.

A policy of sending free annual copies of *Science and Psychoanalysis* to all members of the Academy was adopted, but when Volume III grew in size and cost, questions were raised in Council as to whether a more economical format or a substitute monthly journal was not necessary to avoid raising the Academy's modest dues:

Joseph H. Merin, M.D.
Secretary
Academy of Psychoanalysis

Dear Joe:

Since your letter sounded urgent, I am replying immediately.

My instructions from the Council last May were to continue to edit Volume III in accord with our present arrangements with Grune & Stratton. Therefore, I spent a good deal of the summer working on the third edition of our annual, to be subtitled "Psychoanalysis and Human Values," and sent the manuscript to Grune & Stratton nearly two months ago so that they could get the book out in the best possible format before our May, 1960, meeting. The point is that the Academy officially committed itself to Volume III last May, and that to withdraw from that arrangement now would be not only a breach of good business faith, but would entail a considerable financial loss to a publisher who, largely because of his belief in the Academy, has heretofore taken all the risks, has lost money to date on us, and had hoped to recoup some as the series became established and previous volumes are sold under the stimulus of later ones. The minimal notice acceptable in such contractual arrangements is one year in advance by either party—and we passed that deadline.

But even apart from such considerations, there is no cause for alarm. The facts are:

1. The $12.50 mentioned by Mr. Duncan Mackintosh, managing editor of Grune & Stratton, would represent the *retail* price of each volume if all the material submitted to me had necessarily been published; fortunately, I succeeded in holding the volume to perhaps less than 380 pages, with a corresponding reduction in price.

2. Even so, the Academy has never paid more than 75% of the retail price for any volumes distributed to its membership; i.e., I would estimate roughly that Volume III might cost the Academy not more than $6.50, though I cannot as yet be certain.

3. Last year the council voted to send Volume II to all

Fellows and Associates, but did *not* decide to make this arrangement permanent. In effect, we can discontinue the practice and let the publisher sell directly to our members—thus avoiding any drain on the treasury at all—or give any discount we can afford through treasury subsidy; in either case, the finances of the Academy remain completely within our control.

4. While a journal may be an excellent enterprise for the future—and I would be most happy to collaborate in this in any way the Academy desires—this must be very carefully considered and planned, since it invariably entails financial risks, a long delay in the publication of manuscripts already accumulated for eighteen months, and many questions of future policy. But it hardly offers an immediate solution to the problems at hand.

I shall secure and assemble all available data, and shall do my best to be present at the Council meeting on November 6th.

The proposal for a journal was tabled indefinitely.

A Sub-specialty Board in Psychoanalysis, with a Serendipitous Abortion

An episode, amusing in retrospect, but at the time of serious concern as reflecting the devious political maneuvers—fortunately inept—of certain groups in the American Psychoanalytic Association to undermine the new Academy, is reflected in a file of correspondence with this background:

One day in December, 1959 Dr. Francis Gerty, then president of the American Psychiatric Association—and an old friend on whose behalf (and without his knowledge at the time) I had circularized the APA hierarchy to initiate his nomination and election—informed me of some recent activities of a committee of the American Psychoanalytic Association. This committee had proposed to the American Board of Psychiatry and Neurology* "that a separate Board in Psychoanalysis be set up

*A body officially designated by the APA and the American Medical Association to examine candidates and issue certificates of qualification in the two medical specialties.

in conjunction with the American Psychoanalytic Association" to designate who shall and who shall not "be certified as a qualified Psychoanalyst." This led me to scan the usually boring minutes of a recent APsaA meeting (readily available to me as a "member in good standing") in which I did indeed read that an "Ad Hoc Committee on an Official Accrediting Board" had proposed to the American Board of Examiners that: "The [proposed] Board of Psychoanalysis would be composed of only qualified analysts [so deemed and selected exclusively by the American Psychoanalytic Association] who would have complete freedom to: (a) set standards for eligibility for examination, (b) set examining procedures, (c) approve or disapprove Training Institutes and facilities, and (d) conduct all examinations."

Obviously, this would have given the APsaA virtually complete dictatorship over psychoanalytic training and practice in the United States—a potentially tragic eventuality, particularly in a field greatly in need of unfettered research and scientific progress. Fortunately, this had apparently been recognized by the American Board of Psychiatry and Neurology, which had therefore counter-proposed that the projected Board of Psychoanalysis consist of seven members, *only three of which be appointed by the APsaA.* Whereupon, its Ad Hoc Committee had reported back to the APsaA: "[We] could not afford the risk to [the] standards [of the APsaA] and the possible approval of inadequate training facilities implied in accepting a minority position on the Board."

Nevertheless, since the proposal was still under consideration, I sent the following letter to Dr. David Boyd, secretary of the American Board:

December 15, 1958

Dear Dave:

It has come to my attention as past president and chairman of the executive council of the Academy of Psychoanalysis that the American Psychoanalytic Association, of which I am also a full member, is taking steps to set up a separate American board to examine and certify candidates in psychoanalysis—which, parenthetically, many of us regard not as a separate field, but as a subspecialty of psychiatry and medicine. Since the Academy of Psychoanalysis, as may be seen in the attached roster and a forthcoming supplement, is now comprised of a fellowship of over 450 of the leading psychoanalysts in the country and abroad and, in addition, has enrolled as scientific associates many of those who are heads of departments of psychiatry and prominent teachers and research workers, I respectfully request that the Academy also be consulted as to the advisability, or, if constituted, the format and functioning of any contemplated board of examiners in psychoanalysis.

Dr. Boyd's reply reflected the wisdom of the American board as follows:

December 23, 1958

Dear Jules:

Thank you for your letter of December 15, 1958. I have made this a matter of our records on certification in psychoanalysis.

The present vague and extremely tentative plans envisage the establishment of a Committee on Certification in Psychoanalysis to be set up by the American Board of Psychiatry and Neurology to carry out such certifying functions under the aegis of the parent board. Such a committee would be made up of well-known psychoanalytic educators who are recognized for their contributions to training and who are competent to establish and examine standards of psychoanalytic training and the achievement of psychoanalytic candidates.

At this time I would like formally to request from you a list of possible members for this committee who, in the opinion of you and any of the group you might wish to consult, are eminently qualified for the carrying out of this serious task. It would be very helpful if you would include under each name the reasons for such a suggestion and the achievements of the proposed person. It goes without saying that they must be highly qualified psychoanalysts known for contributions to the field and respected for their educational interests and contributions. They should represent the best in current and future psychoanalytic training and education.

Your cooperation in this will be greatly appreciated by all of us.

Sincerely yours,
David A. Boyd, Jr., M.D.
Secretary-Treasurer

Two follow-up replies:

December 30, 1958

Dear David:

Thank you for your prompt and illuminating reply to my inquiry about a possible sub-specialty board in psychoanalysis. Since all official actions of the Academy must constitutionally reflect the sentiments of its entire fellowship, I shall propose to the executive council of the Academy at its next meeting on January 7, 1959, that it approve my list of properly qualified committee members you request and inform you immediately thereafter.

January 9, 1959

Dear Dr. Boyd:

The executive council of the Academy of Psychoanalysis, at a meeting held in New York January 8, 1959, on my recommendation designated as an Ad Hoc Committee on Certification in Psychoanalysis five fully trained and qualified psychoanalysts who in its judgment would meet your specifications as "well-known psychoanalytic educators recognized for their contributions to training and who are competent to establish and examine standards of psychoanalytic training and the achievement of psychoanalytic candidates." The committee consists of the following:

Dr. Kenneth Appel, Professor and Chairman, Department of Psychiatry, University of Pennsylvania; President of the American Psychoanalytic Association, 1953-1954.

Dr. Roy R. Grinker, Director, Institute for Psychoanalytic and Psychosomatic Training and Research, Chicago.

Dr. John A. P. Millet, Attending Psychiatrist, New York State Psychiatric Institute; Professor of Psychiatry and Director of Psychoanalytic Training, Columbia University.

Dr. William V. Silverberg, Attending and Training Psychoanalyst, College of Medicine, City of New York; President of the Academy of Psychoanalysis, 1958-1959.

Dr. Jules H. Masserman (Chairman), Professor of Neurology and Psychiatry, Northwestern University, Chicago.

Without comment on the chairman, the other committee members are by performance and reputation eminently suitable to act as consultants to the American Board of Psychiatry and Neurology in the question of the advisability of a subspecialty examining board in psychoanalysis, and the personnel and operations of such a board if it were constituted. It was the sentiment of the Academy Council that they should represent the special interests not of the Academy or of any other organization, but rather of the indissoluble fields of psychiatry and psychoanalysis as a whole. We stand ready to meet with the American board and any other designated colleagues in our field at your convenience.

As you also requested, I attach the detailed curriculum vitae of each nominee for your files.

Respectfully,

The Powers–That–Wanted–To–Be in the APsaA were informed of this exchange, and they reacted with various mixtures of incredulity, indignation, and panic. When the balanced position of the American Board was reported to the plenary business meeting of the APsaA in May, 1959, pandemonium ensued: In mounting clamor, clashing recommendations were read from constituent local societies ranging from "tentative acceptance only as a basis for revision" to bitter denunciation of the American Board for its "perfidy." Kurt Eissler, a pillar of isolationist orthodoxy, attacked the Ad Hoc Committee itself for its "disloyalty to the APsaA" as well as for its "bad writing." Finally, so many members of the APsaA began calling each other "subversive," "traitor," and worse that in desperation the chairman adjourned the business meeting and referred the whole matter back to the APsaA executive council. This body in turn again circularized the constituent societies of the APsaA with a document which read in part as follows:

> "At the April, 1959, meetings of the American Psychoanalytic Association, there was great concern and much pressure surrounding the matter. Dr. Herman Serota of Chicago sent a memo to Council members raising several questions:
> 1. Since the Board on Professional Standards of the APsaA has, in fact, been certifying Institutes . . . would it not qualify as a potential "member board" of the Advisory Board for Medical Specialists?
> 2. If the Board on Professional Standards were legally incorporated as a certifying organization could it not become a member of the National Advisory Board? To these questions Dr. Bernard Bandler replied that Dr. Boyd had stated that it is not possible . . . to have an independent organization such as the Board on Professional Standards admitted to membership on the Board of Medical Specialties. The Ad Hoc Committee of the APsaA then reaffirmed its stand as follows:
>
> 1. That there should be a majority representation for the APsaA on a Sub-specialty Board.

2. That the cut-off dates for the grandfather clause should be 1943, i.e., that there would be automatic certification of all members of the APsaA who had graduated from medical school prior to that date.
3. That the Board on Professional Standards of the APsaA was to continue supervision and approval of training facilities and that only such facilities were to be recognized by the Sub-specialty Board as qualifying for its examination.

With manifest sorrow, however, the Ad Hoc Committee also had to report the following:

1. The American Board of Psychiatry and Neurology is planning to set up a Sub-Board in Psychoanalysis whether or not the American Psychoanalytic Association as such is interested.
2. There is no assumption that the APsaA has the right to be directly represented on the Sub-specialty Board, nor is it planned to allot to the APsaA a specified quota of the membership of the Sub-specialty Board.
3. The American Academy of Psychoanalysis . . . will be asked to submit nominations for membership on the Subspecialty Board. The APsaA would be only one of a number of bodies submitting nominations and the American Board of Psychiatry and Neurology reserves all the rights of appointment from among these nominees".

In great concern, the Chicago Psychoanalytic Society called a meeting on October 27, 1959, to act on this report. In anticipation of another display of group panic, I attended in the role of long-lost but possibly salvagable prodigal son. I quote excerpts from the minutes of that meeting:

> President Gitelson expressed the view that the APsaA can still halt further negotiations [with the

> American board] and could perhaps even now withdraw its nominations . . .
>
> Dr. Gerhard Piers agreed that a "sub-board might put psychoanalysis in a subordinate position whereas psychoanalysis does not belong in such a position . . .
>
> Dr. Kligerman read a paragraph from Dr. Boyd's "letter of intention" stating that there is dissatisfaction with the APsaA about its current accreditation activities. Dr. Kligerman questioned whether this statement reflects fact.
>
> Dr. Joan Fleming agreed with Dr. [Roy] Grinker [Sr.] that the theory of psychoanalysis should not be confined; it is a part of a widening body of knowledge. But should training be equally available to anyone who wishes to train or to be trained? With the spreading of psychoanalysis throughout universities and hospitals, the old problem of wildcat training and low standards increases. This should be taken into account in the weighing of issues, and the APsaA should recognize that more and more training will take place in institutions that do not come up to our present standards.
>
> Dr. Heinz Kohut felt that . . . if we accept a sub-committee, we give up some of our prestige. In the near future, there is, therefore, nothing but loss to us because we give up part of our prestige to a new committee.

At this juncture, I considered it opportune as a voting member of the APsaA to help scuttle the whole idea of a Specialty Board in Psychoanalysis. The minutes continue as follows:

> Dr. Masserman expressed the opinion that the discussion had reflected near-unanimity. He proposed this resolution, seconded by Dr. Kepecs: 1. The Chicago Psychoanalytic Society is at this time opposed to the establishment of a Sub-specialty Board in Psychoanalysis. 2. The Chicago Psychoanalytic Society urges the American Psychoanalytic Association to resubmit the question of a Sub-specialty Board in

Psychoanalysis to its component societies and institutes for thorough discussion and for further instruction to the executive council.

Dr. Masserman added that the American Board is not unanimously enthusiastic about this sub-committee and that, if the two leading psychoanalytic organizations opposed a sub-committee, the American Board would drop the idea.

Both resolutions were carried by large majorities!

Nevertheless, because of resolutions sent in by other constituent societies of the APsaA, that body, in a final attempt to bolster its rapidly sagging scientific and professional influence, again petitioned the American Board of Psychiatry and Neurology for a separate certifying body in psychoanalysis, and once more circularized the local societies in support of its action. This time the medical director of the American Psychiatric Association wrote to me as follows:

November 13, 1959

Dear Jules:

It is a matter of common knowledge that consideration has been and continues to be given to the proposed founding of a section of the American Board of Psychiatry and Neurology to be known as the American Board of Psychoanalysis.

I am aware of your interest in this matter and I would be most grateful if your thoughts, motions, ideas and speculations on the pros and cons and the *possible* effects of such an eventuality upon both American psychiatry in general and psychoanalysis in particular were made available to me. Of course I will completely respect your wishes to maintain your anonymity or give you full credit as you prefer.

With warm regards, I remain,

Most sincerely,
Mathew Ross, M.D.
Medical Director

This occasioned another and more vigorous letter to Dr. Boyd, with copies to Dr. Ross and to the Academy council:

October 30, 1959

Dear Dr. Boyd:

It has again come to the attention of the Academy that the American Psychoanalytic Association, noting the growing dissention among its societies and institutes on this question, has distributed among its membership a second circular (copies attached) which raises the following important issues:

1. The document once more represents the Association as the sole arbiter of proper psychoanalytic training in this country, mainly on the basis of the minimum number of hours prescribed for the student in compliance with a numerically pre-set "personal analysis" and a stereotyped curriculum at various psychoanalytic institutes. However, this assumption must be challenged on the basis of the following facts:

A. The quality of this limited scholasticism varies extremely widely from institute to institute, and according to the Association's own confidential reports (by Bandler, Ross, Hamburg, et al.) is seriously inadequate in many.

B. Even in the better institutes, fundamental advances in psychoanalysis related to modern developments in scientific methodology, in communication and transaction theory, in sociology, and in other branches of the behavioral sciences are not only not taught, but are actually forbidden to the enquiring minds of the better students as evidence of their "resistance" and consequent "unanalyzability." It is a conservative estimate that about half of the hours spent by the trainee in many present-day institutes are devoted to a reiteration of theories and practices now only of historical interest, whereas much of the other half would be far better employed in more comprehensive and psychiatrically useful instruction.

C. This mode of doctrinaire and isolated teaching preempts many years of the trainee's time and has often resulted in impairing the breadth of interests, knowledge, and skill of otherwise able and promising young psychiatrists—a circumstance which the examiners of the American Board have repeatedly deplored.

D. In the face of these deficiencies in its pedagogic philosophies and practices, and despite contrary precedents in every other field of medicine, the APsaA has traditionally opposed closer liaison and eventual merging of its training facilities with established medical schools and universities where psychoanalysis could be reintegrated into scientific psychiatry.

2. A second feature of the attached circular from the APsaA is even more disturbing: namely, the Association's deliberate intent to bolster its threatened stranglehold on psychoanalytic training and practice by extending its control to the proposed sub-specialty board in psychoanalysis. This intent is made explicit in passages and self-answered questions such as the following: P.8 "We had set as our goal, appointment of four of the seven Board members by the American Psychoanalytic Association . . . P.13 "What would happen if some future Board of Psychiatry and Neurology was less friendly to the APsaA than the present one and appointed Fellows who were ambivalent or hostile to psychoanalysis?" This question itself is a direct indication that the Association, as of October, 1959, forever equates all psychoanalysis with its own inflexible doctrines and organization . . . P.13 "How can one give an examination in psychoanalysis?" The APsaA answers that the examiner must be "a revered senior analyst" meaning, again, only a member of the APsaA. P.13 "Should we not insist that all members of the American Psychoanalytic Association be automatically certified without any cut-off date at all?" This seems to be the crux of the controversy now raging within the APsaA itself: namely, that most of its members demand automatic certification merely on the basis of membership in the Association and without examination by an unbiased Board as to their actual competence in either psychoanalysis or the parent specialties of psychiatry and medicine.

Precisely to counteract such trends, the Academy of Psychoanalysis was founded in 1955 by academically and internationally recognized leaders in psychoanalysis to promote progress in the field by raising its standards of theory, teaching, practice and research. Since then the Academy has acquired a Fellowship of over 500 fully qualified and carefully selected psychoanalysts, including outstanding teachers and investigators and many psychoanalytically trained chairmen of Departments of Psychiatry. The semiannual meetings and published Proceedings of the Academy (copies attached) have gained international repute, and it may justifiably be said now to have scientific rather than numerical leadership in this subspecialty. However, the Academy has steadfastly refused to become involved in setting up new institutes or arbitrary regulations of training, since it firmly believes that these should be the academic prerogatives of recognized universities and medical schools with duly qualified faculties, and not dictated by any organization desirous of retaining exclusive power and arbitrary control. Ergo, in view of the implicit intent of the American Psychoanalytic Association to encroach upon the essential functions of the American Board of Psychiatry and Neurology in maintaining the high standards of this specialty, the Academy of Psychoanalysis wishes to reaffirm the following principles:

1. The Academy regards psychoanalysis as an integral part of the specialty of psychiatry and neurology, approves of the requirement of a certificate from the American Board of Psychiatry and Neurology for all psychoanalysts, and sees no absolute or urgent need for a Sub-specialty Certificate in Psychoanalysis.

2. Should a Board in Psychoanalysis be constituted, the Academy would request no specially favored or blanket status for its fellows or scientific associates, but would require each to qualify individually.

3. The Academy earnestly endorses the proposed arrangement of having membership of the Sub-specialty board composed *not of representatives, overt or covert, of any "sponsoring body" or political organization whatever,* but of qualified authorities in psychoanalysis irrespective of their affiliation.

4. The Academy recommends that these members of the sub-specialty board be selected exclusively on the grounds of their scientific competence: research and clinical publications, academic rank, breadth of knowledge, and a record of original

and lasting contributions to the field. The Academy, at the Board's request, has submitted a list of such highly qualified individuals to the Board and can suggest others of equal distinction.

5. The Academy of Psychoanalysis, with the full backing of its membership, stands ready to cooperate with the American Board of Psychiatry and Neurology in every other way that would advance the teaching and practice of psychiatry, neurology, and psychoanalysis.

Respectfully submitted,
Jules Masserman,
Past President
Academy of Psychoanalysis

Inevitably, there were reactions of concern from within the Academy itself. Dr. William Silverberg, who succeeded me as President of the Academy, thought my letter "too long, too obviously condemnatory of the APsaA, and perhaps too immodestly laudatory of the Academy." So too, its current President, John Millet, wrote that my letter was "too belligerent": that he had "heard from other sources that my friends Drs. Gerty, Boyd, Branch, et al. could not keep the Board from approving the APsaA's proposal," and that the Academy should threaten "legal action." I replied:

November 13, 1959

William V. Silverberg, M.D.

Dear Bill:

The circular from the American Psychoanalytic Association showed clearly that they wished now, by subversive political methods, to preempt complete control of psychoanalysis in this country and thereby suppress the Academy and all other progressive movements: shall we, then, *not* indict the APsaA for this? We wish all to know that the Academy was founded to counter such influences and eventualities, has been remarkably successful thus far, and should properly be regarded by the Board as a reconstructive force in psychoanalysis and scientific psychiatry—is this "immodest self-praise?" You say that every point in my letter is valid and relevant to the important issues involved—shall we then not marshal them? True, we must avoid innuendos and generalities and make our position justified and explicit—but can this really be done in a paragraph? Actually, I happen to know from personal conversations with Drs. Gerty, Boyd, and Branch—the most influential members of the American Board of Psychiatry and Neurology—that at this crucial juncture they would like a letter as direct, detailed, and unequivocal as the one I sent, and that it would redound to the great advantage of the Academy. I shall let it stand.

November 20, 1959

John A. P. Millet, M.D.

Dear Jack:

Your letter to me does not specify what "other sources" have alarmed the Academy by regarding the situation as "serious," nor how the president (Gerty), secretary (Boyd), and the two other senior members of the American Board of Psychiatry and Neurology you name could be considered as having less than considerable influence on their own seven-member board. Also, I am afraid most readers would regard your proposed note to Dr. Boyd threatening legal action as far more "belligerent" toward the board itself than was any passage in my letter, in which criticisms were certainly directed not against the board but deservedly against the American Psychoanalytic, which had originally raised the issues in question. I urge most strongly that if any "legal consultation" were obtained that it be simply for private advice as to the Academy's rights and defenses under foreseeable contingencies; conversely, any expressed threat to the Board of Psychiatry and

Neurology at this juncture would do the Academy incalculable harm.

The outcome:

December 21, 1959

Frances S. Arkin, M.D.
President, Academy of Psychoanalysis

Dear Fran:

Francis Gerty had lunch with me recently, and confirmed that what we predicted happened: the new Ad Hoc Committee met with the Board on December 12th, made complete fools of themselves and the American Psychoanalytic Association, and fixed it so the whole matter of the subspecialty board will be an essentially dead issue as far as the Board is concerned for at least a couple of decades.

A final fillip from Dr. Boyd:

Dear Jules:

I have your letter of January 7, and I was very pleased to hear from you. You have my permission to quote as extensively as you wish from my letter of December 23, 1958, a copy of which you enclosed. For your own information you may be interested in the fate of this proposal which ended in a dismal disaster.

I worked for weeks drawing up an organizational plan that I felt was very fair and reasonable, offered possibilities of impartial administration, and was not in any way an imposition on the psychoanalytic movement. Francis Gerty and I met again with a large committee from the American Psychoanalytic and negotiated for hours. I was told afterward that all members of the committee swung over in favor of the plan with the exception of two. One did not know why he was opposed but he thought it was safer to be opposed while the other was against any outside nonanalytic control over psychoanalysis. Henry Brosin sat through the negotiations as an observer, and both he and Francis Gerty may be a source of further information for you if you are in need of any. The next day the proposal was presented to the whole American Psychoanalytic by Dr. Bernard Bandler. He was lucky to escape with his life. It was met with very bitter, hostile denunciation and apparently "a new Hitler" was the nicest thing I was called. At any rate, the proposal came out of the American Psychoanalytic deader than the proverbial doornail. I believe that Doug Bond was in on most of the discussion and possibly if you are in need of more information he may be of some help.

It is a blessing to think that I am too old to ever get mixed up in that affair again. If it ever is proposed again someone else had better do it. Personally I would rather attempt to steal a large segment of Jimmy Hoffa's Teamsters Union.

I hope that this gives the desired information, and if I can be of any more help, please let me know. My best to you and your family.

Sincerely yours,
David A. Boyd, Jr., M.D.
Executive Secretary-Treasurer

Dear Dave:

I was present at the meeting of the American Psychoanalytic when Bernard Bandler tried to talk to his incredible colleagues (Hank Brosin wisely refrained), and if it's any comfort to you, what they called each other would make being called a Hitler tantamount to a compliment. I would publish that account in full as a clinical study were it not that (a) I am, *mea culpa,* still a member of the APsaA and would be smeared with my own brush and (b) who would believe that such events

really occurred in a supposedly civilized professional society?
Again with thanks and regards.

Further correspondence proved unnecessary; the APsaA retracted its request for a sub-specialty board, and the entire matter was dropped—nor has it been revived since.

Leadership continued to be important:

June 26, 1961

John A. P. Millet, M.D.
Chairman, Nominating Committee

Dear Jack:

As we both anticipate, the Academy's course under the very able but quite differently orientated administration of Roy Grinker and Sandor Rado is likely to be illuminating and evolutionary, but possibly somewhat strenuous. Since those of us who are devoted to the Academy must look far into the future, as chairman of the nominating committee I would like to submit for your consideration the name of Leon Salzman for President-Elect in 1962. He is well qualified by personality, loyalty, scientific status, executive ability, general popularity—and, indeed, geographic location—to keep disparate elements in our Academy working together, and thereby advance the many important purposes for which the Academy was founded.

When Franz Alexander sent me a copy of a proposed personal letter of protest that some Academy members had not been officially listed as psychoanalysts in a recent issue of the *Directory of the American Psychiatric Association*:

June 27, 1963

Franz Alexander, M.D.

Dear Franz:

Having been occupied elsewhere in the world for seven weeks, I had not seen the Psychiatric "Manpower Bulletin" to which Larry Wolberg refers: I am writing for a copy. However, if only American Psychoanalytic Association members are listed as analysts, this is not a matter for individual protests, but for official action by the executive council of the Academy, which should address an appropriate letter to Dr. Walter Barton, medical director of the APA, requesting that an addendum to the Roster of Psychoanalysts including all fellows of the Academy be published as soon as possible in a supplement to the "Manpower Bulletin." Anything less than this, or any delay in it, would mean our tacit acceptance of the American Psychoanalytic Association's position that only its own members qualify and might cause serious disaffection in the Academy. Conversely, if we proceed correctly, I see no difficulties in having our request granted, especially since those of us making it are already listed and requesting equable treatment for others.

I shall, of course, help all I can from within the APA councils, but it must not be thought that I am the only protagonist of our Academy.

Predictably, as the Academy grew in prestige and influence, it was in corresponding measure regarded as a greater threat to the entrenched American and International Psychoanalytic Associations—so much so that in 1962 Dr. Maxwell Gitelson, president of the International, thought it necessary to publish in the International Journal of Psychoanalysis a "Communication from the President" in which he alleged that the Academy was (a) "a political organization . . . opposed to psychoanalysis," (b) that it was "allied to a subversive European Forum for Psychoanalysis," (c) that it had "no sympathy for the APsaA," (d) that Academy fellows "had not applied to the APsaA" (as, presumably, everyone should), (e) that its scientific associates had had "no training . . . or relationship to Psychoanalysis," and (f) that in general, the Academy being "liberal . . . has never been committed (sic) to Psychoanalysis as such." The only long-range remedy for all this, to quote Gitelson, was to correct "our failure to be uncompromising in the application of our psychoanalytic insight into our authoritarian roles as teachers and educators [so that fewer] of our colleagues and students could find solace for narcissistic injury in alliances in dissident coteries."

Since I was also a life-time member of the International Psychoanalytic Association, the journal of which had a world-wide circulation, this gave me an opportunity to reply as follows for publication in its pages:

Dr. John Sutherland
Editor,
International Journal of Psychoanalysis

To the Editor:

Dr. M. Gitelson's recent "Communication From the President About the Neoanalytic Movement (*Int. J. Psychoanal.* XLIII:3, 1962) seems to require a commentary designed to restore the balance of probity and professional dignity for which your journal has deserved respect. This reply is therefore addressed to your readers rather than to Dr. Gitelson, who in past correspondence has proved to be a nebulous, evasive, and therefore eventually uninteresting protagonist. However, in the particular "Communication" referred to, Dr. Gitelson made his allegations somewhat more explicit than usual, and it is with reference to these that your readers may appreciate the following facts:

The Academy of Psychoanalysis, founded in 1956 by some of the leading psychoanalysts in the United States—nearly all of them members of the International Psychoanalytic Association—has in six years grown so greatly in scientific prestige and influence that:

1. Its Fellowship now includes some of the world's most renowned psychoanalysts: Franz Alexander, Carl Binger, Dex-

ter Bullard, Roy Grinker, Martin Grotjahn, Abraham Kardiner, Judd Marmor, John Millet, George Mohr, Sandor Rado, Janet Rioch, May Romm, William Silverberg, Edith Weigert, *et al.* Five of these have been presidents of the Academy, which now numbers over 500 prominent analysts in both the United States and abroad.

2. Dr. Gitelson correctly notes that many of these Fellows of the Academy are also dues-paying members of the American Psychoanalytic Association and thereby the International; indeed, their number is increasing. However, it is not true, as Dr. Gitelson avers, that they "have no sympathy for the American Psychoanalytic Association"; on the contrary, they feel a deep compassion for, leavened by forbearance with, the current travails of the American Psychoanalytic, and therefore retain their membership and influence in that Association in the hope that, to use Freud's phrase, "the soft voice of the intellect" will eventually resolve its doctrinal, administrative, and pedagogic turmoil.

3. Dr. Gitelson also inveighs against the Academy's acceptance of world-famed authorities in related fields as nonvoting Scientific Associates—a widely sought elective honor which has been reserved for about fourscore of America's leading anthropologists, sociologists, psychiatrists, and other behavioral scientists, including about half of the chairmen of the Departments of Psychiatry in our universities each of whom had rendered outstanding contributions to psychiatry and psychoanalysis. In this connection, it appears incredible that Dr. Gitelson is serious in his implied strictures that analysts should be unique among scientists in *not* being interested in, or avidly receptive of, developments in other disciplines that could advance understanding and skill in their own. Let us trust that our potential friends in these related fields will not take his attitude as representative of all psychoanalysts.

Dr. Gitelson's next allegation is that the Academy is "politically active" and is, therefore, to use two of his favorite panchrestons,* more "tendentious" than "diatrophic"—unless Dr. Gitelson reads the latter term as di-*atrophic.* On the con-

*Garrett Hardin's term for words so protean in their connotations that they are essentially meaningless.

trary, the Constitution of the Academy specifically confines its purposes to research and communication, and to the promotion of psychoanalysis as a scientific discipline; indeed, it expressly excludes the "approval" or "disapproval" of institutes, societies, standards of training, or other preemptive or arbitrary official regulative activities. The only approach to "political" action in which the Academy was ever even distantly involved occurred in 1959 when the American Board of Psychiatry and Neurology, considering the Academy an authoritative and impartial body, sought its advice as to whether or not to establish a Sub-specialty Board of Examiners in Psychoanalysis, and invited the Academy to nominate such examiners if the Board were established. The Academy, after serious deliberation, counselled against the establishment of such a Board, and the wisdom of this advice was later confirmed when the APsaA, which had originated the proposal in the belief that it would have sole control of the Sub-specialty Board, withdrew its petition to the American Board and echoed the Academy's recommendation.

Third, Dr. Gitelson's somewhat free-wheeling accusation that the activities of the Academy constitute "active opposition to psychoanalysis which leave no doubt about the wish to negate its discoveries" must have led to many doubts as to Dr. Gitelson's accuracy of reporting and impartiality of judgment on the part of your readers acquainted with the following facts:

1. The semiannual scientific meetings of the Academy are invariably attended not only by its own fellows and scientific associates but by many other members of the American Psychoanalytic and guests from various scientific societies who desire to learn of fundamental progress in this field.

2. The Academy has been designated as a constitutent body of the American Association for the Advancement of Science, and the two associations, under the chairmanship of the internationally honored Dr. Sandor Rado, are scheduled to hold a joint meeting in Philadelphia on December 26-28, 1962.

3. The scientific proceedings of the Academy, published annually by Grune & Stratton under the series title *Science and Psychoanalysis,* have attained world-wide circulation and acclaim and are being translated into several languages.

4. Basic Book Publishers, contemplating a definitive summation of psychoanalytic knowledge to date, delegated the planning and writing of this organon to the Academy as the most competent and respected scientific organization in the field, and selected as editor Dr. Roy Grinker, Sr., then president of the Academy.

Fourth, and this time a minor but perennially necessary correction of Dr. Gitelson's writings: the Academy had and has no official connection whatever with the so-called International Psychoanalytic Forum.

Finally, Dr. Gitelson's dictum that we must "be uncompromising in the application of our psychoanalytic insight into our authoritarian (sic!) roles as teachers and educators" is so scholastically anachronistic—and so contrary to the free and productive (though always asymptotic) seeking for truth upon which both science and ethics are based—that it would be charitable to regard it as a *lapsus* rather than a credo. Perhaps a trenchant analogy in current history would here be apropos:

The Catholic Church, too, has its Alfredo Cardinal Ottaviani, Secretary of the Supreme Sacred Congregation of the Holy Office, whose coat of arms proudly bears the motto *Semper Idem* and whose creed is "Scripture must be read under ecclesiastical guidance." At the recent Ecumenical Council, progressive elements of the Church, led by Augustine Cardinal Bea, Head of the Secretariat for Promoting Christian Unity, deplored Ottaviani's doctrinal intransigence because it "would close the door to many intellectuals and the outstretched hands of friendship in the old and new world." The Council, cognizant of broader vistas of scholarship and new obligations to humanity, rejected Ottaviani's rigid concepts of "orthodoxy" and followed a greater destiny.

Shall scientific societies seeking knowledge of, and service to mankind in other fields, do less?

Turning to more important matters, invitations such as this could be tendered:

October 25, 1965

Ralph Bunche
Associate Secretary-General
United Nations

Dear Mr. Bunche:

You may recall that last year in my capacity as program chairman of the American Psychiatric Association I invited you to address the annual meeting of that Association in New York in May, 1965; it so happened that you had to be on official duty elsewhere at the time, so that our loss was the world's gain. However, to recoup the former also, I now have the honor to reinvite you to address the Decennial Meeting of the Academy of Psychoanalysis on May 7th or 8th, in Atlantic City, as its most distinguished speaker, on the general subject of "Human Behavior and World Affairs," or on any other topic of your choice.

As an academic and scientific organization we can, of course, offer you only a modest honorarium of five hundred dollars, but it is our hope that your personal welcome as an honored guest and the opportunity to speak through our podium and publications not only to the Academy but also to the scientific world will help persuade you to accept this invitation.

Mr. Bunche accepted—and then came Vietnam. The Academy-APA lecture was given by Senator Eugene McCarthy.

At the current writing, the Academy is comprised of about 800 Fellows, 100 Scientific Associates, and several honorary members, all of high repute. It is their researches, teachings, and writings, and those of their successors, rather than any political or regulative activities, that will continue to determine the Academy's role in the scientific renaissance of American and international psychoanalysis and psychiatry.

9. MY FURTHER EDUCATION IN SCIENCE AND PSYCHOANALYSIS

In 1956, when Dr. Henry Stratton, head of Grune & Stratton, Inc., agreed to publish the annual proceedings of the Academy under the series title of *Science and Psychoanalysis* with myself as editor, some members of the Academy inferred that all papers and discussions read at Academy meetings would automatically appear unedited in these annual proceedings. To rescue the Academy from this fate I had the Council appoint Drs. Roy Grinker of Chicago and David McK. Rioch of Washington as my Associates on the editorial board, and then sent them whatever papers read at Academy meetings that I could not salvage by editing or rewriting, with comments such as the following:

Dear Roy and Dave:

I reread B.'s opus on "Dementia Praecox" with mounting bewilderment replacing my initial amusement. Apart from his sophomoric syntax (which I can edit) and annoyingly recurrent alibis of "insufficient time" to make this or that clear to his palpitating readers (passages I can delete), I have rarely seen a more prolonged display of polysyllabic naïveté and semantic confusion masquerading as an erudite dissertation. If we publish it, philologists, philosophers, psychologists—yea, ethnologists and neurologists, as B. himself smugly predicts, "will certainly be disconcerted"—but whether or not, as he also assumes, they will then come to our Academy meetings to learn "psychoanalytic dynamics," is highly dubious. They may conclude instead that some academicians are outside the realm of rational discourse, and let us all go at that.

I vote rejection, but await your opinions.

The vote became unanimous.

Inevitably, however, a demand that I publish all papers read at Academy meetings again arose in some quarters. My letter to the Academy Council:

Frances Arkin, M.D., President
The Academy of Psychoanalysis

Dear Frances:

Drs. B's and T's complaints to the Council that their papers were not accepted for Volume V are cases in point of how the very considerable work of getting out our annual volume is rendered doubly difficult by the ever-present choice between doing a conscientious job for the Academy, or being popular with everyone while the *Science and Psychoanalysis* series loses its increasingly high standing and wide readership —and eventually its publisher. Faced with this dilemma, I have worked under the following principles:

1. Every other professional organization (including the AMA, APA, ABA, AAAS) recognizes that *not* all of the papers read at its scientific proceedings can be published in its official journal or volume. This is accepted, because, even in the most carefully programmed meetings, papers scheduled to exhibit a speaker or evoke discussion may lack some quality essential in permanent contributions to the published literature, e.g., originality, validity, breadth, or scholarship.

2. Despite the heartening success of our first two volumes,

I did not wish to rely entirely on my own judgment as to the final selection or rejection of papers, since I might become biased or arbitrary. I therefore requested and established a publications committee consisting of one of the most broadly informed and respected men in our Academy, David Rioch, and another with equal qualifications plus long experience as editor-in-chief of the *Archives of General Psychiatry,* Roy Grinker, now our president-elect.

3. The fact remains that the *Science and Psychoanalysis* volumes must be not only important and desirable additions to public and private libraries but also within reasonable size and price if the Academy is to retain its currently excellent arrangements with Grune & Stratton. As my own recognition of this necessity, please note that although I was a scheduled speaker at our last two scientific meetings, not a word of my own, either as a contributor or a discussant, has thus far appeared in our published proceedings, thereby making room for the writings of others, including manuscripts that had to be almost completely rewritten by me.

4. Since the publications committee was constituted, I have submitted every questionable paper to it for editorial review, and have acted on its decisions. During the past three months the Committee decided unanimously that [several papers] did not merit publication unless we wished greatly to lower our scientific and literary standards. Unfortunately, this also eliminated Salzman's excellent discussion of U's paper. The committee's adverse comments, must, of course, be held confidential from the contributors, but if the council wishes, I can relay them in specific instances.

5. It then devolved upon me to soften the rejection as much as I could, one way being to add a personal statement to each contributor that the committee proposed to devote *most* (I did *not* say all) of the next volume to the publication of the two programs on psychoanalytic education Dr. Grinker had arranged. This made it possible to include a few other truly excellent papers—such as Natalie Shainess's rewritten chapter —or even borderline ones such as S's. I know this doesn't quite remove the trauma to some tender sensitivities, but, if the committee and I can stand to strain personal friendships for

the sake of the Academy, contributors should be at least a little loyal in this regard too.

Some weeks ago I requested that the council reaffirm its policies in such matters. Obviously three main courses are possible:

1. To continue our present program of maintaining, within reason and fairness, the high standards of our published proceedings.

2. To reduce these standards, with the inescapable risk of losing status, circulation, and publisher.

3. To retain our standards for the annual volume and establish a separate journal for marginal papers. The latter course, unfortunately, will entail a great financial drain on our treasury, much additional work—and may actually create more complaints and dissentions among contributors than we have now.

All committees, of course, must follow the policies of the Academy, and we shall be glad to be so guided. I am therefore sending a copy of this letter to the members of the council for consideration.

The council reaffirmed that the publications committee retain full editorial discretion to maintain the standards of the proceedings. However, I was also appointed to a committee to consider the feasibility of an Academy journal. I requested Henry Stratton's opinion and he counselled against a journal on both financial and scientific grounds, I replied as follows:

Dear Henry:

Many thanks for your highly informative letter as to what it takes, in the way of financial, administrative, and scientific risks, to publish an Academy journal. The only possible use I could see for it—and it would be an expensive wastebasket—is to take the pressure off *Science and Psychoanalysis* by draining away mediocre or irrelevant Academy papers and leaving only the best on a single topic (e.g. aggression, aging, adolescence, techniques of therapy) for our annual issue of *Science and Psychoanalysis.* Whether or not I would edit the journal would depend on continuing reasonable editorial prerogatives of condensing, revising, or rewriting marginal papers, and rejecting poor ones outright. If, however, the journal is to be only an uncensored outlet for getting diffuse thinking and poor writing into print—as happened with *Biological Psychiatry*—then someone else will have to act as copyboy and mail clerk.

David Rioch concurred:

Dear Jules:

I have read your reports and recommendations with interest, and my admiration for your editorial ability and sound judgment now reaches a new high. I fully concur about not having an Academy journal. The only item I wish something could be done about is that of finances and your being several hundred dollars [perennially] out of pocket.

As always,
David McK. Rioch, M.D.
Director, Div. of Neuropsychiatry
U. S. Army

Roy Grinker also supported my stand by writing directly to the Academy council:

Ralph M. Crowley, M.D.
President
American Academy of Psychoanalysis

Dear Ralph:

Jules has asked me to write you directly regarding the possibility of setting up a journal for the Academy of Psychoanalysis. In the first place, I think that the book should be continued, because under Jules' editorship it has successfully included the best papers presented at the two meetings of the Academy. Even then, it is very difficult to fill the book with good papers. It would be much more difficult to supply sufficiently good papers for a quarterly. Therefore, I would be strongly opposed to publishing a journal, which it seems to me would be a kind of narcissistic gratification for the Academy but would serve no useful purpose. There are too few papers publishable, as you can see when you scan the *Journal of the American Psychoanalytic Association.* I would guess that, other than the papers published in the book, the Academy might have enough material for one issue per year, if one maintained high standards. Additionally, the journal would be troublesome; it would be expensive and it would take a lot of time of any person altruistic enough to do the job.

I hereby register my disapproval of the whole enterprise.

Sincerely yours,
Roy R. Grinker, Sr., M.D.

The idea of a journal was dropped. However, a solution was reached:

Ralph Crowley, M.D.
President
American Academy of Psychoanalysis

Dear Ralph:

Many thanks for your highly clarifying letter, to which I shall try to reply with equal specificity.

1. I am sure the publications Committee will be in complete accord with your assignment of material of current topical interest to a Newsletter, rather than to a new journal, and papers of permanent scientific value to the semi-annual volumes.

2. [To keep the Newsletter itself within reasonable size,]

I shall also be glad to edit and publish in these volumes the proceedings of Academy workshops, seminars, etc.

The problem of an excellent but unsolicited paper:

Russell R. Monroe, M.D.
University of Maryland

Dear Russ:

Your paper "An Existential Elaboration of Adaptational Psychodynamics" poses an editorial dilemma. As you know, I have my own reservations about many phenomenologic and existentialist concepts on the basis of their scientific redundancy and their musically unesthetic fuzziness—which is also the bane of all good poetry.

The trouble is that, on the one hand, your article is an unusually eloquent, clear, and concise statement of a currently much agitated field; whereas, on the other, were we to open these volumes to formal papers not actually read at Academy meetings while we eliminate many that were, the editorial board would be violating council's directives to publish only the best of the annual proceedings, and I would again face the alternatives of lynching or hara-kiri. This would deprive you of a good friend, so for your sake I must return your manuscript, regretfully.

Or a good paper that could be improved:

Nathan W. Ackerman, M.D.

Dear Nate:

My regrets at having had to delay editing your article, but this full APA program chairmanship is now my ninth full-time job, making everything hard to get into a forty-hour day.

Briefly, your style of composition is admirable for lectures, but in the terse, tight volumes of these series would appear in places repetitious enough to make some readers think that you don't trust them to remember what you had already said several times in a preceding paragraph. To avoid this, and to save precious space, I have made certain deletions and condensations which I hope you will accept, since they actually sharpen your points. Please return, retyped, and I shall be glad to publish the revised version.

S. Howard Armstrong: a poignant task

Read in memoriam at the May 5th, 1961 Meeting of the Academy of Psychoanalysis and published in Volume V of the proceedings:

It is meet and proper that we meditate together for a fleeting moment on our departed colleague, but true grief must ever remain a deep and private sorrow.

I shall not review Howard Armstrong's life in detail: his external biography is available in any directory honoring prominent Americans. Yet many of us knew him in many more intimate facets of his rich personality: as a classical scholar and a modern scientist, as a salty sailor and a sensitive esthete, as a dedicated teacher, perceptive investigator, and humble student, as a delightful sophisticate and a devoted husband and father—indeed, as a living representative of the vanishing tradition of Renaissance Man. The Academy has lost one of its most distinguished members, but it is more the measure of our remembrance that those of us who knew him best shall feel his loss longest and most poignantly, and shall have many another moemnt of contemplative regret such as we now, for the last time, tender together to Howard Armstrong.

In the delicate matter of an overlong and involved presidential address:

Leon Salzman, M.D.

Dear Leon:

About this time of year the preparation of the next volume involves the sad editorial task of editing manuscripts so as (a) to maintain not only the scientific but literary quality of *Science and Psychoanalysis* and (b) to get the book into integrated, publishable form. Usually, I do this as an editorial privilege without consulting the authors, even of presidential addresses. Fortunately, I have nearly always received each contributor's thanks not only for condensing his opus so it could be printed within the limited space available, but also for correcting slips of grammar, eliminating redundancies, and clarifying style.

However, in your case, our personally close collaboration leads me to ask your consent for editing and eliminating certain paragraphs in your paper which, though perhaps helpful for emphasis when read aloud, may seem so repetitious when printed as to discourage interest in your message and impair its important impact. No significant thought has been omitted, yet the article is down to printable size, in clearer form. If you approve, please return, retyped as necessary.

Leon heartily approved.

To the author of a desirable paper who wished to withdraw it for publication elsewhere, or revise it as a chapter for a forthcoming treatise on child psychoanalysis:

Robert R. Holt, M.D.
Research Center for Mental Health

Dear Dr. Holt:

I could use a legalistic approach, to wit: "All papers read in full or in part at scientific sessions of the Academy automatically become the property of its annual publication, *Science and Psychoanalysis,* unless expressly released by the editorial board!"

Or I could use the pitch of the encyclopedia salesman, to

wit: *"Science and Psychoanalysis* now has a far wider readership and a much more extensive use as a basic shelf and library reference by behavioral scientists than any other psychoanalytic publication. In fact, even orthodox analysts now read it in furtive privacy or concealed behind their comic books."

Or I could ". . ."—but I won't. Instead, I'll make a professional plea as one appreciataive editor to another, to wit: Your closely reasoned and clearly written manuscript would make a fine introductory chapter to Volume XI of this series on "Concepts of the Ego," scheduled to appear in May, 1967, and would add greatly to the value of the book as a landmark on the road to the clarification of analytic thought and practice. It's about three times as long as any chapter I've previously published, but I see no reason to delete a word. Moreover, you can republish it in your *Contemporary Psychology* text if you wish. Ergo, I shall include it in Volume XI, unless expressly forbidden to do so and send galleys to you in a few weeks.

Holt's excellent paper led off Volume XI.
More appreciation where due:

Harmon S. Ephron, M.D.
New York

Dear Dr. Ephron:

It is a rare pleasure for an editor to receive a paper so topical, replete with thoughtful analyses of relevant content, and so consummately well written as the one by Miss Carrington and yourself. With but a few picayune changes from "will" to "shall" and "diminishment" to "diminution," it will be published, along with Goodenough's discussion, as a prominent feature of Volume XI of this series.

A commentary in the *Journal of the American Medical Association* written by Dr. John King, the associate editor:

"We believe that the extraordinary preface to Vol XI of *Science and Psychoanalysis,* written by the editor, Jules Masserman, will have a quite universal appeal, and we quote it in full":

> Much psychoanalytic writing (I avoid the term literature) emulated medieval scholasticism in postulating how many highflown but impalpable concepts can be made to congregate on the point of a pen. The Ego is one such assemblage of variably angelic (or fallen) notions which the contributors to this volume trace to their mystical re(or de?)ifications and then scrutinize in the light of modern criteria of heuristic, semantic and operational validity. I believe that most readers will agree they have done so with scholarly erudition, literary grace, clinical relevance, and therapeutic significance.

A particularly hirsute hairshirt descended on me during the preparation of Volume XII when a member of the Academy demanded that I publish three unread papers, all of them nearly illiterate. I combined and rewrote two of them and requested approval of the changes. A month later Dr. N returned copies of the originals with a demand for full publication. The subsequent correspondence begins *andante,* rises to a *crescendo furioso* in C sharp minor, and ends in a cadenced *coda:*

Dear Dr. N.:

At the inception of the annual volumes of the Academy, its editorial board, by the direction of the trustees, laid down certain policies which have since assured the success of the series. Three of these policies apply to your contributions to Volume XII, to wit: (1) Each volume must be topical, rather than a diverse collection of discursive writings. (2) Each contribution must be clearly written, stick to its subject, and be brief enough so that the annual issue does not price itself out of the market. (3) In fairness to all contributors, no author may have more than one chapter in any one volume. (4) No issue can be delayed for late contributors, since this places an undue burden on the other authors, the Academy, and the publisher. (5) As in other professional publications, the editorial board is the sole arbiter of the contents of each volume—else chaos would result.

Since the revised versions of the three papers you wish to contribute to Volume XII were sent in over two months past the deadline, I neglected all else to re-edit them immediately so as not to delay the book (the rest of which had to be sent to the publisher weeks ago) a day longer. I then checked my editing with others on the editorial board, who agreed to the following: (1) We cannot publish all three papers, but to save some of your efforts we shall combine Papers II and III as a final commentary to the section on ethology. (2) Your long passages on "psychosomatic medicine" are really irrelevant to the volume on ethology, and must be omitted along with the twenty-odd charts and tables. (3) Your speculative projections of elaborate conferences to be held many years hence must also be omitted from a topical volume. (4) Your Papers II and III, as was your final paper, are again typed in a most peculiar style of capitalization and italics, which no publisher would follow. You will recall that I spent hours correcting the first and second versions of your first paper which had to be sent to Grune & Stratton weeks ago, and I cannot now re-edit and send them still another version. I have once more indicated the very extensive editing also necessary for your other two papers. (5) Since Volume XII could not wait another day, I sent the revisions outlined above to the publisher, where you are welcome to inspect them with the permission of Mr. Duncan Mackintosh. If he thinks it necessary, you may have to retype their combination into printable form; if, on the other hand, you wish not to accept these essential revisions and condensations, you, of course, may withdraw Papers II and III for publication elsewhere.

I am sure you understand that the editorial board must consider not only the integrity of single volumes but the consistency and reputation of the entire series. Such revisions are necessary for many contributors and in no case are they done with personal prejudice; in fact, they are often painfully necessary operations on the efforts of a good friend for the greater good of the Academy. I therefore trust that, whether or not you accept the revisions, you will be not only understanding of, but cooperative with the policies of the Academy.

As to the other kind invitations in your letters, to one who has organized and conducted some four International Psychiatric Congresses, and has had to deal with the realities of travel, finances, and busy Nobelist candidates, your plans sound rather visionary. However, I shall be glad to help in every way I can.

Nine weeks passed:

Dear Dr. N:

Over two months since your first promised date of August 15th, I just received what must now be about your fifth version of Paper I, and new copies of Papers II and III. I shall keep these for our Academy files, but I must in all friendliness point out that, in waiting for, editing, and reediting your contributions, none of which was actually read at the Academy meeting, I have spent more time than with any combination of ten of the twenty-five other contributions to the volume, twenty-three of which were in by the actual deadline of August 1. As I wrote you previously, I combined and edited your last versions of II and III immediately on their receipt and had to send them on to Grune and Stratton to meet the absolute expiration of all possible delay. You are still welcome, with Mr. Mackintosh's permission, to make minor corrections on the edited manuscript now at his office and perhaps, if necessary retype it into proper format and legibility; however, by editorial board decision, it will not be permissable to restore deleted sections or add new ones. Final minor corrections can later also be made in the galley proofs sent to you.

Once again, I trust in your understanding and cooperation.

Dr. N's response was to escalate his demands: He not only wanted us to print Papers II and III as originally written as well as Paper I but he demanded that we turn over to him the selection of papers for the Volume on ethology, permit him to design it, and allow him rather than Grune and Stratton to determine the length and salability of the book. He implied that if this were not done, he not only would withdraw his own papers but he would induce others to do so.

To Dr. Stratton:

Dear Henry:

By now you have probably seen my correspondence with Duncan re Dr. N. If the Academy ever directs me to publish unedited and unexpurgated manuscripts such as he submits I shall, subject only to my contractual obligations of due notice to you, resign as Editor, since I would regard *Science and Psychoanalysis* as no longer worthy either of the Academy or of Grune & Stratton. Meanwhile, I have the unanimous backing of the Editorial Board to proceed as per my editorial directions.

Dear Jules:

I fully agree with your letter of November 9 regarding your correspondence with Dr. N. The Academy and Publisher appointed you as Editor because of the great confidence in your ability; therefore, manuscripts for publication can be accepted only with your approbation, and changes in manuscripts can be made only if you approve them. We, as publishers, have no dealings whatsoever with the contributors.

Dr. Henry M. Stratton

Incredibly, Dr. N yet again reiterated his demands and added threats that he would not only induce all contributors to withdraw their papers but have me "indicted" before the Academy Council. My final reply, in part:

Dear Dr. N:

In the eleven years since the present editorial board was apppointed by the Academy, no contributor has failed to recognize that the board functions without prejudice, fear, or favoritism for the sole purpose of maintaining the high scientific and literary standards of our published Proceedings. The same has been true of over two hundred and fifty world authorities who have contributed to eight volumes of *Current Psychiatric Therapies,* an annual that I alone edit. Indeed, you have been the first to presume that you can dictate the format and contents of an entire volume, including the proposal that even the Presidential Address be deleted to make room for your writings.

I note again both your threats and your invitation to join in another extravagantly projected international seminar on ethology and psychoanalysis. In view of our past dealings, please exclude me from participation in any enterprise with which you are connected. Unreciprocated professional courtesy, editorial forbearance and available time have their limits, so that I must also request that you regard this as our last communication.

After the difficulties and delays thus occasioned, rapport with the publisher's staff needed refurbishing:

Duncan Mackintosh
Editor in Chief
Grune & Stratton, Inc.

Dear Duncan:

I am completely sympathetic with your difficulties in publishing Volume XII of this series, and, though I tried to do what I could, perhaps I could have done more to mitigate them. As always, I had notified every contributor in advance that two copies of his mansucript should be submitted double spaced on opaque paper, that the bibliography must follow the JAMA style, that illustrations must be clear and so on. As always, these strictures had only scattered effects on contributors to *Science and Psychoanalysis,* with the result that I had to concentrate most of my efforts on editing their submissions for content and style, and then assembling them in minimally printable form before the next semiannual meeting rolled around and the task had to be repeated. As you know, Dr. N, one of the less tolerable contributors, particularly delayed Volume XII, and diverted even more available attention and effort from useful editing. Unfortunately also, I do not have free choice of contributors to the *Science and Psychoanalysis* series, since these are foreordained by the Program Committee which selects the participants in the Scientific Meetings; all I can do after that is edit or revise the manuscripts or, as not infrequently necessary, reject some altogether. In contrast, when I alone select the authors as I do for *Current Psychiatric Therapies* and can keep reediting, and returning their contributions for reconsideration and retyping, the results are, I trust, more satisfactory all around.

My thanks for your courtesy and patience.

Appreciations where due:

John P. Spiegel, M.D.
Director, Institute on Aggression
Brandeis University

Dear John:

Your chapter was an intellectual treat and a double pleasure, because, unlike many submitted, it required almost no editing for stylistic clarity and grace. It will be a valued feature of Volume XIII of this series.

Dr. Raymond Sobel
Dartmouth College

Dear Dr. Sobel:

I have just reedited the galleys of your discussion of Jerome Goldsmith's paper, and want once again to express my admiration of its wisdom and delight in its style. It will constitute a memorable closing coda to Volume XV of our Academy proceedings, due out next May.

In contrast, to an authoress who objected to my deleting some flowery introductory tributes to her made by a formal "discussant" of her Academy presentation:

Dear Natalie:

As to your inquiry in re my "great eternal plan" about editing out literary log-rolling, what is involved is not only to save space (although were we to include all the polite preliminary throat-clearings on the part of all discussants, the space required would increase the size and price of the book considerably) but rather what all good editors soon learn: that intelligent readers want to form their own judgments about what they read rather than be told what to think of it; for this and related reasons I have always omitted panegyric commentaries even on my own writings. Since, of course, our proceedings are intended only for intelligent readers, they can judge your (and my?) undoubted excellence on their own as contrasted, say, with the self-adulatory pap of the APsaA journals. In eight syllables: your chapter should speak for itself.

When once more deluged with poor papers after an Academy meeting:

Dr. Harold Kelman, President, Academy of Psychoanalysis
Dr. Sidney Goldensohn, Secretary
Dr. Irving Bieber, Program Chairman

Dear Harold, Sidney, and Irv:

I have thus far reviewed the following manuscripts to be read at our December meeting and have the following comments:

1. "Fetishism and Murder," by R and A. Another one of those essays that derive cosmic inferences from three inconclusive "clinical analyses" of fetishistic murders. In Case One, there are no data that demonstrate any but a coincidental connection between fetishism and murder—and, coincidence is *not* cause. In Case Two, a "highly competent psychiatrist ... terminated his treatment ... when ... this patient committed murder"—a trenchant commentary on this analyst's foresight and competence—although the history supplied does not differ from that of many fetishists who do *not* commit murder. Case Three is a similarly chaotic account until the "diagnosis of schizophrenia" suddenly appears near its end. Again, this most ardent of the three "fetishists" did *not* commit murder. The ensuing discussion likewise attempts to fuse together discrete or incompatible data, and ends typically with a confused statement that, while "murder is unpredictable," the Academy should organize to prevent it! We can, of course, publish such odd essays, but only at the expense of depreciating the scientific status of our Proceedings.

2. In contrast (although I do not personally agree with his concluding formulae about "aggression"), Paul Sebbard's paper on "Fetishism and Sadomasochism" is a balanced, clear, judicial critique of presently inadequate theories, and furnishes sound suggestions as to broader views.

3. Ed Gendel's "Chromosomes and Sex" is factual and pertinent, but obviously needs rewriting for publication (see my letter to him).

4. V. F.'s "Homosexuality in Adolescence" wanders from unmade point to contradictory counterpoint, seems to postulate sets of non-cultural sexual absolutes while trying to remain culturally relativistic, and confuses premises with conclusions; e.g., "normal" sex activity *must* be procreative, ergo "the child must be asexual." The author's theses are that adolescent homosexuality may be (a) regressive, (b) the resultant of heterosexual conflicts in a stimulating but forbidding culture, or (c) the "expression of weak ego" (the epitome of semantic circularity); but all this could have been said in a sentence not much longer than this one—or, if prolixity be insisted upon, in not more than a couple of literate pages.

If these papers are typical of our December scientific sessions, we shall be faced with a perennial dilemma: if we publish all, our reputation as an Academy suffers; if we include only the better ones (and some borderline ones supplemented by corrective discsssions), we'll be accused of being "anti-analytic," or "castrative dictators," etc. Ergo, being both editorially conscientious and desirous of friendly compromise (call it chicken, if you like), I would appreciate having your progress committee bail out the publications committee with your concurrent opinion as to the relative merits of the December papers, and as to whether any, or which of them, really merit a permanent place in our published proceedings. Please give me this consensus as soon as possible so that I might just possibly get Volume XV out in time for our May meeting.

The prerogatives of the editorial board were reconfirmed by the council, and the *Science and Psychoanalysis* volumes have maintained their respected place in the scientific literature.

10. THE SOCIETY OF BIOLOGICAL PSYCHIATRY

The Society of Biological Psychiatry was founded under the leadership of George Thompson and Abram Bennett in 1946 by a group of organically-orientated psychiatrists, neurologists, and neurophysiologists* who felt strongly that American psychiatry was overly preoccupied with mythical or metaphysical fantasies and practices, and had too long neglected the genetic, physiologic, pharmacologic, and pathologic factors in human behavior; ergo, a forum for the adequate interchange of laboraroty research and clinical experience related to the organic etiology and therapy of behavior disorders was sorely needed. I joined the organization soon after its founding, and four years later was nominated president. This created a dilemma described in the following letter:

December 18, 1956

George N. Thompson, M.D.
Secretary
Society of Biological Psychiatry

Dear George:

Your letters present me with a personal problem which,

*Among the most prominent: Percival Bailey, U. of Chicago; Karl Bowman, the University of California; Stanley Cobb of Harvard, Roland McKay of the University of Illinois, and Harry Solomon of Harvard.

since it also concerns the Society, I must share with you and its other officers.

As you may know, for several years I had been greatly concerned about the rapidly declining prestige and academic status of psychoanalysis and the preemption of the field by a highly organized and exclusively powerful group of dogmatic isolationists, yclept the American Psychoanalytic Association. My own efforts and those of some of my friends to correct this situation bore fruit last year in the founding of a new Academy of Psychoanalysis, dedicated to the task of reintegrating psychoanalysis—defined as the study and service of the individual in his cultural-symbolic milieu—with its matrix in medicine and the social sciences. I declined the first presidency of this new Academy; however, I could not conscientiously shirk sharing the tremendous organizational work required to keep it going during its crucial second year, and therefore accepted the post of president-elect with many critical administrative and other constitutional duties. Shortly thereafter, I learned that, again without seeking any of the posts, I had also been elected (a) president of your Society of Biological Psychiatry, for 1957-58, (b) president of the American Society of Group Therapy and Psychodrama, and (c) chairman of the Section on Psychotherapy of the American Psychiatric Association.

The last two posts, though they have many detailed duties, conflict with neither of the others; however, the Biological Society and the Academy must necessarily meet on the same days at San Francisco in 1958. To divide my loyalties and time there would be unthinkable, and I must therefore make a choice influenced by the following reasonable considerations: The Society of Biological Psychiatry is well established, has many exceedingly capable men available for its officers, and is already surprisingly well run by its perennial secretary George Thompson. In contrast, the Academy, though it is filling a long-felt need and therefore has been very well received (250 fellows and scientific associates the first year) is still in its formative stages and must depend for another year or two on intensive work by its founders. Despite my equal devotion to the organization and purposes of the Biological Society, it may therefore be best that Joseph Wortis or some other deserving officer take precedence over me for the presidency until I can relinquish my duties to the Academy in May, 1958. After that date, should the Society so desire, I shall be happy to devote my main attention to the post of its president, councillor or any other function it assigns me. If however, the Society decides that the precedent of officer progression must be followed, I shall do whatever I can in 1957-1958.

The Society chose to override these reservations. As part of my initial duties as president, I arranged to honor Dr. Percival Bailey with a life membership on his sixty-fifth birthday and appointed the best program committee I could find, with Lester Rudy as chairman:

September 19, 1957

Lester H. Rudy, M.D.
Superintendent
Galesburg State Research Hospital

Dear Les:

Thanks for your acceptance. We both understand that in many ways, perhaps justifiably, the Society is George Thompson's special preserve, but you have full rights to take your own initiative or to join with George in inviting speakers, arranging schedules and even setting precedents. Please do.

The Academy of Psychoanalysis is rapidly becoming a major influence in the American behavioral sciences in a way even I had not dared to hope, but its many ramifications (for example, representation on the American Board of Neurology and Psychiatry) and mushrooming activities must take much of my time—including frequent trips out of town. So, too, I shall of necessity be preoccupied with Academy affairs in San Francisco, I can entrust you with the May meeting, and of course I'll arrange to give the "Presidential Address" somehow (in appropriately techno-scientific language and with impressively illegible slides) no matter when the dates are fixed.

I'll talk to Percival at the next governor's authority meeting, and give him a preveiw of the certificate I'm having prepared for him.

My next service to the Society was to inquire whether Henry Stratton would publish its annual proceedings, which he agreed to do if, as in the case of the Academy, I would undertake to edit them.

February 12, 1958

Dr. George N. Thompson
Secretary, Society of Biological Psychiatry

Dear George:

The program of the Society of Biological Psychiatry this year sounds so excellent that it cries for publication in a single volume, simply entitled *Biological Psychiatry.* As current editor of *Progress in Psychotherapy* and *Science and Psychoanalysis,* I have excellent relationships with Henry Stratton of Grune & Stratton; without committing our society in any way, I shall explore the possibility of his publishing such a volume.

Parenthetically, please note that a presidential address should not shoulder any of the excellent papers off the program. Indeed, I shall be most happy to confine my remarks to an after-dinner speech entitled "Say Id Isn't So, with Music," with obligatos on the violin and viola which I shall play. After this, I shall silently fade away. However, if you want a formal address replete with slides and arpeggios, its title will be "Norms, Neurotics, and Nepenthics."

My heartiest congratulations to you, Les Rudy, and all for your excellent work.

Henry Stratton responded favorably to the list of papers planned for *Biological Psychiatry.* Ergo:

March 20, 1958

George N. Thompson, M.D.

Dear George:

In accord with the favorable reactions of various council members to our recent correspondence, I arranged a second conference yesterday here in Chicago with Dr. Henry Stratton of the publishing house of Grune & Stratton. Henry not only confirmed his offer to publish this year's proceedings of our Society at his own publishing risk, but urged that the volume appear soon after the meeting (within a few weeks if possible) for a number of reasons. Among these were: that we would have priority on the desirable title *Biologic Psychiatry* for the projected series of annual volumes; that there is currently a need and demand for the early appearance of the first of such a series; and that it would be well to collect and edit the manuscripts to be read at the meeting as soon as practicable.

There is one more point I could propose to the Council: that the first volume should be dedicated to you, with an appropriate tribute and frontispiece as a token of the Society's appreciation of your indispensable service. I am sending copies of this letter to the Council to elicit their personal wishes on this point also.

June 15, 1958

Dr. Henry Stratton

Dear Henry:

After spending most of my cruise time aboard the Naiad in rejecting, editing, and integrating manuscripts, and reducing the incredible number of illustrations to reasonable proportions, I believe I have your new volume on *Biological Psychiatry* in almost acceptable shape. I need merely the approval of some authors for the revisions and condensations I have made, and then the manuscripts will be in your office.

One delicate point: in view of George Thompson's yeoman services to the Society (co-founder and perennial secretary), I got the Council to agree to dedicate the first volume not to me, but to him. Whereupon, he sent along his picture for a frontispiece. If policy permits, please print it.

In any case, herewith the rough draft of a preface, the last part of which has direct reference to a Dr. Henry Stratton in whom you may be interested. I shall welcome any suggestion on this, too.

Best of summers, and I shall look forward to seeing you in Rome—though I am afraid that on the Wednesday of your party, Christine and I must be on our way to Greece. Best from both of us.

The first volume of *Biological Psychiatry,* with a dedication to George Thompson, co-founder of the Society, was assembled, accepted by Grune & Stratton, and widely advertised by them in advance to promote a successful initial sale. However, this may have prompted President-elect Dr. Joseph Wortis to object that I had become a "private editor of too many publications," that no one should "preempt" the editorship of *Biological Psychiatry,* that its name should be changed to *The Proceedings of the Society of Biological Psychiatry,* and that each succeeding president should "anonymously" edit the current issue in collaboration with "a publications committee." This occasioned the following correspondence, relatively polite at first:

July 23, 1958

Dear Dr. Wortis:

To correct possible misapprehensions and review some facts relevant to your recent letters:

1. None of the volumes I have thus far worked on—or intend to—have been, as you for some reason, put it, "privately edited." Specifically, *Progress in Psychotherapy* is based on the transactions of the APA section on psychotherapy; Dr. Moreno and I were directed by the APA to expand these proceedings into a succession of annual volumes, and they have become a

highly successful series in only four years. So also, *Science and Psychoanalysis* records the transactions of the Academy of Psychoanalysis, the executive council of which also appointed me editor. Both volumes bear full acknowledgement of their affiliations as does our own volume on *Biological Psychiatry;* indeed, the rough draft of the preface which I sent to the publications committee makes this explicit.

2. On the other hand, any publisher will tell you that to handicap *any* book with the title "Transactions of (with a date and an anonymous editorship)" will immediately convert it into the equivalent of a house organ, cut its general sale drastically, make the publication economically unfeasible, and thereby defeat any educational purposes beyond its own society.

3. There are excellent precedents for mutually satisfactory and generally advantageous arrangements among societies and publishers (e.g., between Saunders and the Mayo Clinics; or between Grune & Stratton and the American Psychopathological Association, the Academy of Psychoanalysis and the APA section on psychotherapy) on the basis that one or at most two editors be held responsible by both the publisher and thc society for producing an integrated annual volume of scientific merit and wide professional appeal. As directed by our council in 1957, I investigated various possibilities for publishing the proceedings of our own society and succeeded in getting a most advantageous offer from Grune and Stratton. You will remember that the executive council approved this choice of publisher, the title *Biological Psychiatry,* and appointed me editor of the 1958 volume. This was confirmed at a formal business meeting of the society where, you may recall, considerable satisfaction was expressed over various features of the plan: an attractive yearly volume, dignified advertising and distribution, and no cost or risk to the society, including editorial expenses which always exceed "royalties" for at least five years, and which, therefore, I offered to bear personally. The general format of the 1958 volume, including its dedication to George Thompson, was thus determined by the society. It may, of course, be changed if, during your prospective term as president, the council wishes

to revise its action and, incidentally, contravene its contract with Grune & Stratton.

4. In any case, from considerable experience, I know how much time, trouble, and effort were connected with the proper editorship of a volume of this kind: for example, just the preliminary work of editing and letter-writing has already taken many hours a day and, more recently, two solid weeks of my "vacation." The rest of the revisions, reorganizations, substitutions, retypings, discussions, illustrations, filing, galleys, page-proofs, index, etc., etc., yet ahead, will take much more of my time and about half that of a secretary for a period of about three months. I made the investment knowingly so that we could get the series started, but, frankly, I have no intention of continuing the editorial assignment a moment longer than the Society directs that I do so. Therefore, to provide continuity, I suggested a Publications Committee, which I have consulted and followed on all matters of policy. For the sake of the success of future volumes, I hope that the present format will be continued with only favorable modifications and under the aegis of only one or two future editors since no committee can effectively divide the job.

5. Finally, your own suggestion that you substitute for the paper you actually gave at our spring meeting another unpublished one given a year ago may establish a dangerous precedent for other authors who may wish to avoid preparing acceptable and original papers for our meetings. However, in view of your position as current president of the Society, and with the consent of the publications committee, the substitution may be made in this instance.

6. I am still negotiating with the AMA as directed by the Society to secure separate *Index Medicus* listings for each contributor. This has been contrary to their established policy on similar volumes, but I happen to be personally acquainted with the *JAMA* editorial staff, and perhaps I can arrange it; I will let the committee know of the results as soon as possible.

Finally, I hope that the notes of pique and polemic which, for the first time in many years of affiliation with the society, you seem to have introduced into its correspondence, are (a) inadvertent, (b) transient and, therefore, (c) will call for no further reviews such as this. For the sake of the society, let's keep it a friendly as well as a scientific organization.

The letter had little effect—something I would have anticipated had I known Dr. Wortis better. Indeed, he tried personally to induce Grune & Stratton to change the title, format, and contents of the book, and so confused and alienated the staff and so long delayed the processing and printing of the manuscript that Henry Stratton appealed to me either for final directives or for abrogation of the Society's contract with him.

As chairman of the executive council of the Society, I then circularized the council as follows:

October 6, 1958

To the Council and the Editorial Committee
Society of Biological Psychiatry:

I am in receipt of yet another proposal from Joseph Wortis that we again change the format [of our annual volume of *Biological Psychiatry*] originally agreed upon by the council, the membership of the society, Grune & Stratton, and myself. You will recall that the title page was to specify, and the preface and text elaborate the fact that the volume is a record of the proceedings of the society; indeed, a history of the society is included in the preface. However, for the sake of a far wider advertising appeal and sale we had also agreed (a) to call the volume by the simple but comprehensive title *Biological Psychiatry* with a subtitle, the year, and principal theme, (b) to have successive editors' names appear as customary on the cover, and the membership of the editorial board on the face sheet in tribute to the society's choice and the tremendous work involved, and (c) to avoid any format leading to the impression that the book is merely the minutes of a society meeting and therefore of interest only to its membership.

I am prepared, of course, to accept any new directions from the council and committee, and to request Grune & Stratton to agree, but in the absence of such changed directives, I shall proceed according to our original plans until changes are officially made, not arbitrarily by any single member but only by the editorial board—and, I personally hope, a new editor.

I somewhat wearily again attach my previous correspondence with Dr. Wortis for your ready reference, and shall be happy to hear your wishes on the subject.

The first volume of *Biological Psychiatry* appeared and was well reviewed and received. George Thompson expressed the gratitude of the society, and I replied:

May 20, 1959

Dear George:

Thank you for your very kind comments on the editing of *Biological Psychiatry.* The work was gratifying since I hoped to serve not only my friends in the society, but also the interests of neuropsychiatric teaching and research in general. And, as I said in the preface, any scientific precedent the book may set or any success it may attain will be attributable not to its editor, but to the many excellent contributors whose work I assembled.

As to my editorial costs: you remember that at the 1958 meeting I myself proposed to the society that my expenses be covered out of accruing royalties; this meant specifically that I would take all the financial risks (the book would have to sell about 1800 copies before the 10% royalty would cover secretarial costs alone), and that thereafter I would assign to the society in perpetuum any excess over my initial expenses.

As the Society's next president, Dr. Wortis assumed the editorship and despite his previously expressed sentiments, persisted in retaining it. The results:

Dear Jules:

With regard to *Biological Psychiatry,* I am afraid that I will have to disassociate myself from the society. The sales of [the later editions of] this book do not warrant its publication.

Sincerely yours,
Dr. Henry M. Stratton

The series is now published elsewhere on partial subsidy as a collection of abstracts; fortunately, the Society itself, under the return of more able leadership, has continued to prosper.

11. PSYCHODRAMATIC VENTURES AND MISADVENTURES

In 1954 Dr. Frieda Fromm-Reichmann, author of classic contributions to the therapy of schizophrenia and one of the most gentle, clear-thinking, and progressive of psychoanalysts, joined with Jacob L. Moreno, assertive and preemptive originator of psychodrama, in organizing a section on psychotherapy as part of the annual meeting of the American Psychiatric Association. At the first business session of the Section Dr. Fromm-Reichmann was elected its chairman, I its vice-chairman, and Dr. Moreno, secretary. The first transactions of the section were of such quality that Henry Stratton offered to publish them with Drs. Fromm-Reichmann and Moreno as editors, and to continue them as an annual if their scientific standards were maintained. At the second meeting of the Section, I was elected to succeed Dr. Fromm-Reichmann as Chairman, at which time she also requested that, since she had already experienced various difficulties as coeditor with Dr. Moreno, I replace her in that capacity also. It was one of her last requests: her death within a few months was an incalculable loss to American psychiatry.

The Section on Psychotherapy prospered; invited experts presented papers which were discerningly discussed, and the audiences grew until within two years its sessions were those best attended at the annual APA meetings. Soon, however, complications arose, to wit:

At the third annual meeting of the section I declined re-election as chairman in the belief that this leadership should change at least every two years. This policy was adopted, and Lewis Wolberg was elected chairman, Jerome Frank vice-chairman, and Leon Salzman secretary to replace Moreno. This pleased everyone except Moreno, who made it obvious that he had somehow planned to be a permanent officer and policy-maker of the section.

In 1959, Moreno and I were invited to represent American Psychiatry at the First Czechoslovak International Psychiatric Congress, where I was to give an opening address intended to foster perhaps the first direct rapprochement in a generation between American and Soviet-oriented psychiatry. In essence, I spoke as follows:

We of the West employ three major approaches to the understanding of human behavior: the historic-philosophic, the interdisciplinary-scientific and the comparative-experimental. In this we are in obvious accord with our Soviet colleagues, since they, too, see man as the product of ethnic and politico-economic evolution, study him currently by means of every one of the interrelated social sciences, and investigate even his highest neural functions in the objective experimental tradition of Sechenov and Pavlov. Many of us in the West know this because we follow the Russian scientific literature—in fact, the U.S. government subsidizes its translation—and because some of our leading neurophysiologists (e.g., Grey Walter, Horace Magoun) had exchanged or were planning to exchange visits with Russians of the caliber of A. I. Oparin, A. Luria, and the late, great Professor Bykov. Neurology is hardly a neglected science among leading psychiatrists in the West (e. g., David Rioch, Percival Bailey, Ben Boshes, Roy Grinker), and even our orthodox psychoanalysts profess respect for Freud's basically biologic orientations despite the fact that no two of them have ever really agreed on a tangible definition of psychoanalysis. So also, since Freud himself kept changing his theories and methods of therapy, "Freudianism" is too impalpable a concept to bear much attack.

Currently, most properly trained psychoanalysts regard their subspecialty as only (a) a special method of research into each patient's energy systems, personality development, unique concepts and values, and characteristic transactive patterns, (b) a constantly improving but ever tentative set of correlated postulates about human behavior, and (c) an individually adaptable, rather protean and essentially socially oriented mode of interpersonal therapy. Indeed, what we actually refer to by our somewhat unfortunate term "psychology" is the integrated study of man's total adaptations to his material and cultural milieu, whereas our Russian colleagues really mean the same when they use the perhaps equally abstract concepts of "primary and secondary signals," "higher cortical analyzers and effector systems" or "conflicts between excitatory and inhibitory radiations." As to ancillary experimental approaches, I wished to present not only my own work but that of Gantt, Liddell, Pribram, Delgado, Mirsky, and others that equaled in rigor and objectivity the classic experiments of Pavlov and, like his, led to certain basic biodynamic concepts of behavior that best fulfilled the criteria of breadth, economy, and predictability required of truly scientific formulations. Certainly the best psychiatric therapy everywhere utilized every available physical and environmental means to restore personal happiness and social usefulness. Excluding irrelevant economic or political considerations, then, it might well be that many of the differences between Eastern and Western psychiatric thought consisted in the choice of words rather than in operational referents; in any case, we of the West, and perhaps all of those present, hoped that the Congress would help remove this semantic handicap to greater rapport and collaboration among us.

My talk ended the first day's session, and despite the courteously prolonged applause, there was no way of ascertaining whether it had been received as an admission of and retreat from Western confusions and weaknesses, as a challenge to conflict, or as what it was meant to be: a sincere offer to leave clanking arms and tattered standards behind in outmoded battlements, lower the drawbridges, and meet on common ground for friendly scientific concourse. That it was taken in all these ways—but fortunately mainly in the third sense by most of the leading Russian delegates—became apparent as the Congress progressed.

The first indication of this beginning rapprochement occurred at a roundtable discussion on "Concepts of Neurosis" scheduled that evening. When asked to contribute to the discussion, I reviewed the neuropathologic connotations of the terms "neurosis" and "psychosis" from Cullen and Feuchtersleben through the kaleidoscopic meanings of Kahlbaum, Charcot, Freud, Sullivan, Fromm, Jaspers, and then back again through Eysenck and Guilyarovsky to recently renewed Russian assertions that "neuroses are simply a disease of the higher nervous system." I stated that we could agree even with this if the term disease were taken quite literally to mean a "dis-ease" or disruptive un-easiness experienced by an individual under circumstances that he had somehow come to regard as stressful and threatening. In such conditions (or, in Pavlovian terms, with such "conditioning"), the subject would be called "neurotic" if he reacted with greater physiologic (autoplastic or "psychosomatic") and social-transactional (alloplastic) disturbances than, by cultural relativity, were thought to be necessary or appropriate by most observers, yet not sufficiently severe in intensity and duration ("psychotic") to justify forced isolation and treatment. However, in view of the current expansion of the term "neurosis" to cover so many viewpoints, vectors, and contingencies, perhaps we would sooner or later abandon it as no longer of etiologic, diagnostic, or prognostic value, much as we no longer accepted the previously literal meanings of Hippocrates' "frenzy," Kahlbaum's "vesania," Galen's "hysteria," or Prichard's "moral insanity." Instead, much as the physicists outgrew concepts such as "phlogiston" or "cosmic ether" and progressively sharpened their lexicon, so should we also to suit more *dynamic, transactional,* and scientific concepts of behavior and its vicissitudes.

Perhaps this discussion constituted a bit of a gambit, since I knew that in other sections of the Soviet literature neuroses were considered to be subdivisible—again by analogy to animal experimental observations by Shenger-Krestovnikova and others—into definite categories of neurasthenia, psychasthenia, and hysteria, whereas my presentation of predominant Western views had implied a partial challenge to this position. But the general reaction was most gratifying: When a psychiatrist from one of the Eastern countries, apparently for the ears of his Party bosses back home, began criticizing me as obscurantist, unscientific, misleading, deviationistic, idealistic, and, as ultimate epithets, a religious capitalist and imperialist, he was peremptorily silenced by the chairman, himself a highly placed Communist, as being completely out of accord with the scientific and fraternal spirit of the Congress. The chairman's remarks were fully translated into the five languages of the Congress and were soundly applauded as an edict that this type of political and *ad hominem* polemic would no longer be countenanced.

Unfortunately, this cordiality did not remain unstrained; occasional speakers from countries under Soviet influence thought it necessary once again to disparage Western psychiatry as "decadent," "bourgeois," and "imperalistic." Even more regrettably, Moreno in his address half way through the Congress asserted that all forms of psychotherapy were merely deviant offshoots of psychodrama and, apparently in all seriousness, proposed that, in accordance with psychodrama techniques, the United States "reverse roles" with Russia and "become communist for a year" while during this interval the USSR "becomes democratic." In reply R. A. Zachepitski of Leningrad merely remarked that in the USSR they had indeed explored the usefulness of psychodrama, and had decided to rename it "psychocomedy."

When Dr. Moreno and I returned to the U.S., additional differences between us grew onerous. He circulated a letter and questionnaire among APA members as to whether they did not wish, in effect, to restore his control over the Section on Psychotherapy by establishing an "Executive Committee" with himself in permanent charge of Section programs. He also persisted in attempting to devote a major portion of each annual issue of *Progress in Psychotherapy* to articles written by his disciples on psychodrama, some of which approached illiteracy. This occasioned considerable correspondence during the preparation of the first three volumes which culminated in the increasing acrimony of the letters I reproduce here:*

January 3, 1957

Dear Jack:

I am afraid I must repeat some fundamental conditions of our joint editorship, to wit: I am on the consulting editorial staff of quite a number of publications, including those of the American Medical and the American Psychiatric Associations, and I know of no editor who relinquishes the right (as you suggest we do) to reject a manuscript, invited or not, either before or after requested modification. Any surrender of this editorial privilege would be certain to lower the standards of any publication. Your own proposed policy of invariably publishing first revisions must also entail this: what if, for instance, Schultz refuses to change his manuscript at all (as Cosin did) or "revises" it but leaves it still scientifically unacceptable? Must we then print it? Actually we have only one ultimate means of control: ultimate rejection.

Since you wish to use my own case as an example, let us do so. In the last twenty years I have published over eight score papers in leading journals of neurology, psychiatry, and psychoanalysis in 5 languages. In only ten of these, revisions were requested and made satisfactorily; in five more, we could not agree, and the paper was withdrawn, to be published elsewhere. If our authors' papers are worth while, their work is certainly not wasted: they can do the same. But if their writings are trash, we have no greater obligation to publish them than does any other journal.

This last is a crucial point: I did not recommend rejection of the "contributions" of Schultz, Kempf, Perls, and Frankl because they were "poorly written," but because their ideas were pompous, bombastic, self-contradictory nonsense. Gantt's paper was poorly written, too, but though I disagreed

*Without Dr. Moreno's permission, I cannot reprint his letters to me, but since I tried to reply to them as objectively and respectfully as possible, their content may be inferred.

with nearly everything he said, I deleted only one paragraph because the rest presented a consistent and empiric, though doctrinaire, point of view. Cosin's opus was long-winded and repetitious, but I took the trouble to edit it because he had much that was original, valuable, and practical. The same for Kurt Goldstein, on which I also spent considerable time—and then approved for publication.

As to letters to authors, I am afraid I must object a bit to the format used in your sample to Goldstein in one respect: the reference to me as "an editor on my staff." I realize that Goldstein is your friend, as Gantt, Cosin, and many others I edited severely (for example, Rascovsky) are mine. But if I must write to them, I shall say that "the editorial board of the *Progress* have agreed on these alterations"—a more dignified and unitary collaborative statement, and one less likely to result in personal inquiries and complaints. And if Rascovsky, whom I had solicited, refuses my suggested recommendations, "the board" can and should decline publication.

Now as to a fresh start for Volume III: If I am to continue as co-editor (and not, like Frieda, drop out because of misunderstandings of unsatisfactory policies), we should agree on these points: (1) A joint choice of all contributors, including those assigned to write "critical reviews." (2) All authors must understand that they are *invited to submit* articles in the usual scientific fashion for editing before acceptance—or, if mutual agreement cannot be reached, withdrawal or rejection. (3) Correspondence with authors also must be mutually acceptable. (4) The final contents of the book must be approved by both of us in page proof.

I believe the above is what Frieda wanted, too. But even if she did not—and much as I like and respect her—my name is not Frieda. It is still

Your friend,
Jules

January 18, 1957

Dear Jack:

My first impulse on reading several pages of Nic Waal's paeon of praise to Nic Waal was to discard it completely. My second, in view of possible commitments on your part, was to cut it down by four-fifths, which I proceeded to do. However, on rereading the manuscript I had to return to my first conclusion: the report on Scandinavian psychiatry is (a) intolerably biased, (b) incomplete (it leaves out Bergen and other centers in Norway, the world-famous work on alcoholism by Martensen-Larson and Jacobsen in Denmark, Sögren's studies on Swedish epileptics, etc.), and to my personal knowledge is (c) inaccurate in the rest of its contents. I recommend returning it to Dr. Waal with a tactful letter requesting complete revision for the 1958 *Progress*—if necessary, with the collaboration of men such as Evang in Norway, Sögren in Sweden, or others who know what is really going on outside of Waal's limited circle. To publish the report in its present form, even if put in literate English, would offend nine of ten psychiatrists in Scandinavia, and I prefer not to. The most we can do, if we are irretrievably committed, is to publish only the section on Norway as edited.

June 7, 1957

Dear Jack:

Your letter is a little puzzling, since some of its points are contrary to our previous understandings, to wit:

1. I am not at all certain that either of us, apart from selection and editing, has a mission to "write an evaluation of the contributions of our authors each year," particularly reports from foreign fields. In fact, apart from acceptance, revision, or rejection, this is usually *not* done by editors of other yearbooks, since authors may well resent such "evaluations" without opportunities for reexplanation or rebuttal. And we may offend and alienate many.

2. Each of us, as previously agreed, should *not* write authors or pass on manuscripts independently; this violates the

intent and spirit of co-editorship, and may lead to misunderstanding and confusion and cross-purposes. Instead, each invitation should be agreed to and signed by both of us, and all editorial changes be similarly bilateral. Please note that, as an example I sent the letter requesting Bartemeier to revise his manuscript to you for approval and signature.

3. As to which of our offices should send them, I thought that you had arranged for a larger share of the royalties to cover these expenses in New York. However, if you want me to arrange to pay for part or all of this work, I shall be glad to do so.

October 7, 1957

Dear Jack:

I began by trying to edit S. Lebovici's *Psychoanalytical Psychodrama,* but after a few pages decided that the translation was not only atrocious, but that the paper itself was so involved, confused and either trite or obscure that the publication would in no way benefit Lebovici, psychodrama, analysis, yourself or the *Progress.* If you want a try at making some sense out of this chaos I shall be happy to review the result; otherwise, I suggest return of the French original with our regrets that it is "not quite suitable for Volume III."

October 27, 1958

Dear Jack:

I am much more concerned about the continued excellence and reputation of the *Progress* series than I am about Victor Frankl's feelings; moreover, if we do not make more explicit to him what we want and he sends us another unacceptable effusion, and we again reject it, we will offend him much more. I therefore am perfectly willing in this exceptional case for you to send him both letters: yours signed only by you, and mine signed by myself. He can then do as he likes: either write a scientifically literate article or be angry only at me—a fate I can easily bear.

December 2, 1958

Dear Jack:

I must insist that I review the final version of the whole *Progress* manuscript, since only then can I judge the inclusion and the best order of the chapters (since I have sent you all my edited copies), derive a table of contents with the most appropriate headings, write a preface especially suitable to Volume IV, and perform other final editorial duties. If you continue to insist otherwise, I shall have to direct Henry Stratton not to publish the volume until he has sent it to me—a most disagreeable step. I hope, of course, that this will not be necessary.

August 17, 1959

Dear Dr. Moreno:

Your circular to the membership of the APA Section on Psychotherapy is seriously in error on a number of counts, among them:

When you and I completed our term of office as secretary and chairman respectively, we likewise terminated all influence over the affairs of the Section except as co-editors of the annual *Progress in Psychotherapy* which may or may not publish the section's proceedings. Even so, neither of us need be consulted about its programs.

There is not and never was a so-called "committee of the section"; like other sections, its affairs—consisting solely of arranging for the annual scientific program—are by APA tradition left to its duly elected chairman, vice-chairman, and secretary. Drs. Wolberg, Frank, and Salzman, the current officers of the section, could therefore have arranged its 1960 program unilaterally by virtue of their office; instead, they correctly sought and obtained the guidance of the membership.

The business meetings of the Section have always been run openly and democratically by members sufficiently interested to be present. The one which you skipped was attended by about a hundred people, and the joint meeting with the Academy of Psychoanalysis was proposed from the floor and passed almost unanimously. It was there made explicit also that the 1960 meeting should constitute no precedent as to future joint meetings with the Academy or any other organization. However, since the section desired an objective survey of modern trends in analytic theory and therapy, this single joint meeting with a leading scientific organization in the field was judged to be highly desirable. Contrary to your allegations, the section has always been and, by all present indications, will continue to be broad, eclectic and integrative in its orientations. This you must accept as co-editor of its proceedings.

Finally, you must also have been aware that the executive council of the APA has approved the entire procedure as correct and in accord with APA administrative and scientific policies.

In view of these and other considerations, your circular is misleading and perhaps deliberately calculated to cast discredit not only on the officers and active members of the Section, but on the Academy of Psychoanalysis and the Executive Council of the American Psychiatric Association as well. In the past, out of respect for your contributions to psychiatry, I have excused as well-intentioned idiosyncrasies many of your previous similar actions; however, this one cannot be condoned. As a member of the section and the APA, you are entitled to any survey of opinion you may wish to make, but I am constrained to say that unless you correct the false impressions your circular may create in those unacquainted with the facts, I, like others before me, shall consider it necessary publicly to dissociate myself from you in every respect.

cc: Lewis Wolberg, M.D.
Jerome Frank, M.D.
Leon Salzman, M.D.
William Malamud, M.D.
C. Hardin Branch, M.D.
John Donnelly, M.D.
Joseph Merin, M.D.

September 2, 1959

Dear Dr. Moreno:

I regret that your responses to my letter of August 17th have been unsatisfactory. Since I do not propose to descend to the vituperation of your note of August 20th, I can only restate my position and necessary decisions as follows:

Any competent judge of "opinion polls" would conclude at a glance that the questionnaire you circulated on August 10th to the entire APA membership was prejudiced and misleading, and that therefore the response to it could not represent a properly informed and considered consensus of the membership. Parenthetically, your statement that by August 24th you had received and tabulated "a large percentage" of 1300 replies on a midsummer mailing a scant two weeks previously is chronologically and statistically very remarkable; even so, in view of the skew in your questions, the vote you report actually *endorses* the actions of the Section in arranging its own scientific programs.

In your letter to me you make more dubious assertions, such as "the business meetings of the Section are not properly announced" when it is a matter of record that a notice as to their time, place and purpose is clearly printed each year in the APA section program.

Finally, even if your alleged grievances [about not being re-elected permanent secretary] had been fully justified, you disdained the proper procedures of open discussion at either the section or general business meetings of the APA, appeals to the program or other committees, proposals to the APA Council and officers for revision of Section procedures, or the many other ethical and constitutional recourses open to all APA members. Instead, you chose unilaterally to disseminate misinformation and create dissention in a manner that is not compatible with allegiance to the democratic and scientific principles of the APA. I have always believed in frank and open action; therefore, please be advised: (a) That I wish my name removed from all listings as "consultant," "associate editor," or in any other capacity from all publications of the Beacon Press and any others under your aegis. (b) That, while I shall fulfill my current obligations to Grune & Stratton with regard to the 1960 edition of *Progress in Psychotherapy,* I shall notify Dr. Stratton that after this issue, I cannot continue with you as co-editor. (c) That whereas I do not intend to circularize the section, I shall make this correspondence available to its officers to use as they judge best.

Again regretfully

In accordance with my commitment to Grune & Stratton that I would complete the 1960 edition of *Progress in Psychotherapy* in my terminal year as co-editor with Dr. Moreno, I continued to correspond with him editorially as per the following:

January 4, 1960

Dear Dr. Moreno:

I have read your own chapter for our final volume. My comments: Your opinion of my status in American psychiatry and psychoanalysis is of no particular moment, but your paragraph about me on p. 11 that I am not an "official" psychoanalyst has implications for an otherwise uninformed reader which would be contrary to facts. The latter are: There is no "official school" of psychoanalysis in this or any other country, any more than your own group therapy methods are "official." As to qualifications, I have been fully trained in the Chicago Psychoanalytic Institute, am a fully accredited member of the Chicago, American, and International Psychoanalytic Associations, and am a fully accredited training analyst—the highest "official" professional recognition attainable in the field. Moreover, the Academy of Psychoanalysis, of which I am a past president, has already achieved more academic status than any other organization in the sense of scientific and administrative influence. We should delete any portion of any contribution to the *Progress*—including my own writings—that could be shown to be demonstrably untrue or misleading; by this editorial rule, your paragraph should be omitted.

P. 17: The paragraph lauding Mrs. Moreno while derogating Mrs. Masserman is in such exceedingly poor social taste that I must also insist on its deletion.

P. 18: The passage advocating a "reversal of political roles" between the U.S. and the U.S.S.R. is not only extremely undiplomatic but could be interpreted as frankly seditionist; therefore, it will not appear in any publication with which I am connected. Since Grune & Stratton could also be legally involved, I am sending your chapter to Dr. Stratton for direct discussion with you as to his possible liability. Section VII of your paper might also offend so many Jews that I would regret having it thought I gave it editorial sanction.

I am likewise not in accord with either the style or the content of other portions of your chapter, but consider them less misleading or dangerous and can therefore abide by our past arrangement not to edit each other's chapters where such considerations do not apply. The passages I specified, however, must be edited.

Regretfully

On inquiry, Dr. Clarence Farrar, editor of the *American Journal of Psychiatry,* denied that Dr. Moreno had exclusive rights to publish all papers read in the Section on Psychotherapy and promised that he would release to me specific permission for each paper, as requested and deemed appropriate in the future. My correspondence with Moreno thereafter was limited to his fervent condemnation of my report of the Czech Congress we had jointly attended, and my reply:

January 13, 1960

Dear Dr. Moreno:

Since you seem unable to think or write above the level of personal vilification, it is probably useless to repeat that your opinions of me are of no moment or even interest to anyone important in our field, and least of all me. For the record, however, I may inform you that contrary to your statements that I distorted my account of the Czech Congress, and in accordance with ethics and courteous forethought, I sent my report to the Congress secretary and other Congress officials irrespective of their past sympathies, and all of them not only approved my version as completely in accord with the verbatim Congress transactions, but complimented the friendliness, accuracy, and style of the article. The Canadian guest, Eric Wittkow of Montreal, also read a draft and wrote me in a similar vein. I have likewise been deeply gratified by a flood of spontaneous personal accolades and invitations to lecture in several eastern European countries received from many who attended the Congress, including the leaders of the Soviet and allied delegations, and I have recently received a final enthusiastic endorsement of my role as Western representative and mediator, made after a personal follow-up survey in Czechoslovakia by Dr. Frank Fremont-Smith and Dr. John Rees, respectively president and director of the World Federation of Mental Health.

I could only wish that you had been as careful in checking the imprint of your own actions abroad and the possible effects of your present writing. Instead, you followed the format of the chapter I sent you weeks ago, but unfortunately, not its objectivity, spirit, or intent.

However, neither facts nor appeals to reason seem to be effective, so I must inform you that Dr. Stratton has instructed his staff not to send the book to the printers without a final endorsement directly from me of all of its contents, including your own contributions. Further, to save you a form of embarrassment to which I would not wish to subject any former colleague, I again advise you not to exceed Dr. Stratton's or my own patience by further innuendos, personal attacks, spurious bargainings, or attempts at unilateral maneuvers. Conversely, if you wish to return to rational editorial collaboration, we can fulfill our joint contracts for Volume V somewhere near our promised schedule.

January 18, 1960

Dr. Eugene Wolf
General Secretary, Czech Psychiatric Congress
Prague, Czechoslovakia

Dear Eugene:

Many thanks for your letter; I am happy indeed over the official reactions to the Congress. I shall send the reprints I promised to several of the Soviet psychiatrists who requested them including Myasishchev, and shall also ask Academician Koupernik for a reprint of his excellent presentation of Russian thought.

Parenthetically, in my travels south after Prague I learned first-hand of Moreno's behavior in Jugoslavia and elsewhere, and did what I could to repair the damage. More recently I had to read his own fantastically misrepresentative accounts of his prestige and influence in what he wished to publish as an introduction to Volume V of the *Progress in Psychotherapy* series, including his self-evaluation as "by far the most influential figure" at the Congress, and his advocacy of "collective role-reversal," i.e., that the U.S. "adopt ten years of Communism" while the USSR "try democracy" before changing back. Rest assured that this final insult to everyone's intelligence will *not* be published, even if it means no Volume V and the co-editorship of Masserman and Moreno officially dissolved.

January 27, 1960

Dear Jules,

Your letter of the 18th arrived a day after I had received an incomplete draft of Dr. Moreno's introduction to the *Progress* volume with a request for my comments. In the covering note he refers to having sent me a complete draft some time back; this, however, never reached me. Thus I had grounds to anticipate some of the contents of your letter, but nonetheless I read it with much regret.

Dr. Moreno's introduction has, of course, shaken me. The only logical conclusion that can be drawn from my lengthy reply to him is that he would do well to omit the Jesenik

Congress entirely from his report. I was, therefore, greatly relieved to learn from you that you have decided to exercise your co-editorial veto on his report on Czechoslovakia altogether; . . . for this would [be in accord with] the very spirit and aim of the Jesenik Congress and the follow-ups we hope for.

Eugene Wolf,
General Secretary of the
Czechoslovak Congress

The results: Grune & Stratton discontinued the *Progress in Psychotherapy* volumes and in 1961 initiated another series entitled *Current Psychiatric Therapies* with myself as sole editor, but with other tribulations to be recounted in a separate chapter.

12. CURRENT PSYCHIATRIC THERAPIES

My most enduring, demanding, and eventually most gratifying editorial endeavors were devoted to the annual issues of *Current Psychiatric Therapies*, a series instituted on the demise of my co-editorship with Dr. Jacob Moreno of the unlamented *Progress* series also published by Grune & Stratton. Now only carefully selected authors, each a literate authority in some psychiatric subspecialty, were sent the following forms accompanied by a personalized invitation for each to contribute a chapter to later annual volumes.

Dear Dr.__________:

The publishing house of Grune & Stratton has commissioned me to edit a series of volumes entitled *Current Psychiatric Therapies*, embodying the following features: *Special contributions* individually solicited from experts in therapeutic subspecialties both in the United States and abroad. *Annual summaries* of the current advances in various modes and techniques of therapy to be prepared by selected authorities in brief psychotherapy, hypnotherapy, psychoanalysis, existentialist and related schools, group methods with ancillary modalities, family care, psychopharmacology, advanced institutional and community rehabilitative practices, and other developments of theoretical and clinical importance. *Condensations,* with the consent of the editorial board of the *American Journal of Psychiatry* or other professional periodicals, of the best papers on psychiatric therapy presented at the APA or other scientific meetings. *Reviews* prepared by the editor of special advances on topics not otherwise covered in each issue.

As you may know, in the past few years the series has attained worldwide circulation and achieved a position as a progressive reference in the field. I trust I may therefore take the privilege of inviting you to contribute to the 1961 volume of *Current Psychiatric Therapies* as specified below: (1) Preparation of a chapter of approximately ______ words on the topic ________. (2) A review of approximately ______ words on recent advances in the field of ____________. (3) A condensation of your paper entitled __________ as presented at the recent meeting of the __________.

Manuscripts are due by November 1, 19—, but will be welcomed earlier if possible.

There can be no monetary compensation other than two complimentary copies of the volume and the availability of reprints. However, we hope that you will accept this opportunity to communicate with your colleagues in psychiatry, in other medical specialties and in related sciences everywhere who will value your authoritative contribution. For your convenience, a suggestions sheet, an acceptance form, and a return envelope are enclosed.

With best personal regards.

Suggestions for Contributors to Current Therapies in Psychiatry

Limitations on the length designated for each contribution have the following purposes: (a) to promote the presentation of each subject in clear, pithy, easily readable, and readily reviewable form (b) to keep the annual volume within convenient reference size and (c) to make possible a price range that will insure the widest distribution to the medical and allied professions. Your chapter may then be organized as follows: (1) *Introductory material,* confined to a definition of the field and the terms employed. (2) *Historical reviews* and discussions of the literature, kept to an informative minimum. (3) *Therapeutic procedures* should constitute the major theme of each chapter; ergo, the author's original or special techniques should be described as clearly and specifically as possible. (4) *Case presentations* need illustrate only the clinical points of issue. (5) *Results,* both immediate and long-term, should be indicated wherever available. (6) *Discussions and summaries* are superfluous in a chapter written with brevity and balance. (7) Bibliographic references may be appended in brief JAMA form.

Corrections and Proofs: Manuscripts may be altered by each contributor even after submission up to the printer's deadline, and minor changes can subsequently be made in the proofs.

Style: Every contributor has been selected because of his literary as well as his professional skills, and is therefore aware that good writing is characterized by simplicity, clarity, and logical progression, and avoids obscurity, redundancy, and overgeneralization; nevertheless, within these parameters the editor will respect and preserve each contributor's personal style as his inalienable prerogative.

A sampling of subsequent editorial correspondence:

September 18, 1962

Harley C. Shands, M.D.
Professor of Psychiatry
State University of New York

Dear Harley:

May I make the following suggestions as to your otherwise immaculate manuscript?

P 2-3: To call psychotherapy "outside the scientific . . . pale" because of its "dyadic transactional complications" would be to relegate physics there also (*vide* Heisenberg, Dirac, et al.), since no one can study an atomic particle without influencing it. Your strictures may therefore need some modification.

P 3: "Art," which you contrast to "science" is defined by Webster as skill derived from experience—ergo, also "scientific."

P 5: The repeated quotations of Freud call for more specific references to his writings. James' religious "conversion" has also been compared to modern "brainwashing" by Jerome Frank, who might be credited here.

P 8: You describe psychotherapy as though it were a jockeying for dominance, but it need *not* be a zero-sum game.

P 10: Isn't a person's "self" or "identity" *whatever* he is currently doing or thinking? Isn't it time to abandon this vacuous shibboleth of "Selfhood?" Glad to have you do it.

P 12-14: The relevance to psychotherapy of your long discussion of role-playing is a bit obscure until p.15. Can this be clarified earlier?

P 16: "Emotional" is repeatedly contrasted with "intellectual," but the meaningful differences are never specified—if indeed they can be.

P 17: Again the "role" is made discrete from the "self"—though many think them mainly different in spelling.

I make these suggestions and the few pencil notes on the manuscript only because you requested a bit of critical dialectic; please use them in any revision as you wish.

October 18, 1962

Nathan W. Ackerman, M.D.

Dear Nate:

I have again edited out passages such as "interwoven . . . parallel activities"—since such esoteric geometry would seem possible only in an Einstein tensor matrix. Also, the interview excerpt, while certainly demonstrating four-square family animosity, gives no leads to the unsophisticated reader as to its therapeutic purposes or techniques—hence does not help the cause of an annual volume that promises prepaid information on How To Do It. However, I'll publish the rest and, if you like, include another interview which is more explicitly therapeutic if you send one on.

October 31, 1962

Iago Galdston, M.D.

Dear Iago:

Sorry, old boy, but in justice to the justified expectations of the large and growing readership of this series, I can accept this paper for Volume III only if you care to amend it as follows:

1. Please purge it of paragraph after paragraph of pretentiously pompous phonemes about "phenomenology," the portent of which is nowhere made clear. I have indicated some of the passages that would be judged either vacuous or redundant by any discerning reader.

2. Define your central concept of "ontologic thrust," which apparently can now be interpreted as connoting anything from etiology through predeterminism and teleology to an eschatologic mystique.

3. Either furnish some operationally comprehensible instances of what you are talking about, or leave the reader to wonder whether the fancy language was really worth the cost of the chapter or the pay of the editor.

I would rather have you refer to our previous correspondence and discuss this frankly now than have me edit the article and you be horrified by the truncated proofs. I hope you will amend rather than withdraw the paper, but in the latter case I trust we can continue to talk in friendly fashion about all else.

In contrast:

November 2, 1962

Stephen Fleck, M.D.
Yale University

Dear Stephen:

My sincere thanks for an article written with clarity and high intellectual grace. Rest assured it will be a feature of Volume III.

Best regards, and very sincerely.

An annual invitation that invariably produced an introductory chapter by the current president of the American Psychiatric Association:

December 20, 1966

Lawrence Kolb, M.D.
Columbia College of Physicians
and Surgeons

Dear Larry:

As you probably know, it has been an unbroken tradition since the inception of this series nine years ago that the president-elect of the APA write the introductory chapter on any topic related to psychiatric therapy he chooses—and as briefly or as extensively as he wishes. I know the many other commitments the office entails, but if you can send me any manuscript you select—or a revision of a previous one—by November 1st of 1967, it will again be an honored feature of Volume VIII, due to be at hand at the time of your inauguration in May, 1968.

I attach forms supplied to other invitees for the sake of completeness—not that they apply to your contribution. With best of personal Season's Greetings.

To a colleague who requested advice as to how he could initiate and edit a parallel series on industrial psychiatry:

February 24, 1967

Ralph T. Collins, M.D.
Rochester, New York

Dear Ralph:

Your inquiry is most complimentary, but is somewhat akin

to asking me how I go about being a psychiatrist while avoiding the multiple mistakes and perennial pitfalls of the profession. In short, after 15 years of hard work at it, I know it would take a fair-sized book to answer your questions, and perhaps some day I'll write that volume. Meanwhile, perhaps we can meet somewhere for an evening (a usual device is to invite each other for a lecture—or to take time at the May APA) where I can have the sample forms, letters, proofs, etc., and go over all the techniques, troubles and triumphs of editorship with you. Let's arrange it, and I'll look forward to it.

Reply to a friend who submitted an unsolicited travelogue "for publication in one of the many books you edit."

Leo H. Bartemeier, M.D.
Medical Director
The Seton Psychiatric Institute
Baltimore, Maryland

Dear Leo:

Your ms. leaves me in a quandary, especially since it is a clear, literate, modest, and gracefully written description of your trip to Brazil and Peru. While I indeed edit two annuals, my dilemma is this: The *Science and Psychoanalysis* series is, by edict of the Academy, limited to papers read at its annual meetings, and the *Current Psychiatric Therapies* annuals are, by contract with the publisher, devoted exclusively to descriptions of new techniques of treatment in psychiatry, mostly here, or occasionally abroad.

This last gives us the only opening, to wit: could you please partially revise your article by leaving out dinner accounts, etc., but so that it would deal more specifically with topics as to why Kleinian psychoanalysis is preferred in Latin America and how it differs in techniques and results?—Or what the interpersonal techniques of the Peruvian *curanderos* can really teach us about influencing patients by spells and potions more magical than we use? I would then not only be able to publish it in Volume IX of this series, but would be happy to do so.

If, however, you want to have this charming opus printed as is, I rather think that Eric Wittkower would be glad to have it for his more suitable *Transcultural Psychiatry Quarterly*. Alternatively, a university publication would appreciate its literary quality, as witness the *Northwestern Quarterly* reprint of a similar account I wrote some years ago.

To an author who insisted on a second extensive revision of his galley proofs:

Dear Dr. M________:

Your chapter with Dr. N for *Current Psychiatric Therapies* required much initial editing; and now, regrettably, your very extensive revisions of the galley proofs would: (1) cost you several hundred dollars for a complete reset of type; (2) add nothing significant to the content; (3) impair the value of the article, by restoring redundancies, and grammatical and stylistic errors.

I have, therefore, directed Grune & Stratton to let the galleys stand as is. If, however, this is not satisfactory to you, please notify them and me immediately so that your chapter can be removed from Volume XI, and your names removed from the roster of contributors.

The manuscript was published as edited.

To a world-famous authority who submitted a chapter on cerebral electrophysics which might be recognized as highly relevant to psychotherapy—a generation hence:

W. Grey Walter, M.D.
Burden Neurological Institute
Stoke Lane, Stapleton
Bristol, England

Dear Grey:

Your erudite manuscript is (a) too long, (b) not concordant with the purpose of the series, which is to prescribe specific *current* techniques of therapy, (c) far in advance of its time, and (d) likely to evoke reminders from many readers that my editorial function is to keep the series "practical." I'll therefore gladly publish it in Volume VI, with deep appreciation of its originality, forethought, and eventual scientific import.

With thanks, personal regards, and my hope to see you again soon.

Preface to Current Psychiatric Therapies, Volume VIII, 1968

This volume—heaven forgive—marks the thirty-first book I have authored or edited. I have, accordingly, also written a score and ten prefaces—each time with growing wonder as to why any one of them was required. Certainly not to preview the subject and organization of any volume; the intelligent reader—and no other is ever invited—would have seen the title, could glance through the table of contents, or better, survey the index for that information. So also, without any prefatorial celebration, the roster of contributors would indicate that each author was known to be among the most authoritative and literate in his specialty, including the president of the American Psychiatric Association, who writes the traditional introductory chapter.

Why, then, a preface? Mainly, it appears, to give the editor a page or two to introject his own literary style and professional prejudices. Since, *mea culpa,* I have already done so on thirty previous occasions I shall, with heartfelt thanks to all who continue to help write, print, and distribute these issues, herewith take a sabbatical.

A soft plea to another friend who had been nominated President-elect of the American Psychiatric Association, and who, probably because of an intercurrent hospitalization, had not submitted his presidential chapter in time for the 1969 Volume of *Current Psychiatric Therapies.*

December 4, 1968

Raymond W. Waggoner, M.D.
University of Michigan

Dear Ray:

There may have been a secretarial slip-up somewhere, or the infinitely more important consideration of your recovery from your recent illness may have interfered, but I hope you will recall that I spoke and wrote to you about the fact that every APA president-elect since the founding of this series of annual volumes eight years ago has contributed the honorary introductory chapter. As you know, the series has since attained international distribution, and judging by favorable reviews and many adoptions by teaching institutions, has achieved a most gratifying scientific reputation. Since I am now preparing Volume IX for publication, may I request that you continue this tradition? I attach the invitation and suggestion forms usually sent to other invitees only to emphasize that these conditions do *not* apply to you; indeed, any manuscript of any length related to psychiatry will do, including one already published that you feel needs a renewed and wider readership, in which case I will also arrange reprint permission. But please send the manuscript or reprint as soon as possible so that the volume may, as is usual, be released by the time of the May meeting.

An excellent essay on *Psychiatry in the Modern World* was received within a few days.

As in the *Science and Psychoanalysis* series, the collaboration of the publisher's staff—even though at times over-meticulous—had to be welcomed and maintained:

December 14, 1967

D. R. Castle
Grune & Stratton, Inc.

Dear Miss Castle:

I greatly appreciate your concern about keeping the bibliographies in the CPT series completely consistent in form; however, herewith my own sentiments on such matters. As a fairly experienced writer and editor, I am deeply concerned about content, style, clarity, validity, originality, grace, etc. in what I write or edit—but far less about bibliographic addenda. Indeed, I am not greatly agitated even when the titles of the articles referred to are omitted (as in *Science* and many other top-drawer publications); as long as journal, year, and page are given in any order, anyone really interested can find the source. Nor do I suffer deeply when the style of the reference lists varies from volume to volume—few people really care, and their obsessions would not change the intrinsic value of any chapter.

By these more pragmatic criteria, T's bibliography is quite adequate; nevertheless, I have requested that he revise the format in accordance with JAMA style. Should he be unwilling or unable to do so in time, use his present form as returned herewith and please do *not* delay Volume IX further.

Parenthetically, since Dr. T lives in New York, much time could have been saved had you but picked up the phone and made your request directly; you have my permission to do so in future similar instances.

A final intriguing exchange:

December 3, 1968

Victor Bloom, M.D.
951 E. Lafayette Street
Detroit, Michigan 48207

Dear Dr. Bloom:

You will recall that my invitation to you to write a chapter for the CPT series on prevention of suicide specified about 2500 words and was accompanied by a Suggestion to Authors form indicating that the volumes, as their name implied, were manuals of therapeutic techniques rather than journals of clinical research or theory. As to the latter, it is now fairly well accepted that, without recourse to outmoded periphrastic jargon, suicide may occur as an escape from (and revenge for) poignant familial or social rejections—a point you could repeat more briefly. Would you, then, rewrite your article so that, within the necessary limitations of space, you describe more specifically the dyadic milieu and social therapy required to restore necessary modicums of hope and interpersonal security to the potential suicide (p. 15 ff)? Since you write clearly when not worrying about your self-image as a classical analyst, I am sure you can do so, and if I receive a suitable revision before December 15, I shall be glad to publish it. Parenthetically, by applying humanstic common sense rather than recondite circularities about "masochism," "Thanatos," etc., I have had not a single suicide in 35 years of intensive and varied hospital and private (including modern progressive psychoanalytic) practice. But since I edit these volumes rather than write them, I shall look forward to your version.

With thanks and regards.

December 9, 1968

Dear Dr. Masserman,

Enclosed is my paper, again all 4500 words of it. I'm sorry I agreed a long time ago to revise it down to 2500 words—at the time I did not appreciate what it entailed, how much of the substance of the paper would be sacrificed. I also did not realize that *General Concepts in Therapy* was a manual of therapeutic technique, nor did my reviewing several issues give me that impression. In fact reading several issues gave me the distinct impression that you allowed some authors great breadth and latitude. If you do not wish to extend this license to me, that is your privilege and your choice. You speak of "necessary limitations of space." I must assume that you decide what is "necessary," because some issues of *Current Concepts* are fat, and some are thin. If I am naive about the publishing business, so be it. I must deal with them, but they must deal with me. I do not intend to write a list of prescribed techniques for the treatment of suicidal patients which is not backed up by clinical material as evidence for my conclusions. The reader, you assume, grants me the clinical background because Jules Masserman selected me as an "expert." The hell with that jazz.

You have some nerve accusing me of "outmoded periphrastic jargon." I had to resort to the dictionary for "periphrastic" and "recondite." So you, practicing a "progressive psychoanalytic" (the rest of us practicing regressive therapy, of course), using "humanistic common sense," got away with no suicides in 35 years. I take off my hat to you. You ought to write it up and let the rest of us know how you perform these miracles. "Recondite" refers to concealment. (Thank you for teaching me a new word.) My paper is meant to reveal, not to conceal. If you have that opinion of my paper, you should not have asked me for any version of it. I do not see psychoanlaytic theory as "outmoded"; unpopular, now—yes, difficult to swallow—yes; a narcissistic threat, yes. I bet you hate it that Freud came up with this stuff before you did. Let me venture a mild "wild analytic" interpretation with you, since you feel so free to criticize me.

I understand you are a "card-carrying" psychoanalyst, progressive, of course. How the hell did you think you derived the "humanistic common sense" that you have? Do you think you were born with it? Do you think you do not irrevocably and unconsciously see people a bit more realistically and clearly, because of your psychoanalytic training and analysis? . . . Here is my paper, take it or leave it.

Victor Bloom

December 31, 1968

Dr. Victor Bloom
951 E. Lafayette Street
Detroit, Michigan

Dear Dr. Bloom:

Since you wished it, I reread your manuscript. Again the case reports in the first 15 pages of your manuscript deal with clinical data so well known that they hardly need rehearsal, and you would not wish to confine your contribution to the relatively sound though over-generalized recommendations on your remaining pages 15 to 20. Nor in view of the title and explicit purpose of *this* series, do I quite understand the import of your "reviewing of several issues" of a publication purportedly called "General Concepts of Therapy."

All in all, judging from the vituperative (a word you can look up in any high school dictionary) tone of your letter, it would seem that we would both be happier if you published your article in some more analytically (dys?-)oriented journal; I am therefore returning your manuscript with thanks for a somewhat amusing editorial episode. Indeed, since I am currently reviewing the vices, vicissitudes, and victimizations of editorship for a forthcoming book, I would be happy to exchange permissions with you to publish our relevant correspondence, deleting the profanity in yours.

Dr. Bloom returned the above letter with quite conciliatory marginal notes to the effect that he had been unreasonably angry over the "attack on psychoanalysis" but that since his ideas were original, he again requested that his paper be published immediately, rewritten by me or "my editorial assistants" so that it could "save a few lives." I replied:

Dear Dr. Bloom:

I appreciate your marginal comments. Regrettably, Volume IX of *Current Psychiatric Therapies* is already full and in press, and even if this were not so, I would not personally (and

I have no "assistants") presume to condense, let alone rewrite your chapter. Nor can I relinquish my conscience or intelligence as a rational (please, not "rationalized") scientist to be as constructively critical of the vacuities and circularities of much analytic jargon as I am of the inadequacies of our nosology, the naivetes of Behaviorism, the pretentious mystiques of Existentialism, or other current meanderings in our behavioral pseudosciences. But as a responsible and, I believe, generally respected editor, I am perfectly willing to publish the writings of those who think otherwise, provided they are presented in lucid form and with direct reference to useful psychiatric techniques.

I am, therefore, glad to renew my invitation to you to rewrite your chapter for Volume X of this series, and enclose once again the routine forms for your files while keeping the other copy of your manuscript for my own.

October 22, 1969

Dear Dr. Masserman:

Enclosed is a copy of my paper on prevention of suicide. Again, thank you for giving me the opportunity to givc my ideas a wider audience.

This year I am able to condense my paper to less than 2500 words, as you requested. As the job is now completed, I look back on my stubborn reluctance to do so and my demand that you publish the overblown original paper "as is" as foolish and neurotic.

The present paper is lean, trim, muscular, rid of its excess baggage—which was pure fat. Thanks for sticking to your guns, whatever the reason.

I am awaiting publication of your chapter on coping with varieties of neurotic or otherwise "prima donna" authors.

Sincerely,
Vic Bloom

October 29, 1969

Dear Dr. Bloom:

My thanks for your letter and for your chapter, now concise, clear, and constructive. I may publish the former in my memoirs, but the latter will certainly appear in Volume X of *Current Psychiatric Therapies.*

In 1966, I proposed to the American Psychiatric Association and to the Academy of Psychoanalysis that Dr. Henry Stratton, in view of his outstanding contributions to both fields, be made an honorary fellow of both associations. When both societies approved, Duncan Mackintosh, executive editor of Grune (a mythical partner) & Stratton, Inc., and I arranged a surprise luncheon at which both honors would be bestowed by the respective presidents. Officers of both associations were present, and there were brief speeches by Harvey Tompkins (APA president-elect), Henry Brosin (APA president-elect-elect), Robert Felix and Dan Blain (APA past presidents), Sandor Rado and myself (Grune & Stratton authors). The occasion was, I think, quite memorable.

A characteristic follow-up from Henry:

May 25, 1966

Jules Masserman, M.D.
8 South Michigan Boulevard
Chicago, Illinois

Dear Jules:

First, I want to thank you for your letter of May 13, the mimeographed form from the APA, and the copies of the letters which you wrote to so many people in order to bestow on me the Honorary Fellowship. There are hardly any words to express my thanks and appreciation. Even a brother could not have done a better job. We have been friends for many years and I do value this friendship. Jules, I have many honorary memberships in medical societies, and I am a life member in several others. But it gave me great satisfaction, and I owe it all to you. Again, many many thanks!

As ever yours,
Dr. Henry M. Stratton
(Publisher, *Progress in Psychotherapy, Science and Psychoanalysis, Current Psychiatric Therapies, Psychiatry, East and West, et seq.*)

13. ADDITIONAL AUTISMS OF AUTHORSHIP

A bit of retrospection: By 1942, six years after coming to the University of Chicago, I had published some fifty articles, mostly technical reports (plus motion pictures) of work on cerebrospinal hydrodynamics and on the neurophysiology of animal behavior. They included only two major clinical studies: one on epilepsy and the other a follow-up of the results of psychiatric treatment at the University of Chicago and elsewhere—a research project which, though it could not claim statistical precision in a multifactorial field, nevertheless indicated that no one had succeeded much better by any method than had Esquirol who, in 1836, had reported that about a third of his patients "treated with simple kindness" recovered, a third improved, and a third remained unchanged or got worse. It was, therefore, time to write my first Book which would indicate that I was, after all, not only a feline, canine, or primate psychologist, but also a Clinical Psychiatrist or, even better, an Anointed Psychoanalyst—a status pinnacle at the time. As mentioned in Chapter 3, in 1942, I wrote a monograph on the relevance of my animal work to human conduct, entitled it somewhat pretentiously *Behavior and Neuroses*, and submitted it to the University of Chicago Press.* I recall the elation

*This early work is reviewed in Chapter 21.

with which I acknowledged my first publisher's contract; later correspondence, however, indicates some dampening of enthusiasm:

September 28, 1945

Mr. Rollin Hemens
Comptroller, University Press

Dear Mr. Hemens:

In the contract for my book, *Behavior and Neurosis,* which you published in 1943, there is a clause to the effect that I would be furnished each year with a statement of sales or royalties due. Undoubtedly, through some clerical oversight, I have never received such notices. Since, aside from the minor question of royalies, I am interested in the sales of the volume to date, I would appreciate such a statement at the convenience of your office.

Neither statements nor royalties appeared. *Behavior and Neuroses* finally exhausted its third reprinting by the University of Chicago Press and was shelved until republished as a "classic" by the Hafner Publishing Co. in 1964. However, after the appearance of my *Principles of Dynamic Psychiatry* in 1946, offers from other publishers became gratifyingly, but sometimes embarrassingly, frequent. Sample replies:

April 14, 1950

Arthur J. Rosenthal, Jr.
President
Basic Books, Inc.

Dear Mr. Rosenthal:

Thank you for your kind comments about my "sparkling writing" in the *Scientific American* and your offer of a free choice of title, content, and style for a proposed book. As to the former, anything illuminated by even a tiny glimmer of light may seem to "sparkle" these days when the pervading fog in our field is so oppressively dense. As to your proposition, I would like nothing better than to write a blithely serious "book on psychiatry for intelligent lay readers," even though my *Practice of Dynamic Psychiatry,* for want of time, has remained unrevised for three years. Perhaps, like Beethoven, I should alternate portentous and bucolic works. I shall give the matter as serious consideration as any of which I am capable while sailing my yawl this summer. And just possibly—as in two previous years—have a book written at the end of the cruise.

September 25, 1956

Silvano Arieti, M.D.
Editor, American Handbook
of Psychiatry

Dear Dr. Arieti:

Your letter raises an old problem that troubles my scientific and literary conscience: Namely, how often am I justified in repeating myself in print? True, I have never written two papers quite alike, but the fact remains that I have summarized my integrative "Biodynamic Approaches to Psychiatry" in various ways since 1940, and only a year ago published a half-million-word book on the subject called *Practice of Dynamic Psychiatry.* Of course, some of my ideas may have cleared or even developed a bit since then, but hardly enough quite to call for yet another review. I can therefore accept your kind invitation only on the proviso that, although I shall include much new work by myself and others, my chapter must necessarily repeat many of the concepts and practices I have previously presented, and perhaps even in an accustomed choice of words I have found to be most economical and effective. If this is acceptable, I shall do the best I can.

The invitation was repeated, and I wrote the chapter for Arieti's *Handbook.*

The psychiatrist, being wishfully but imprudently thought

to possess near-oracular wisdom, is often called upon to speak and write on almost any conceivable subject for lay audiences. An intercurrent adventure as author-editor concerned a project under the auspices of the American Medical Association to distribute to a puzzled and palpitating lay public a weekly newsletter on mental health, each issue being devoted to some topic such as "Is a Nervous Breakdown Serious?" "What Can Be Cured by Hypnotism?" or some such common concern.

Herewith my introduction, and three sample letters:

An Introduction, an Explanation, and an Invitation

These letters are going to be concerned with your personal problems—your troubles and your satisfactions, your intimate loves and hates and the difficulties in your life that may stand in the way of your success and happiness. But to be really helpful in such matters, we shall not confine ourselves to vague generalizations and moralistic sermons, although, of course, we shall often have to discuss the necessity for complying with laws and customs. The main purpose of the letters, however, will be to deal with your personal difficulties, and to furnish the best understanding and the most specific advice that modern psychiatry, psychoanalysis, and mental hygiene can offer. It may be well, then, first to state in simple language what these sciences consist of and how they can be of direct use to you.

First, exactly what is psychiatry and just who is a psychiatrist? Up to only a few years ago, psychiatry was limited to the study of so-called mental diseases, and these were thought to be due to "weakness of the nervous system," or to infections and poisons that affected the brain. Mental disorders were therefore thought to be mainly physical in origin, with the addition that people also feared that they were hereditary, dreaded them as a family "disgrace," and thought they were incurable. Psychiatrists still believe that bodily health is helpful—though not essential—to mental happiness, and for this reason, all qualified psychiatrists must also be graduated as doctors of medicine before undertaking the five or more years of special study necessary to make them specialists. Unfortunately, it is true that psychiatric disorders are still very common: One person in twelve enters a mental institution sometime during his life, and more hospital beds (200,000 in the U.S.) are required for this purpose alone than for all other diseases combined.

Fortunately, recent advances in psychiatry have revealed various forms of treatment which are effective in many disorders formerly thought to be incurable. But perhaps the greatest contribution that psychiatry has made has been to provide a deeper understanding of man's nature, his intellectual and emotional growth, and the ways in which he adapts to the strains of life so as to achieve stability and contentment. To make the service as useful as possible, special letters will be devoted to answering inquiries from readers who have personal problems of general interest. You are therefore welcome to write the AMA outlining your own problems and requesting information about their solution. In doing so, you may rest assured that your identity and confidences will be completely respected, and that your inquiries will be answered as soon as practicable.

The Convenience of a "Nervous Breakdown"

One characteristic that most clearly distinguishes Homo sapiens from other animals is a readiness to blame his misbehavior on mysterious influences beyond his control and to demand that these be removed by others. In one sense we can be proud of such mutual dependence, since it implies our hope that we can trust each other to be humane: *i.e.*, civilized. But our addiction to the ancient art of the alibi also means that we often like to deny our responsibilities or misuse our privileges. And in this penchant for prevarication, the so-called nervous breakdown is a perennial problem.

And how did this fascinating fiction get started?

Twenty-three hundred years ago Hippocrates, a famous Greek still revered as the father of medicine, observed that the ladies of his day had long since developed a striking capacity to get their way by staging histrionic tantrums or, when necessary, dramatic faints. Hippocrates, as the progenitor of a long line of physicians and gentlemen, professed to overlook the fact that many of his charming patients cast such "spells" in obvious attempts to evade some unpleasant situation, elicit sympathy and service, and so exert control over those about them. Instead, the Greek word for it was "hysterical," which courteously implied that the feminine furors were caused by a supposed "wandering of the uterus" (Greek, *hysteros*). True, Hippocrates tempered his chivalry and saved his scientific sanity by prescribing some fairly drastic treatments designed to convince both the uterus and its owner that they had better resume their rightful place and function; nevertheless, for four-score and seven generations the gentle verbal deception was taken quite literally. In fact, it was not until the turn of the present century that Charcot, a great French neurologist, could convince people that since "hysterical" behavior also occurred in men, it obviously could not be attributed solely to unscheduled uterine peregrinations in the zone of the interior.

True, many physicians had doubted that fanciful theory long before, but had substituted other physical explanations just as absurd. For example, Galen, who lived in the second century A.D., thought that when yellow bile (Greek, *khole*), black bile (*melas*), blood (*sanguis*), or phlegm (*phlegma*) predominated in the body, the person became correspondingly choleric (irritable), melancholic (sad), sanguine (happy), or phlegmatic (dull). A millenium and a half later William Cullen first used the word *neurosis* to mean striking and unexplained deviations in behavior, but again theorized that these must be caused by undetected diseases of the nervous system. A hundred years ago, George Beard coined the even more attractive euphemism *neurasthenia*—a pseudo-medical term that became understandably popular among all who were eager to attribute their evasiveness, contrariness or ill temper to "nervous exhaustion" from "overwork," and who wished thereby to justify periods of rest, escape, and special indulgence. Sigmund Freud himself added to the confusion by proposing that some forms of neurasthenia were "actual neuroses" due to "nervous exhaustion" from various sexual inhibitions, deviations, or excesses. Freud later withdrew this explanation, but the ever eager public merely added an intriguing erotic aura to the notion of "nervousness" and "nervous breakdown."

There is, then, a widespread misconception that almost

every disturbance of feeling and function: anxiety, depression, restlessness, insomnia, sexual dissatisfactions, stomach ulcer, high blood pressure, and a hundred other—may be due to some subtle physical damage to or "breakdown" of the nervous system. And yet there is hardly a shred of verifiable medical evidence for this popular notion. Among the thousands of experts who have tried for decades to find structural or chemical alterations in the body which might *cause* (rather than accompany) neurotic behavior, there are few men of scientific status who claim to have found such changes, and even these claims are seriously questioned. Direct medical evidence is also negative; for example, during the Korean encounter the prolonged physical and emotional stresses which our soldiers suffered certainly produced many severe "combat neuroses"—and yet no damage to the nervous system was ever found, and the symptoms disappeared rapidly under treatment by such simple methods as a few days of rest, good food, skillful recultivation of group morale and a desire to return to duty. On the other hand, research studies in my own and other laboratories during the last twenty years have demonstrated that nearly all forms of neuroses can be induced merely by subjecting an animal or human subject to vital but seemingly insoluble problems of adjustment, and that the neurotic reactions disappear when these problems are solved.

A "nervous breakdown," then, is a *dis-ease* only in the broadest sense of the term: a state in which the subject literally feels intensely un-easy or anxious about troublesome life situations. When the problems are mild and easily resolved, the symptoms of tension and vague depression rapidly disappear. However, when the troubles are regarded as overwhelming the person concerned—or perhaps over-concerned—may exaggerate or distort reality, make excessive demands upon those about him, find refuge in illness or seek forgetfulness and confusion (miscalled "tranquillization") through drugs or drink. In an important sense even chronic alcoholism can no more be considered a true "physical disease" than can thumb-sucking or excessive eating—though both forms of self-indulgence may eventually *produce* serious bodily deformities which are then a *result* rather than a cause of the original disorder.

In essence, then, neurotic behavior, although it may be face-saving and escapist to those who practice it, cannot really be attributed to constitutional defects or physical disease. Nor, by the same token can it ever be cured by diets, massages, or drugs—or vacations or divorces. Instead, so-called nervousness simply means a state of serious maladaptation in one's relations with the world, the important people in it and the future here and hereafter; correspondingly, a "cure" can be affected only when the difficulties in adjustment are clarified and resolved. Fortunately, this can usually be done through one's own intelligent efforts, or with the aid of family, friends, minister, or private physician. It is only when these fail that the counsel and guidance of a psychiatrist or psychoanalyst become necessary.

Sexual Maladjustments in Marriage: An Introduction

We have all inevitably been concerned with the many problems of marriage—our own, or those of our friends. You probably know that one marriage in about every five now ends in divorce, and that this rate is expected to increase. However, even these disturbing statistics do not reveal the actual amount of marital unhappiness that exists today in all walks of life. Many couples secretly long to separate, but continue to suffer an almost intolerable existence together because of financial necessity, social pressures, concern for their children—or just sheer inertia. Others try to forget their unhappiness by throwing themselves hectically into all sorts of social diversions, although these turn out to give them little real pleasure. Some try to escape by indulging in furtive extramarital affairs—which generally also end badly—or by taking to drink and drugs. Many others crowd the waiting rooms of poorly trained "marital counsellors" or even seek advice from newspapers or radio commentators; others, with better judgment, consult experienced ministers or qualified physicians and psychiatrists. The point however, is this: About four persons out of five who seek counsel complain that the greatest handicap to their contentment in marriage lies in what they generally call "sexual incompatibility."

Are, then, poor sexual adjustments in marriage so very

common? The answer is yes, since, much as it may be regretted, unfaithfulness by one or both parties occurs in about half of all marriages, and about one wife in three never experiences what she would like to conceive to be "a really satisfactory climax." But it should also be noted that since it has become the fashion these days to talk freely about sex, many couples blame all of their troubles altogether on sexual causes. Yet in many cases, sexual dissatisfactions may themselves be traced to deeper and more disruptive incompatibilities between husband and wife. For instance a wife, rightly or wrongly, may feel that her husband is uncouth, dislikes her friends, earns just enough for marginal support but makes no effort to furnish her with the little pleasures or luxuries of life, or is inconsiderate in a multitude of ways. In such circumstances, she may submit to her husband's embraces, but whether she is conscious of it or not, her accumulated disappointments and resentments will make her cold and unresponsive. As a result, her husband's ardor is chilled and neither she nor he experiences any depth of satisfaction. On the other hand, a husband may regard his wife as thoughtless, selfish, unsympathetic, undutiful, or whatever, and reacts to his interpretation of the situation by wishing more than ever to assert his "authority" and "teach her a lesson." Consequently, he may become abrupt and demanding when his wife is indisposed, and so create a situation in which every attempt comes to be regarded by both partners as a battle of wills, rather than as a mutually pleasurable consummation of a happy union. Such couples often come to the psychiatrist with the mistaken idea that if only he would give them definite "instructions" on sexual techniques (each generally accuses the other of willful ignorance in the matter), all their problems would be solved, and an impending separation or divorce would be averted. Unfortunately, it can now be seen that in most such cases, it is the will and not the way that is mainly at fault, and that in such instances both husband and wife must analyze and readjust their attitudes toward each other in many relationships other than the sexual before lasting compatibilities can be achieved. In fact, if such a couple can be helped to straighten out their cumulative familial, financial, social, recreational, and other disagreements, their needs for each other are gradually restored, and their sexual difficulties disappear as earned love returns. This beginning commentary is important because in the current flood of sensational literature on sex in marriage, much of which is little more than pornography in the guise of so-called marital advice, it is often forgotten that when two people live together in almost every conceivable way during the 168-hour marital week, how they feel about each other does not altogether depend on the relatively few minutes they spend in merely physical contact.

Nevertheless, the fact remains that pleasurable sexual relations should for many years be a part of every successful marriage, and that even when other adjustments are satisfactory, marital happiness can be seriously impaired if not destroyed by sexual incompatibilities. Moreover, in many cases in which this is true, such incompatibilities arise from sheer ignorance or neglect of simple but effective methods for increasing the natural pleasures of sexual arousal and coitus.

Here, however, some people may begin to protest. Some may say that such "intimate" affairs are not to be discussed in public. Others may insist that intercourse can never be sanctioned for mere bodily pleasure, but only for the purpose of begetting children. To the first objection it may be pointed out that until recently venereal diseases, too, were considered to be "intimate" affairs, but that after the U.S. Public Health Service began to insist on the publication of frank information about them in the press, much unnecessary sorrow has been avoided. The objection to bodily pleasure in intercourse also springs from a related source: Namely, that somehow sexuality must be considered as animal-like, debasing, "evil" and therefore its discussion conflicts with ethical or religious principles. True, the religious conviction that sexual intercourse is natural only if it is intended to result in the conception of children must be fully respected. But even for adherents of this belief, there is no reason why the sex act should not be so conducted as to give the maximum of natural pleasure to both parties, particularly since it has been shown that under such circumstances successful conception and contented parenthood are most likely to result. Certainly, we do not penalize ourselves in this way in other spheres of living. For instance, we eat to sustain life—yet we do not think it "unnatural" to stimulate our appetite and aid our digestion by making the food we eat varied and palatable. Clothes, too, were originally designed mainly to furnish warmth and protection, yet most religions permit us to make our clothes interesting and attractive. Similarly, there is no real reason why the natural purposes of sexual intercourse in marriage should not be served by making the sex act as complete and pleasurable as possible, especially since this contributes greatly to the contentment of both partners and also—for their children's sake—the happiness and stability of the home.

Hypnotism and "Auto-suggestion"

Hypnosis was known to the ancient Hindu and Egyptian priests, who employed it in religious rites designed to influence the ignorant and gullible. Since then, various forms of hypnosis have been used in attempts to treat nervous disorders, either by charlatans such as Greatrakes who made a fortune in the seventeenth century by "stroking" imaginary diseases from the body, or by misinformed enthusiasts such as Mesmer who believed they were dealing with "animal magnetism." One of the first and greatest of clinicans who conducted studies of hypnotism, August Bernheim, summed up his findings in two aphorisms: "There is nothing we can do with hypnosis that cannot be done more effectively and with less danger by other methods," and "It is a wise hypnotist that knows who is 'hypnotizing' whom." I teach my physicians undergoing speciality training in psychiatry the various methods of inducing the relaxed, compliant rapport called hypnosis, mainly to remove its intriguing mystique. Nearly all authorities now agree that hypnotism should be used only by well-trained physicians, who can control its effects and combine it with other esential forms of treatment; in fact, many psychiatrists believe that even under such circumstances the long term psychologic complications of hypnotism almost always outweigh its transient advantages. In addition, there is virtual agreement among experienced psychiatrists that the various forms of "auto-suggestion" as advocated by Coue, Salter, and others are either completely ineffective, or else they make the person who practices them progressively more neurotic by encouraging self-preoccupation, unrealistic thinking, and false beliefs.

Sound medical advice to people with personality problems is as follows: Avoid self-administered mumbo-jumbo as you would avoid taking advertised patent-medicines to cure an undiagnosed illness. If you have difficulties in familial, sexual, occupational, or other adjustments beyond your own capacities to correct, seek advice from those adequately trained and experienced: your minister, your physician, or an expert personnel counsellor. If these cannot handle your problems, they will refer you to a psychiatrist or psychoanalyst who can.

An article invited—and rejected—by an avant-garde magazine:

The Theatre of the Absurd and the Absurdity of Clothes

In Ionesco's play *The Chairs,* an aging couple enacts a fantasy in which all the Great of their time, up to and including the Emperor, crowd into their home to hear their Ultimate Message to the World, as finally delivered by a completely inarticulate orator. There are only three actors in this parody on geriatric futility, and as a compliment to the imagery of a perceptive audience, the play can be presented on a stage completely bare even of the imaginary chairs for the imaginary guests. Since every adult viewer can even more easily discern the dying bodies beneath the preposterous posturings, should not also the actors be bare? Are not their superfluous clothes as absurd as an unnecessarily cluttered stage? Is it not one purpose of modern art, as part of a new humanitarian Renaissance, to discard outmoded restrictions and gaucheries? But to make such questions less "academic"—in the emerging sense of the fatuous—let us examine more closely what we mean by the term "absurd."

The word is derived from Latin *ab-surdum,* meaning disparate or incongruous. In this respect the plays of Ionesco, Beckett, Albee, Genet, or the classical Plautus are no more "absurd" than the paintings of Picasso, or the poetry of Daumal or Desnos, or the music of Bartok, Berg, or Babbitt. Many other insightful artists, writers, and composers are currently engaged in stripping man's nature of its artificial or hypocritical facade of harmony, rhyme, and reason. So also in the intellectual sphere the philosophies of Husserl, Sartre, and Camus, and the neotheologies of Buber and Tillich reflect man's confusions, contradictions, and the futilities of his earthly existence—although they prescribe no antidotes save clarity and courage—or the ultimate absurdity of illogical "faith." Paradoxically, all of these trends are in accord both with Tertullian's resigned *Credo, quia absurdum est,* and Thomas Hobbes' addendum, "Man has the sole privilege of absurdity, to which no other living creature is subject." Indeed, perhaps the essential function of modern "education" is *not* to abolish our irrationality of thought and behavior—a Sisyphean task—but to modify our individual absurdities so that they will transiently conform with the "normal" absurdities of our social milieu until we can change them all for the better.

Traditions: Like other ostensibly avant-garde movements, indeed, the "Theatre of the Absurd" is but one modern expression of ancient modes of primal imagery. The *theatrum mimus*—a derisive, often improvised commentary on current follies in which the hero is depicted as a *moros* or *stupidus*—was popular in classical Greece. Nude beauty was worshiped—and pompously panoplied politicians and stuffy sages ridiculed. What could be more delightfully impertinent than the pre-Freudian analytic episode in *The Clouds,* in which Aristophanes has a fat, bald Socrates, literally suspended "up in the air" in a basket, insist that his supplicant Strepsiades free-associate on a couch until he discloses his unconscious wish to have the moon in his pocket "so that he could stop its waning and would not have to pay his monthly bills?" Sannio (In-sane), the correspondingly foolish philosopher of Roman Comedy, evolved through the *Zanni* of the Italian *Commedia dell'arte* into our English *Zany.* In the German *Fastnachtspiele* human vices, first personfied as fiends and devils, evolved into the clowns and jesters that enlivened the plays of Shakespeare and Molière. So also do we now cherish the Chaplins, the Laurel and Hardys, the W. C. Fieldses, and the Harpo Marxes, who lend an ambience of profoundly significant absurdity to every scene they inhabit. "Delight in nonsense," wrote Freud, as though it were news, "has its roots in the feeling of freedom we enjoy when we are able to abandon the straightjacket of the unconscious," and Ernst Kris added, "Wit is a thin ledge above an abyss of anxiety." T. S. Eliot put it more trenchantly:

Go, go, go
Said the bird
Human kind
Cannot stand much reality

Throughout the ages, then, playwrights deliberately filled the stage with the disconcerting clichés, the significant non-sequiturs, and the frenetic fantasies of dreams, and thus anticipated the "modern" Theatre of the Absurd. Strindberg introduced his "Dream Play" with: "On a slight groundwork of reality, imagination spins and weaves new patterns made up of memories, experiences, unfettered fancies, absurdities and improvisations. The characters split, double and multiply; they evaporate, crystallize, scatter and converge. But a single consciousness holds sway over them all—that of the dreamer. For him there are no secrets, no incongruities, no scruples, no laws."

Wrote Martin Esslin: "Human beings . . . who are no longer aware of [the true] state of affairs and its disintegrating effect on their personalities are brought face to face with a heightened representation of this schizophrenic universe. . . . The audience . . . by being made to see that the world has become absurd, . . . takes the first step in coming to terms with reality."

The poetic poignancy of the mobile Rorschachs of the modern theatre, then, resides in this: that each viewer can have his own unique set of percepts and responses to derive and treasure. Let us review some of these possible interpretations:

The Zoo Story, premiered in Berlin on September 28, 1959, was Albee's first play. In it Peter (the Rock?) may represent entrenched middle-class stolidity strangely fascinated by a disillusioned, contemptuous Jerry (Jeremiah?) who, after eluding his landlady (society) and its vicious guardian (the Dog) accosts Peter on a Park Bench, offering atavistic nonconformity (the Zoo Story) and penetrates Peter's smug privacy; however, he thus threatens to preempt Peter's prior Establishment (the Bench) and thereby precipitates a quarrel that leads to Jerry's demise, after which Peter flees in terror with his cherished Book of Fictions. The play can thus be briefed in a single sentence, but its connotations as to the eternal conflict between *bourgoisie* and *beatnik* are endless.

Beckett's *Endgame,* which opened in London in 1957, is a more dolorous decrescendo of death. All that moves and hopes is destroyed. The aged expire with discarded indignity in ashcans; the middle generation in blind inertia; and the young in dependent rage—and all humanity ends, again in the words of T. S. Eliot, "not with a bang but a whimper."

But what does all this macabre morbidity and avid absurdity have to do with the erotic aspects of nudity that are also invading our arts, our writings, our movies, and our plays? The factor of frankness has already been mentioned, but perhaps a deeper motivation is this: In an age when the touted miracles of technology are turning our earth not into a Utopia but into a stinking, momentarily exploding globe, when old economic and social systems are rapidly disintegrating, and when the myths of the old animistic religions no longer assure us of eternal ecstasy in a celestial penthouse, men—and women—may turn to the unconcealed pleasures and togetherness, however transient, of sexuality. But since physical coitus is neither continuously available nor possible (especially to exhausted or aging males who can no longer take yes for an answer), the indirect and implied promises and anticipations of the act are all the more welcome. Ergo, near-nudity for both sexes is acceptable on beaches where every pastime but swimming is allowed, topless and now bottomless dancers perform for dining couples in nightclubs as "previews of attractions to come," and even more pervasive are the titillating semi-exposures of current street and evening clothes.

On the latter subject, I was recently invited to be a guest expert (ex-pert *may* be translated as not-pertinent) on a television program during which I was supposed to be primed to explain why male animals were so splendidly decorated by nature to attract the female, whereas a man's clothes are more sober and can only within limits even express his personality? I replied, in an appropriately Bowdlerized fashion, somewhat as follows:

To begin with, it is not true that our male animal cousins wear their glorious panoplies of colors or furs just to attract the female of their species: that allegation is literally only for the birds. Even there, the display of fine feathers is much more often designed to assert male virility in the larger sense of territorial possession and dominance, much as in our own societies of noble savages: (*e.g.*, African Ashanti, Plains Indians, or U.S. Marines): the uniform grows more gorgeous with higher rank and power. So also male attire can be more easily modified for other communicative or utilitarian purposes: the rumpled professorial tweed suggests that its wearer has time only for thoughts more transcendently esoteric than erratic or erotic, whereas the thoughtfully prearranged permanent crease in the flannels of a business executive provides a non-telltale lap for secretaries. But since men's sexual nidus is relatively concentrated amidships (a region traditionally uncovered by a pubic bay in his outer garments or suggestively emphasized by modern versions of the medieval pudenal bag or pod), male fashions need change only slowly.

In contrast, since a woman's charms are tridimensionally distributed, she needs changing fashions to display all her intriguing aspects, and thus avoid the lurking specter of male ennui, especially in some of our surfeited split-level suburbias. Ergo, the perennial variations throughout the Western world between plunging necklines and soaring hems (often dictated by designers not certain of their own sex and therefore perceptive of both views) express the sibilant, sisterly slogan: "Women of the West Unite; You have Nothing to Lose but Your Chastity Belts."

Nevertheless, customs and costumes vary independently with time, place and culture: For a millennium Minoan nymphs displayed their breasts as unself-consciously as Samoans did until recently, and Spartan maids and youths exercised innocently together in the nude much as the co-educational Japanese bathe now. On the male side, connotations between clothes and customs were never high. During an ostensibly moralistic century, men's costumes were more foppishly elaborate than were women's—and as to hair styles, Lord Raleigh and George Washington (not to mention Samson) wore their hair longer than any Hashbury Hippie—many of whom, parenthetically, do not advocate free love as ardently or as inclusively as did our own Benjamin Franklin, who, dressed in his simple woolens at the French Court, was truly a wolf in sheep's clothing. Nevertheless, raiment, or the lack of it, has always occasioned interesting comment, from the nihilistic Fable of the Emperor's Clothes to *bon mots* such as Robert Herrick's:

> *"A sweet disorder in the dress*
> *Kindles in clothes a wantonness."*

—vis à vis Shakespeare in *King Lear:*

> *"Through tattered clothes small vices do appear*
> *Robes and furred gowns hide all."*

But perhaps the most enduring aphorisms are anonymous: e.g., "Clothes make the man"—lately given an intriguing semantic twist by the modern double-entendre of "make." Or, in another happy paraphrase, even our children chant:

> *"Mother, may I be in the swim?*
> *Yes, my darling daughter*
> *Hang your clothes on a hickory limb*
> *But don't go near the water."*

In effect, human habiliments and human habits have ever varied with whim and whimsey. But in our time, when the quantum theory has also signified a discontinuously qualitative jump into an Age of Anxiety, the bitter absurdities of our lives, as bared in our graphic and performing arts, are scarcely mitigated by our frenetic flights into the clothed or unclothed eroticisms of our current turmoil.

From nudity and absurdity it was an easy step to a clinical study of more pressing problems, to wit:

*The Vagaries and Virtues of American Youth**

Long before Plato quoted Socrates on the subject, it had become customary for the elders of each era to deplore the physical, esthetic, civic, military and moral degeneration of the youth of their time. In this tradition—and in almost the same terms—do we today also deride our love children, flower-people, hippies, boo-hoo disciples, pot-, speed-, and acid-heads and other current descendants of the late unlamented Beatniks. This original term, as formerly adopted by them with defiant avidity, basically implied an accusatory assumption on their part of having been "beaten" into martyrdom—an attitude particularly irritating to those of us who regarded many of them as poseurs who, if anything, had been pretty well spoiled by foolishly overpermissive parents and an excessively indulgent milieu. But the Beatnik insisted that his pose be loudly advertised and trumpeted; ergo, the term and its derivatives also came to connote glaring gaucheries in dress (soiled jackets or shapeless sweaters over miniskirts, or dirty pants tapering to sloppy sandals), strange coiffures (tangled highrise or hip-length hirsutism), variably obnoxious speech and manners ("You cubes from No-wheresville don't make the scene with us cool cats in camp, Daddy-O"), social irresponsibility (contemptuous rejection of schooling, work, and familial, economic and civic duties as intolerably "square"—without offering presumably more rounded substitutes); execrable esthetics (raucous cacophony miscalled music, stereotyped jerks, athetoid movements or clonic convulsions miscalled dance; or monstrous montages miscalled art); an abuse of nepenthic and so-called psychedelic drugs (from alcohol, through dexedrene-and-barbiturate "goof balls," to marihuana, mescaline and LSD), and finally, aberrant eroticism (brazen exhibitionism, flagrant fetishisms, public promiscuities and defiant deviations in sexual techniques, objects and partners) miscalled "love."

Sociocultural Perspectives: It is, perhaps, this last set of

*Reprinted from Masserman, J. H. *A Transcultural Psychiatric Approach,* New York. Grune & Stratton, Inc., 1969.

contraventions of our supposedly cherished customs that most often troubles us—especially, perhaps, certain aging and envious male elders who may be finding it more libidinally difficult to take a disconcerting and unexpected female assent. But this consideration of asocial or antisocial sexual behavior brings into sharper focus two much broader issues of fundamental importance, to wit: (1) Who—at what time, in what place, in what culture, and with what authority—is to define what patterns of interpersonal behavior, sexual or other, are to be regarded as "normal," "idiosyncratic," "Beatnik," Hippie "neurotic," or, for that matter, "psychotic"? And (2) are there special circumstances in our own time, place and culture that so impinge on our younger generation as to make definite judgments currently all the more difficult?

Culture and Sex: Using the special case of sexuality as but one parameter among many other variables, let us first consider the range of permissible libidinal expression in other times and places, thus furnishing broader contexts for our own. In cultural terms erotism per se (i.e., apart from concurrent complications of rivalry, conquest, dominance, etc.) can play a partial role in the genesis or expression of neurotic conflicts only in the relatively few societies which adhere to a sexually repressive Judeo-Christian tradition; in most others, a seminar on sex practices would be regarded as about on a par with a conference on the culinary arts. Indeed, in more than one culture, the latter are considered somewhat more private and socially significant; for example, the contemporary Souno Indians of the Amazon headwaters, as did the classic Etruscans, copulate openly, but would be shamed into exile if caught eating in public. In the Islamic world, where Omar Halebis' Laws of Love is considered a literary masterpiece as well as a manual of erotica blessed of Allah, many a Turk or Bedouin could easily shame our brashest Beatnik in the enthusiasm with which he would discuss the size of his phallus and the range and objects of his amatory exploits with anyone at any time.

In the modern East Jacobus Sutor, a French army surgeon who studied the subject avidly found some Hindu sects to be ". . . as lascivious as the monkey. . . . Every wife betrays her husband whenever she can, if she finds pleasure or amusement in it. . . . There are few virgins above the age of 10, the hymenal membrane having been stretched or worn away by the little Hindu girl's repeated contact with brothers, cousins and others" (l'Ethnologie du Senses Génitale, Paris, 1935).

In storied Cathay, Wong Shih'cheng, in *The Golden Lotus*, put it thus, "The world is based upon continuous interaction between the male and female principles, therefore one cannot say that anything so done is out of depravity, or that any sexual passion is evil."* The term "anything" in the above quotation is comprehensive enough to include, as Edwards and Masters point out in considerable detail, nearly every conceivable variation of sexual technique, partner and orifice, including cross-species intercourse among pastoral and agrarian peoples openly practiced throughout Africa, India, Asia and Polynesia; indeed, in only a few Western cultures can terms such as "polymorphous perverse sexuality," "carnal sin," etc. have any deprecatory meaning. Such considerations may have led the Sufist poet Haji' Abdu'l-Yezdi to write:

There is no Good, there is no Bad
These are the whims of mortal will
What works me well, that I call good
What harms or hurts I hold ill
They change with place, they shift with race
And, in the veriest span of time
Each Vice has worn a Virtue's crown
All good was banned as Sin or Crime
All faith is false, all Faith is true
Truth is the shattered mirror strewn
In myriad bits, while each believes
His little bit the whole to own . . .
Thy faith, why false? My faith, why true?
'Tis all the work of Mine,
Only the foolish love of self
Makes the Mine excel the Thine.

Quoted by Sir Richard Burton

In full justice, not everyone in the Western world, Beatnik or not, has continued to jitter over Jeremiah, to pore over the

*Paraphrased from Clement Egerton, London, Routledge & Kegan Paul.

platitudes of Plato (who personally preferred pederasty) or stand in awe of Aristotle and Augustine. More virile voices have been heard, even in Judeo-Christian history: from doubly venerable King David, who proudly served 18 wives plus numerous concubines (and by cuckolding Uriah, with Bathsheba fathered Solomon to write his lustful Song of Songs), down the ages through the unchaste Chaucer, the boisterous Boccaccio and ribald Rabelais, to the D. H. Lawrences and Norman Mailers of modern times.

And since we are down to the here and now, let us consider the examples of sexual hypocrisy we elders furnish our youth when they witness the frenetic mate-combinations, permutations and divorces in our split-level suburbias, or read of flourishing organizations called "Swingers" in some American cities composed of thousands of married couples who, in this modern age of technology, utilize computerized matching to guarantee that their sexual exchange of marital partners every weekend would be mutually satisfactory.

Stresses on Modern Youth: But even if we put not only the sexual but all other patterns of deviant behavior in such comparative historical and social contexts, the second of our two questions still remains: are there special circumstances in our own time, place, and culture that especially influence some of our youth toward the extremes that we berate as Beatnik? We cannot here encompass all the genetic and early experiential factors that predestine personality even in early childhood, but let us briefly review, as seemingly more germane to our subject, those that profoundly affect our offspring from adolescence through early adulthood—and incidentally note what can be done by us to correct various deviations of conduct during each period.

Adolescence: Modern personality theory no longer takes seriously Freud's dictum that basic character development is virtually complete when the so-called Oedipus complex (fear of castration by the father in punishment of childhood desires for maternal incest) is reawakened at puberty, and either satisfactorily resolved or again repressed to constitute the unconscious source of both normal conduct and neurotic deviations. Instead, we now recognize that the crucial years between puberty and the arbitrary ages of legal "adulthood" constitute an all-important period during which the adolescent must seek and acquire what, as academically trademarked by Erik Erikson, is currently called "identity." In our almost incredibly intricate culture, with its multitudes of familial, occupational, esthetic, economic, political and other intertwined socio-transactional relationships, this acquisition of an adequately multiadaptive, yet unique, individuality is an increasingly difficult task even for the most intelligent and talented of our youth, especially when our present methods of education ill prepare them for a world of such technical and social complexity. The late adolescent may spread himself thin trying to be simultaneously a dutiful child, a brilliant scholar, a winning athlete, a popular leader, a potent lover, a seductive nymph, a cynical sophisticate, a social reformer, a blasé escapist, an avant-garde esthete, a cryptic mystic and a dozen other incompatible alter egos. The result is often a fragile superficiality ("identity diffusion") in each role, or at worst, chaos and "anomic" breakdown in all. Ergo, interim or permanent, partial or complete failures of adaptation occur which may take the following forms.

Regressions: There may be a return to familial or other dependencies, as expressed in deliberate failures at school or minor delinquencies requiring repeated interventions and "succorances" by parents or guardians. These perennial "protectors" and "rescuers" may protest loudly, but are often secretly happy to retain pre-emptive custody and control of their precious and perennial child, whatever his age. On the other hand, if familial hegemony seems neither practicable nor attractive, the late adolescent or young adult may seek other securities in a peer group which offers support through common patterns of dress and conduct, idiomatic modes of speech, stereotyped musical and other esthetic tastes, escapist hideouts in shacks or "pads," exploratory sexuality and pseudosophisticated talk of avant-garde cynicism, social protest or naive nihilism. Fortunately most such peer cliques and groupings are either harmless or actually beneficial as interim experiences throughout youth—and indeed may continue into adulthood in the form of fraternities and societies with their prescribed insignia, secret handclasps, passwords and rituals, professions of high social purpose and, not too infrequently, real public service. Ergo, we need to become seriously concerned only when an adolescent becomes so immersed in "extracurricular activities" as to neglect his education, physical health and broader social development, or when he selects a group that advocates "sports. which endanger others ("chicken" dueling, drag racing), or promotes public obscenity, sexual arrogance and physical violence.

Sexual Promiscuity: As we have seen, the connotations of "promiscuity" vary widely even among Western cultures: as one more example, in the Scandinavian countries, teenagers in the upper social strata are expected to have lovers and mistresses, an estimated 40 per cent of pregnancies are conceived outside of marriage and all children born out of wedlock may be raised without onus of illegitimacy. In our own country, sexual customs are changing rapidly under pressure from our iconoclastic youth; formal "dating," often encouraged by upper-middle-class parents, now frequently begins at puberty; "going steady" with a succession of 2- and 3-month partners is a status symbol in many a juvenile group, and may involve "necking" or "petting" (including fondling of breasts and genitals) or "making out" to the extent of sexual intercourse. If and when these practices become even more widely and frankly accepted, the adolescent's fears of social reprisal will correspondingly diminish, but because of the inherent uncertainties and insecurities of this age period in our culture the poignant rivalries, jealousies, disappointments and reactive hostilities involved may continue to give rise to idiosyncratic behavior.

Pre(mature)-Marital Counselling: More marraiges are being contracted near the minimal age limits by couples who, under the guise of undertaking mutual marital responsibilities, are again seeking dependent securities, social approbation of sexual license and variously rationalized escapes from the necessity of more thorough preparations for adult relationships. Under these circumstances disappointments and dissatisfactions are inevitable and give rise to intense anxieties, depressions or periods of diffuse restlessness with accompanying insomnia and somatic dysfunctions, more attempts at relief through drugs and alcohol, and sexual frigidity or impotence, usually limited to the spouse. It is of medical relevance that partners in a poorly planned and conducted marriage, after a few days to as many decades of recurrent crises, may come to psychiatrists or "marital counsellors" with the plea that if only their "sexual problems" can be solved, including their needs for escapist or covertly punitive extramarital or homosexual adventures, then their marriage "could still somehow be worked out." As noted, a specific request is often made for instruction in "sexual techniques," in the illusory belief, which the counsellor should *not* share, that this would form a solid base for marital compatibility.

But all of these predisposing circumstances are outweighed by a far more overwhelming apprehension, in that many of our perceptive youth simply fear that *they have no future worth having unless our current social order is promptly and radically changed by peaceful or, if necessary, by violent means.* With our country now dominated politically and economically by a firmly institutionalized military-industrial-trade-union complex that demands 80 billion dollars a year of our national budget and consumes over 12 per cent of our total national product; with a standing army of 3½ million men and women, hundreds of thousands of whom in Viet Nam are commanded to commit unspeakable acts of civilian destruction for which we ourselves at Nuremberg condemned and executed Nazi criminals; with the most intensive and least discriminating program of "peacetime" military conscription in the history of any democratic country constituting an unpredictable hazard to every young man's future; with the odds for global nuclear destruction estimated to about 1 in 3 by 1990, about even by 2000 and greatly increased by the recent decisions of our War (née Defense) Department—is it indeed any wonder that thousands of our youth, whatever their "race," "class" or other convictions, and who are not escaping to Canada or Scandinavia, consider their currently prescribed educational and other disciplines as a preparation for death rather than for life, and labor under a sense of not-so-quiet desperation—let us face it—that may well result in revolution?

Triple-Bonded Beatniks: This, then, is but a brief resumé of some of the current strains on our youth—stresses that incidentally produced the species *"Beatnik"*— a word which, like *Sputnik*, is remotely Slavic for fellow-traveller, far out. But just as Sputniks can take different orbits, Beatniks can also follow differing courses to different landings. Three of the most easily recognizable of these orbits may, in progressively lesser degrees of dysrhythmia or asynchronicity, be characterized as the Off-Beatniks, Down-Beatniks and Up-Beatniks.

The Off-Beatniks: These we have already considered as the more seriously erratic, troubled and troublesome misfits, disharmonious with their own milieu and, despite their pretensions, contributing little that is truly constructive or even original to our culture. But perhaps we can derive a thin twofold comfort from their presence: first, that our enemies as well as our friends must share them—indeed, I have personally seen their almost stereotyped visages on both sides of the so-called Iron and Bamboo Curtains; and second, that almost everywhere their extreme behavior is more often than not a sobering example to the more sensible youth who will really direct our future.

The Down-Beatniks: This describes the more consistent noncomformists who more articulately and rationally condemn the inequalities and injustices of our societies and, often with some courage and justification, rebel against them—sometimes to the extent of outraging our sensibilities, occasionally violating essential provisions of our social and legal codes. The prognosis here is often favorable: with further maturity and increasing wisdom most of them become good citizens, competent parents, and sometimes even staunch Republicans.

The Up-Beatniks: This group, even with their occasional beards, tresses, play-readings, placards, proclamations and protest marches, are the best of the lot; basically earnest, energetic, intelligent and well-intentioned, they are a not inconsiderable help in prodding us oldsters to review our smug hypocrisies and revise our medieval customs and conduct—though sometimes we cannot help wishing that, in view of our doddering age and failing mentalities, they would be just a bit less strident, pressing and impatient. Or, in the technical language of their lesser peers, "Like, look, man, quit bugging us too much!"

Socio-Pharmacology: Let us now consider another of our prime social concerns: the tendency of our youth toward the excessive use of harmful drugs. This raises three fundamental questions: (1) Why are the drugs used? (2) What harm can they do? (3) What can we do about the individual and social difficulties so engendered?

Man's Ur-Illusory Faiths: The first question is the most searching of the three, since it probes the deepest roots of human behavior. Current vagaries of our youth not only in their pharmacologic, but also in social and religious conduct may be better understood in the broader context of what I have essayed to call the ultimate *Ur*-illusions of all men of all ages at all sentient times, namely:

First, that far from being a highly vulnerable conglomerate of perishable proteins, we are—or soon will be—omniscient, omnipotent and immortal beings ready to conquer the cosmos.

Second, that we are also just about to graduate from 3 million years of feral fear and ferocity to become truly civilized and trustworthy social partners.

And third, that the mind of man can really attain not only insight into, but implicit control over, the transcendent and the divine.

In essence, these have ever been man's eternal aspirations, and his vain but restless seekings to realize them constitute his tragic history. Here, however, we can hardly take more than another fleeting glance at how youth's current frustrations in all three spheres tend to foster not only a recourse to nepenthic drugs, but also to the accompanying escapist patterns of social and psychiatric concern we have already touched upon. Let us consider the three *Ur*-stresses in turn.

Technological: It is becoming painfully apparent that our vaunted sciences and mechanical skills, while increasing our mobility and longevity, are also rapidly making the air, water and environs of our centers of industrial "civilization" more or less uninhabitable through chemical pollution and, as we have seen, perhaps soon by nuclear obliteration. Ergo, those of us in America who can afford it escape, moderately fortified with alcohol and tranquilizers, progressively to the further suburbs, to the Virgin Islands or to New Zealand, whereas our less solvent youth repair, with their supplies of less expensive, more rapidly active and longer lasting LSD* to hippie colonies such as the Haight-Ashbury or Tamalpais districts of San Francisco, or to Walden-type rural pads or remote Indian reservations.

Social: In our current semi-civilization (where we must profess to be friends but be ever prepared for latent rivalries and enmities) we can hardly wonder that some of the disillusioned among us, as has been done by Utopia-seekers throughout history,† set up enclaves of sexual freedom, shared parenthood and communal property, and take methedrine or other supposed aphrodisiacs to enhance such relationships.

Theo-philosophical: Finally, we can also appreciate why, as our futile factories and frenetic fraternization fail us, we might turn to ever-farther-out fantasies and escapist illusions. Some of our self-styled intelligentsia thus become preoccupied with Zen and its quest for *satori,* or seek Nirvanas under Eastern mystics such as the Maharishi Maresh Yogi or become lost in the impenetrable jargon of Germanic existentialism; so also, our equally idle but less affluent youth seek their dereistic escapes through marihuana, LSD or even more vividly deleriogenic drugs such as dimethyltryptamine (DMT**), with or without the esoteric mentorship of gurus or of Boo Hoos of various pretensions or degrees of exhibitionism up to that of the recently notorious Timothy Leary.

*Daniel Freedman points out that LSD, possibly by "binding" serotinin and slowing the metabolism of other catechol-amines at distal synapses, impairs traumatic recall and apprehensive anticipation and thereby enhances "the immediacy of the now."

†For example, the Sabbatai Zevi in seventeenth-century Jerusalem who regarded sin as essential to salvation, or the Brethren of the Free Spirit who, in colonies throughout Europe, have for centuries praised and practiced the ecstacies of free thought, shared property and communal sex, enhanced then as now by the serotonin-like indole Yohimbine (Hallek). As Moynihan points out, compared to such preachments the Port Huron Protocols of the New Left are conservative indeed. Nevertheless, some of the statistics of the "new morality" are a bit disconcerting; gonorrhea is showing an annual 6 per cent rise; at the present rate, 1 of every 6 girls now age 13 can expect to be illegitimately pregnant before 20, and half of those in Chicago will be pregnant again within 18 months. (MedicalWorld News 8:64-68, March, 1967).

**Twenty-five centuries before LSD, the Upanishads contained the following passage: "As you practice meditation you may see in vision forms resembling snow, crystal, wind, smoke, fire, lightning, fireflies, the sun, the moon. These are signs that you are on your way to the revelation of Brahman. You will realize that the Self is separate from the Body and will not be affected by disease, old age or death." Who, then or now, really needed or needs LSD?

Are Psychedelics Harmful? The answer to this second thematic question obviously depends on who votes what way on which drugs are supposed to be psychedelic: i.e., "mind-expanding" or "inspirational." Long before DeQuiney wrote his "confessions," Lao-tzu praised the narcotizing "poppy of philosophy," Galen prescribed Samian clay (perhaps containing lithium) to meliorate melancholy and clear consciousness, and in the Western World our Navajo and Pottawatomie Indians had traditionally greeted the Great Spirit with peyote and mescal. In more recent times, Stephen Foster claimed he could not compose his songs, nor Edgar Allen Poe his poetry, without the activating alchemy of alcohol. For that matter, Freud was long convinced of the inspirational properties of cocaine, and Churchill insisted that he wrote and spoke best under the optimum synergism of nicotine and ethereal spirits. As physicians we know full well that not only cocaine, but excessive smoking and drinking are harmful; nevertheless, most of us still believe that a cocktail and a cigar make us feel more alert, imaginative and creative.* The use of nepenthics then is, like our sexual mores, a relative rather than an absolute issue, and it is mainly by sheer numbers that we consumers of alcohol and ataractics outvote and condemn the votaries of other drugs which, speaking from the standpoint of over-all comprehensive social welfare, are considerably less disruptive.

But cannot objections be raised to this form of medical sophistry on the ground that LSD, DMT, intravenous mephedrine and other "psychedelics" are *individually* far more dangerous than the other pharmacologic toxins alluded to? Even before Sydney Cohen's prospective review of his controlled 5-year follow-up study of the physical and psychologic effects of LSD and other substances, we can safely infer from present

*Such magico-religious-psychedelic beliefs pervade many foreign subcultures as well as our local enclaves of pot-smokers and acid-heads. As but one other example, Jan Ehrenwald (From Medicine Man to Freud, New York, Dell, 1956, p. 77) quotes Albert Schweitzer as follows: "[Secret societies of the Negroes of Labarene drug themselves with the plant *iboga*] in order to reach a state [in which they] are content with the knowledge that they have risen above the ordinary condition of humanity. By means of this ecstasy they get to know the other, the truer world compared to which the daily world is nothing more than an illusion. White men occasionally have themselves initiated into the secret societies and become faithful and absolute believers."

evidence that the drug is definitely treacherous.* Thus Ungerleider et al., reported that "bad trips" in the Los Angeles area immediately or as recurrences long after ingestion of LSD (cf. Smart, and Frosch et al. 1968) now exceed hospital facilities even for emergency care, that chlorpromazine is far from a reliable antidote for LSD toxicosis and that unpredictable suicides (Keeler), homicides and psychoses requiring months of hospitalization (Ungerleider and Fisher, 1966) are becoming tragically frequent.† Worst of all, some LSD users tend to become ardent proseletyzers of the young and gullible to join their ranks. Nor may the effects end with the users; Irwin and Egoscue have detected in vivo chromosomal abnormalities in LSD habitues which can endanger the welfare of future generations. Although this last effect has been questioned by Laughman et al., and by Warkany and Takacs, the total threat of the psychedelics certainly cannot be viewed with equanimity.

And yet all this must be taken in the sober context of other human vicissitudes. Of the 70 million Americans who use alcohol, no less than 5 million drink it to harmful excess; in addition, we take 13 billion doses of amphetamines and barbiturates annually. Nor can we forget the untold tons of so-called tranquilizers, ataractics and antidepressants we avidly consume with or without benefit of prescription, especially since, as Esrig and others warn, either directly or during withdrawal, they can induce convulsions, delirium and death. In further amelioration of the psychedelic problem, Freedman and Jaffe estimate that the great majority of those who try LSD never take a second dose whereas, according to Cohen, the minimum lethal dose of the drug is so great that in one case 15,000 micrograms given with homicidal intent were not fatal. Nevertheless, despite the rationalizations of those avid for them, no drug has been shown to be of any objective aid in

*Laurea reports that 13 per cent of LSD users experience "overwhelming panic," 12 per cent become violent, 9 per cent suicidal and 10 per cent "require extended hospitalization." According to a survey reported in the *San Francisco Examiner and Chronicle* on January 12, 1969 (p. 18): About one sixth of San Mateo County high school students use "speed" and more than a third have tried hallucinogens and "goof balls." Drug arrests have increased 1448 per cent in eight years, 324 per cent in the last 6 months.

†Laurea, Fink and others have published similar reports.

creativity, and carefully controlled studies* have proved that none of the psychedelics is really useful in any form of physical or psychiatric therapy except possibly for the dying patient (Kast). Since, on the other hand the psychedelics do have unpredictable and sometimes devastating side effects, the moral justification of their use "to expand the horizons of the human mind" is wishfully illusory and medically dangerous.

To a follow-up inquiry from a New Jersey matron as to "what *was* going on in our split-level suburbias":

Dear Mrs. W.:

Obviously, I cannot relay confidential details, but you are most welcome to conduct your own clinical (from the Greek root *klinikos,* bed or couch) research.

With best wishes.

Radio and Television:

Psychiatrists called upon to write radio and TV scripts designed to enlighten the public on the causes and treatment of human failures have to consider topical and popular appeal, simplicity and clarity of language, and many other factors, including accuracy and professional ethics. On a radio series sponsored by the American Medical Association on the general topic of "The Family and the Child," one episode, entitled the "Murder of Intelligence," was intended to caution parents against the premature exploitation of their children. For this, I dramatized the case of Boris Sidis, a famous psychologist in his time, who so pressed his brilliant son William to achieve premature fame that, the boy lapsed eventually into tragic mediocrity. My concluding comments on the murder of intelligence:

Every person has his own natural, spontaneous rate of physical, intellectual, and emotional development. No one of these three aspects of growth can be artificially hurried with-

*Contrast Heard (1963) with Van Dusen et al. (1966) and Smart (1968).

out serious danger to happiness and social usefulness. A poignant illustration of this tragedy is the story of William James Sidis whose father Boris, a famous psychologist of the last generation, carried away by overconfidence in his own theories of child development, forced his son, who was indeed potentially a genius, into interests and activities beyond his emotional development. The result was that the boy had no opportunity to develop his skills *at his own pace via* toys, games, and peer relationships through the usual phases of childhood and adolescence. At first the boy seemed to confirm the validity of his father's theories. William learned four languages, entered Harvard at fourteen, and became a brilliant mathematician; however, this precociousness soon had contrary results. The boy became subject to severe depressions and turned away from human relationships, and when he was old enough to throw off the authority of his parents, he rebelled completely. The arts and sciences made him ill. He fled from responsibility, from friendships, from everything except a morose desire to live alone. His chief interest was the hobby of collecting streetcar transfers, which he carried to absurd lengths. He quit jobs when he was recognized as the former boy prodigy and bitterly resented all efforts to return him to the academic life that had once absorbed him. In his forties, he was a clerk in the Massachusetts Department of Unemployment Compensation, earning sixteen dollars a week.

These are the dangers which threaten any child whose parents are impatient with normal growth and development and who, believing that *their* child is unique, deprive it of normal childhood. Nature has provided childhood for a purpose. We tamper with it at our own and our child's peril.

An intercurrent undertaking entitled *Modern Concepts of Psychoanalysis* under my co-editorship with Dr. Leon Salzman of Washington, D. C. eventually emerged from a welter of correspondence and was published by the Philosophical Library.

October 17, 1960

Dear Leon:

If we are to make any publisher's list by the spring of 1961, we must have the *Modern Concepts* manuscript reviewed, edited, and accepted by early January. I therefore have spent the weekend reading the papers submitted thus far, and herewith my comments on them, alphabetically by authors:

I.H.—"Object-Relation Theory and Ego-Theory": an overlong horror myth of the "introjected bad mother" (Little Red's grandmother eating the wolf variety) but with less interesting *dramatis personae.* If we want these aspects of British cultism represented, the least we can do is ask (the author) to condense his peregrinations to not more than 15 pages—a generous allowance of our readers' patience. Frankly, I don't know anyone outside London or Leeds who would, literally or symbolically, buy this Kleinian Nachtmusik.

I.L.—"Modern Concepts in Psychoanalysis": Begins here on earth among real people and recognizable realities, but quickly zooms to the cerulean stratosphere above left field, where it gets quite lost from mortal view; in fact, after page 15 the text becomes almost incomprehensible. We cannot publish this material in any book that wishes to be indexed under either "science" or "psychoanalysis." We must ask I., for his sake as well as our own, for a rewrite.

Carney Landis—"Viewpoint of an Experimental Psychologist": Superficial criticisms of Freud on the basis of the outmoded concepts of experimental psychology (dated circa 1920-40). More modern, comprehensive, and constructive criticisms have been published, but what he writes is still relevant.

Judd Marmor—"A Reevaluation of Certain Aspects of Psychoanalytic Theory and Practice": Powerful and effective medicine despite Marmorial delayed-action sugarcoating. Judd has never written better, and his and Ruesch's articles, if not too diluted by pap elsewhere, could make the book.

Ashley Montagu—"Man and Human Nature": A smart-alecky and overdramatized jeremiad. I have edited it extensively (in easily erasable red pencil) but it needs more; also retyping. Can possibly be used as condensed and revised.

Jurgen Ruesch—A surpassingly deep and clear thinker who has produced a superb review, comprehensive in content and elegant in style. Accept; hardly a word needing alteration.

Edith Weigert—"The Nature of Sympathy in the Art of Psychotherapy": A euphoniously written paper, full of her characteristically high-minded ambiguities. On one sample page (7) not a single key term (e.g., emotion, empathy, positive, negative, contagion, etc.) is defined, with the result that the whole has the effect of impalpable mood music—ending unresolved in the atonal chord of "autonomy"—itself vaguely depreciated two pages later. However, the paper is saved when Edith returns to clinical eloquence after page 14, and can therefore be used.

The question of a publisher is becoming daily a more difficult one. Saunders is busily engaged with the second edition of my revised *Principles*, and does not usually publish compendia. However, if you agree, I can inquire of Henry or Saunders as to their interest, and we can go on from there.

An example of the courteous hypocrisy demanded of editors:

October 17, 1960

Dear Dr. E. X.______:

We greatly regret that, after conferences with prospective publishers, we must change the contents of our projected volume on *Modern Concepts of Psychoanalysis* so that your own excellent contribution would be out of context. We are therefore releasing it to you with our sincere thanks for your courtesies.

The volume was published by the Philosophical Library Press, reprinted in England, issued again here in paperback, and achieved fair success.

Next came my *Modern Therapy of Personality Disorders* with this preface:

A professor of psychiatry is a man of many sorrows—not the least of which is that his staff and he must spend a great deal of time in *un*teaching. This is necessary because many advanced students of medicine, social work, psychology, sociology, nursing, and related disciplines seem to have learned, back in their early college days, so much about human behavior that either was hidden almost inextricably in outmoded technical Kraepelinian, Pavlovian, Freudian or Rogerian jargon—or else simply wasn't so.

It therefore seemed an act of mercy to all concerned to write this review—brief, yet hopefully clear and comprehensive—of more modern approaches to an understanding of human conduct: its biologic roots, its development, its vicissitudes, and the interrelated physiologic, individual, and social methods of correcting undesirable deviations and restoring optimum happiness and creativity.

May it be received in the kindly spirit in which it was written.

Valued appraisals:

October 10, 1966

Dear Jules:

My mail today contained among many items something that I truly value. I am, of course, referring to your beautiful little volume entitled *Modern Therapy of Personality Disorders.* It is indeed a masterful job and one that we will make sure that our residents read during the first week that they start their residency with us.

Edward M. Litin, M.D.
Chairman, Department of Psychiatry
Mayo Clinic, Rochester, Minnesota

October 18, 1966

Dear Jules:

On returning from lunch, I found on my desk the *Modern Therapy of Personality Disorders.* I am simply astonished—

even at first glance—at the clarity and scholarship that you succeed in compressing into 117 brief pages. I hope to learn not only in substance, but something about style.

It is a remarkable accomplishment and I am putting it beside our tome as an object lession and inspiration. Many thanks.

Best Wishes,
Daniel X. Freedman, M.D.
Professor and Chairman of Psychiatry
University of Chicago

Preliminary to the publication of *Psychiatry, East and West* (cf. Chapter 20):

August 12, 1968

Dr. Henry Stratton
Grune & Stratton, Inc.

Dear Henry:

Since you have become not only an Honorary Fellow of the APA but also its acknowledged chronicler, I am sending you herewith the Proceedings of the Association's Fifth International Psychiatric Conference, entitled *Transcultural Problems of Youth,* to which I invited the reputedly leading experts from a dozen typical socio-economic cultures around the world. The topic is certainly of universal interest and, by editing the transcript for the apparently inevitable prolixities, redundancies, vague speculations, and empty *recherché* with which too many writers padded their presentations, I have reduced the manuscript from over five hundred pages to its present 140-page readable size.

Please glance over the text and advise. Meanwhile, our very best to you.

The book was accepted by Dr. Stratton with a gentle reminder that its publication would probably profit neither of us —if finances alone rather than international considerations were at stake. My letter to the Executive Editor:

September 22, 1967

Duncan Mackintosh
Vice President
Grune & Stratton, Inc.

Dear Duncan:

I appreciate Dr. Henry Stratton's generous acceptance of this brief manuscript, but as an old friend I would not have offered it to you if I did not really believe that it is a fairly valuable contribution to the literature. This may be so for a number of reasons, among them the following:

1. It deals with a topic of intense current interest in many fields: i.e., psychiatric theory and practice in differing sociocultural-political systems, particularly those under Communist regimes.

2. It considers these influences not only in Russia but in Poland, East Germany, Czechoslovakia, Hungary, and Rumania and also in border countries, such as Turkey and Greece.

3. It traces the remarkable progress of Communist psychiatry through four successive International Conferences on Psychiatry and contrasts it with concurrent developments in Britain, France, Israel, and the United States.

4. It presents these developments not as the hurried, partial, and possibly prejudiced impressions of foreign visitors, but as reviews by representative authorities native to and thoroughly acquainted with each country.

5. The comments by colleagues from other lands, East and West, are edited down from about 600 diffuse transcript pages to about 60 trenchant ones—without, I hope, complete sacrifice of spontaneity.

6. These interchanges were further focused and clarified in the final clinical conference by mutual concentration on actual patients openly interviewed by psychiatrists from East

and West and then discussed as to diagnosis, prognosis, and therapy—with concurrent comments from a select professional audience.

I shall of course leave the format in your expert hands, but I would be perfectly willing to have it published in paperback as inexpensively as possible, thus promoting greater distribution and—I hope—eventually more profit for Grune & Stratton.

Soon after, I published a monograph on "The Biodynamic Roots of Human Behavior." The first page of the preface:

Picture a scene some fifteen years ago in my basement animal laboratory at Northwestern University Medical School. The *dramatis personae* consist of a psychoanalyst on a Dante-esque trip to the nether regions of science, myself, and a cebus monkey named Sisyphus. Some months ago Sisyphus had been subjected to several unexpected encounters with a mechanical snake exhibited simultaneously with a conditioned food reward, and had developed persistent feeding inhibitions, multiple phobias, severe gastro-intestinal and sexual dysfunctions, peculiar stereotypies, and "dereistic" patterns such as eating wholly imaginary food or maintaining cataleptic posture for hours at a time. The monkey is silent, but the other two characters speak:

Visiting Psychoanalyst (after observing Sisyphus somewhat disapprovingly for a few minutes): "And is this what you call an 'experimental neurosis?' "

I (with polite trepidation) "Well . . . operationally, yes. The phenomena you see seem to be analogous to those we call neurotic or even psychotic in the human, and can quite predictably be induced by controlled experimental techniques . . ."

Psychoanalyst (patronizingly) "But I can easily demonstrate that this animal *does not* have a neurosis!"

I (humbly): "Please do."

Psychoanalyst (pedagogically) "All we have to do is use basic analytic concepts. Can a monkey know its own father?"

I (reflectively) "Well, half its DNA *is* paternal, but I don't suppose Sisyphus can ever be induced to admit it."

Psychoanalyst (patiently): "You see, you are already defensive. But if this monkey never knew its own father, can it have an Oedipus complex?"

I (puzzled, as usual): "But none of us—including Oedipus—can ever really be sure who *was* his father."

Psychoanalyst (triumphantly): "Nevertheless, if you had ever been thoroughly analyzed, you would *know* that despite the fact that the toy snake was a phallic threat to the monkey, in the absence of an Oedipus complex there can be no neurosis!"

Sisyphus moans softly . . .

I (*sotto voce*): " *Non erat demonstrandum. Et non credo, quia absurdum est.* "

Sisyphus moans softly . . .

This scene, fantastic in recall, nevertheless occurred almost literally as described even though innumerable observations in field and laboratory, as clearly reported, had shown (a) that many patterns of behavior previously thought to be exclusively human (for example, familial loyalty, peer alliances, altruism) could be elicited in laboratory animals or observed in animals in their feral state; (b) that the dynamics of much deviant conduct could be traced not only to conflicts of attraction and aversion, but also to impasses of positive choice or to any stresses that exceeded the animal's genetic or learned capacities for adequate prediction and adaptation; and (c) that our own had, with significant clinical relevance, explored the rationale of the physical, dyadic, and group modalities of "therapy" that could modify or reverse the neurotic process.

Comments on this opus:

January 23, 1969

Dear Jules:

Your "The Biodynamic Roots of Human Behavior" is certainly a very much needed and excellent addition to the literature on the subject of psychiatry. You can be classed as one of the outstanding thinkers in psychiatry not only here in our country but in the world.

Again many thanks and warm personal regards.

Richard H. Young, M.D.
Dean, Medical School
Northwestern University

A more protracted and whimsical coda sent me in manuscript by Arnold Mandel, Professor and Chairman of Psychiatry at the new La Jolla campus of the University of California, was eventually published in *Social Psychiatry* under the title "Jules Masserman—The Last of the Red Hot Mammas":

> The Fiskes and the Vanderbilts, even the Watsons and the Averys are gone. In their place are management teams and computers, technicians and statistics (who knows the name of the group that made Xerox go?). In the same way, gone are the Jolsons, the Garlands, and the Gables. The smash this season on the tube was Laugh In; a highly complex piece of tickle that ostensibly had stars (Rowan and Martin) but entertained with a cascade of unidentifiable people doing intricately timed bits with a "mad" producer-director and a team of television experts punching the control cards. Polling teams produced instant feed-back correctives for next week's game plan. It appears that the cult of the charismatic character is gone . . .
>
> Much in the same way, it appears that the frontiers in research and theory in psychiatry have gone through a rather radical transition in the past decade, away from magnetic personalities and ideas to a more anonymous accrual of small bits of information by less stellar but larger groups of research teams. It would seem appropriate, upon the recent publication of a book by a Sophie Tucker [of psychiatry] ("the last of the red-hot mammas") to review briefly the historical

context which seems to make the man and his theory more meaningful.

Most of us in psychiatry can trace the history of the ideas of our field with the same methods used by the genealogist. Progressions from the charismatic "greats" have substituted for the history of findings and ideas that characterize other fields of scientific endeavor. Kuhn, in a recent essay, has used the history of physics in the 18th and 19th century to define a cause of change in theory and method in a field: the anomalous finding . . . In psychiatry, it appears that in the past the transitions depended on the emergence of a figure who wrote, talked, and socialized while manifesting that mystical set of properties that make for leadership. Such a person would need intelligence, curiosity, breadth, courage, and sufficient psychosocial valence to reach into the growing body of psychiatry and be heard. . . . Often a dabbler in various peripheral fields (ethology, neurophysiology, biochemistry, animal experimental behavior), the owner of this rare voice would occasionally launch himself into a lifelong attempt to broaden, change, feed-back on, and influence a progression of theory from Freud that moved down the generations of psychiatrists with the same social force (and probably the same dynamics) as a theory of social behavior moved from Abraham, to Isaac, to Jacob. The price . . . was pretty great. These too few fresh voices were often disenfranchized (informally, of course—like segregation in California) by many of their institutional connections. The basic science establishment viewed their findings with a monumental lack of enthusiasm; their data were seen as limited either by its manifestations of technological lag (after all, who can be an expert in everything) or by overdrawn conclusions (desperate efforts to stretch experimental findings into the realm of human behavior theory). The psychodynamicists responded to these voices as bearers of nonapplicable trivia ("What does this mean about treating my patients?"), and the psychoanalytic institutes disavowed their title of psychoanalyst.

It seems to me that both Jules Masserman and his recent book, *The Biodynamic Roots of Human Behavior,* are most appropriately seen through this view of psychiatric history. His was one of these early, wonderfully fresh voices; his has been a lifelong attempt to keep the scientific findings of related fields alive in psychiatric theory; his role has included intense personal involvement with academic ideals and the encouragement of the young psychiatric investigator to work in the laboratory; he went (and goes) there himself. And, at the same time, he continued to allow himself to be [involved] with clinical patients and teaching and attempted to find rapprochement between these activities. He was doing this when it was a lot tougher than it is now . . . Jules Masserman was a pioneer in an era of charismatic transition who pointed the way toward modern academic psychiatry through the sheer strength of his intellect, personality, and perseverance. And yet, he is not finished.

His recent book is an elegant essay that weaves biological and behavioral concerns into a pattern of theory consonant with many if not most of modern psychodynamic thinking. Using material from history, political science, literature, zoology, anthropology, bacteriology, architecture, information processing, neurophysiology, ethology, neuroanatomy, psychopharmacology, experimental animal behavior, developmental psychologoy, family dynamics, and physics (I may have left out a few), he derives his "biodynamic theory." Following a delightful mock (?) interview with a "straw analyst" who refused to accept an induced syndrome of multiple phobias, sexual dysfunction, and bizzare behavior in a monkey as a possible model for human neurosis, Masserman puts up a hard to refute series of arguments as to the applicability of observations from ethology and what he calls "comparative biodynamics" (forgive him—

he means animal experiments) to an understanding of the psychodynamics and psychopathology of man.

He then elaborates systematic definitions (with pertinent references) of various concepts from other fields—the ingredients for his later "biodynamic" concoction. From ethology he brings the reader instinct, social releaser, and imprinting; from neurophysiological neuroanatomy, he brings the oral, aggressive and sexual features of the limbic-hypothalamic system; from molecular biology he presents (every clinical field needs a Sol Hurok for the basic sciences) DNA and biorhythmicity; from developmental psychology, he presents the influence of early infantile experience; and from information processing theory, he describes experiments that have used this model. He follows this mélange with a description of interesting ethological and comparative experimental aspects of the behavior of creatures at various levels of the evolutionary scale, noting similarities between these and the human predicament (he had protected himself in the introduction from potential accusations of anthropomorphizing by reducing us all to the limits of a "Kantian mind"). In his concluding section on human values, he lists what he calls the three "*Ur*" values that he feels are goals for all man . . . Even after all the pleas for a comparative view, he admits we humans are "on beyond zebra" after all (to borrow from Dr. Seuss).

What is the purpose of such a theory (and theorizer)? I think that both in the past decades and perhaps even today (as a mopping-up operation), this man and his work: (1) Keeps psychiatry broadly concerned; (2) Helps legitimatize research and scholarship in many fields as pertinent to psychiatry; (3) Inspires young psychiatrists to look into various other disciplines by both making them exciting and not too far afield from their specialty; (4) Helps purely psychodynamic psychiatrists feel "scientific" and at the same time goads them into reading other fields (a good psychotherapist, he contributes some narcissistic supplies before making a dystonic interpretation); (5) Makes for lots of intellectual fun.

Though I suspect he doesn't need encouragement to write more books, please let every year continue to bring us another Masserman Book.

When I send Dr. Mandell *this* book, I shall autograph it:

Dear Ernie,

Herewith another. Possibly the last.

14. ISPI: THE BIRTH AND GROWTH OF A RESIDENCY TRAINING PROGRAM

On June 22, 1957, Governor William G. Stratton appointed me to the nine-man Illinois Research and Training Authority, charged with dispensing a million dollars annually in support of selected projects "for teaching and investigation as part of an overall program designed to promote the mental health of the citizens of Illinois." Part of this program was the opening in Chicago of the new thirty-million dollar Illinois State Psychiatric Institute (ISPI), whereupon my first act as Authority member was to recommend as its director Dr. Lester Rudy, a former student of mine who also happened to be the most able young administrator in the State. His first act was to put me in a somewhat difficult position by requesting that I be director of education for the new Institute—difficult because I was already co-chairman of psychiatry at Northwestern, because there were seven residency training programs at other schools and institutes in Chicago, and because I already had a plethora of clinical, research, administrative, and editorial commitments. Nevertheless, I accepted on these conditions:

1. That the Institute cooperate closely with, rather than compete against, these other programs.
2. That this collaboration be effected through an advisory

body consisting of representatives from each of the other schools.

3. That each of the schools undertake to supervise the clinical services on one floor of the Institute, to rotate its residents through these services, and to cooperate in the overall training program of the institute by appointing instructors and consultants from its faculty.

4. That the Institute's own training program be truly comprehensive and pedagogically progressive.

5. That I develop and administer the program on a part-time basis until it was well established, after which a full-time successor would be found.

When the official notice of appointment came from Dr. Otto Bettag, then State Director of Public Welfare, I sent an acceptance with an addendum as follows:

Dear Dr. Bettag:

I am, of course, gratified by your telephone notification and the departmental news release announcing my appointment as director of education of the Illinois Psychiatric Institute. However, since to date we have had no opportunity to discuss the nature and duties of this appointment and since these should also be determined and supervised by a properly constituted Advisory Board of the Institute, I respectfully submit that my acceptance should be contingent on the following:

1. The selection of an Advisory Board, which I hope will include Dr. Francis Gerty, Dr. Roy Grinker, Dr. Percival Bailey, Dr. John Madden, Dr. Ben Boshes, and others who have long done fundamental work in planning and implementing the Institute, and whose continued services would be essential to its success.

2. The approval by the Advisory Board of all the key appointments to the Institute, no matter how well qualified the candidates may appear to be. As to my own appointment, if and when the Board prefers full-time service or another appointee, I shall be glad to withdraw, or to serve in any other designated capacity.

3. The approval by the Board of all programs and plans

submitted to it by officers of the Institute, particularly with regard to basic policies of clinical service, research, and education. I shall prepare detailed plans for the training program, including recruitment of residents, university collaboration in teaching, service rotation through state hospitals, etc., but I could not proceed with any program—nor would I desire to—without the approval, confidence and collaboration of the Board, and of the universities and institutes it will represent.

Again, I am gratified by the Department's confidence in me, and submit the above so that we may begin our work in a manner best calculated to achieve the purpose we all share with you: to make the new Institute of maximal service to the State and outstanding in its field in the nation.

With a personal addendum:

August 18, 1958

Dear Otto:

Herewith the official letter, with this private note to assure you it is intended in the friendliest of spirits and solely for the best interests of the Institute. As to the details of my own appointment, may I suggest:

1. That you make it about 1/3 time since, though I'll actually be spending much more than this over-all on the many duties involved, that form of appointment would avoid any criticism of my not being physically present at the Institute eight to ten hours every day.

2. That the salary be at a level to seem fair to the administration and the public. For comparison, I may submit that my combined annual salary from the Veterans Administration to supervise training at the Downey VA Hospital with personal attendance only one day per week is $7,500 plus supplementary consultant's fees from the Great Lakes Naval Hospital. Actually, I am resigned to the fact that my new duties as Director of Education at the Institute will take sufficiently more time out of my private practice, writing, lecture fees, etc. to reduce my total income to a considerable extent in which case a few

hundred more or less in my state salary would not make enough difference to compensate for possible criticism of the Department.

But suspend all these concerns for a bit, and have a swell time on your trip abroad.

The first task was to prepare a brochure that would best describe the new Institute and its associated facilities, outline my projected training program and thus attract qualified trainees. The Prologue to the first edition read as follows:

> For over half a century, medical and educational leaders in Illinois have been planning an institute which would combine the most modern facilities and resources for care, treatment and rehabilitation of the mentally ill, for psychiatric and other training of personnel to serve in this field, and for research relating to mental health and mental illness.
>
> This plan has been translated into reality. The Illinois State Psychiatric Institute, located in the state's famed medical center in Chicago, is a striking symbol of the cooperation among the medical and educational professions in the State of Illinois.
>
> The Institute, containing facilities for the care and treatment of 320 mental patients and linking them to comprehensive programs in psychiatric training, education and research fulfills a triple function. It is the physical product of the combined wisdom and experience of experts in many fields, and has invited international attention to progress in the field of mental health.
>
> Operated by the Illinois Department of Public Welfare, the Institute joins within its walls separate divisions staffed by the psychiatric faculties of seven post-graduate schools of psychiatry, and the Chicago Psychoanalytic Institute, thus offering to those seeking it advanced education that compares favorably with that available anywhere.
>
> The training program will furnish the didactic and laboratory instruction and supervised experi-

> ence designed to qualify the candidate for the professionally competent and socially responsible practice of psychiatry, and interest him in the dignity and satisfactions of the clinical, research, teaching, and administrative careers available to him in the Illinois Department of Public Welfare and related institutions.

There then followed descriptions of these facilities, outlines of courses, lists of outstanding instructors recruited from the five university facilities, modes, and hours of individualized clinical supervision, qualifications for various levels of training, scale of stipends, and not of least importance, provisions for the aid in finding housing, recreation, and schooling for children.

The Advisory Board, later called the Psychiatric Council, was duly instituted, and on December 1, 1958, I submitted a tentative outline of a proposed schedule for training. It follows:

Interim Report of Plans for Residency Training

1. *Purposes of Submission:* This schedule has been prepared sufficiently in advance of the opening of the Institute for the following reasons: (a) So that it may be revised in accordance with the suggestions of the advisory body; (b) To acquaint consultants and other appointees from the universities and institutes with the projected organization of the program; (c) To submit, in revised form, to the certification committees of the AMA and the American Board of Neurology and Psychiatry in order to obtain approval and appropriate listing in the AMA directory of approved residencies. (d) For distribution, with other information, to prospective trainees.

2. *First Year:*

Distribution of Time: The scheduled work week consists of about 45 hours, exclusive of emergency duty estimated about twice monthly; this should leave the trainee sufficient leisure for reading, thought, and/or familial or other life. Of the assigned 45 hours, about 12 per week are spent in didactic courses as indicated; the remaining 33 are for direct or supervised clinical service to patients. The academic year of three trimesters parallels the schedules of the participating universities and institutes, so that the summer quarter may be devoted to make-up study, service, and necessary vacations for residents, consultants, and staff. Residents beginning work in July will be given preliminary orientation courses. Tuesdays are kept relatively free to permit everyone interested to spend the day with prominent invited lecturers to be scheduled once monthly or so. It is hoped that the Illinois Psychiatric, Chicago Neurological and Chicago Psychoanalytic Institutes and other societies will also take advantage of our auditorium to hold their meetings at the Institute, thus affording additional learning opportunities for our residents and staff.

Progression of Courses: Those essential to the initial orientation of the resident (neurologic and psychiatric examination, diagnosis, hospital therapy, and other procedures) are scheduled early, with theoretical elaborations presented in later contexts.

Lectures: All Institute residents will be assigned to all training courses and seminars; other residents are welcome, but may or may not be assigned to these by their respective services. Trainees in psychology, social work, nursing, etc. may attend after proper arrangements with their respective training supervisors.

All didactic courses will be given by full-timc or half-time personnel from the staff of the Institute or the IJR, thus assuring competence and continuity as well as budgetary economy. The lectures are so distributed as not to overburden any single instructor, yet enlisting the active interest and participation of as many as possible in the program.

Assignment of Residents to Ward Work and Supervision: The residents of the universities and institutes rotating through the Institute will be under the direct supervision of their service directors and consultants appointed by the respective university or institute. Psychiatric Institute residents assigned by agreement to rotate for a semester through a service will also be under the supervision of that service. In this way each resident can profit not only from group rounds and seminars, but from individualized case supervision for diagnosis and continued therapy from two to four hours per week.

OPD: The schedule provides for outpatient department service available for all residents on Monday and Wednesday afternoons, so that they may be given supervised experience in (a) consultant outpatient work; (b) individual follow-up, especially for patients previously hospitalized on their service; and (c) family therapy.

3. *Second Year:* Insofar as practicable, it is planned to have all residents in the current Department of Public Welfare Training Program spend at least one trimester of experience at the Institute before being reassigned for one year of service and further clinical training at a State Hospital. (In those of our state hospitals not at present approved by the Board, the maximum period is six months.)

4. *Third Year:* There is no immediate urgency for a detailed schedule of the third year of training, but the following is envisioned:

Courses: (a) Review and advanced courses in neuroanatomy, physiology, neurology, and neurosurgical indications. (b) Further training in the theories and methods of various schools. (c) Review and advanced courses in drug and shock therapies. (d) Forensic and Industrial Psychiatry. (e) Recent developments: Existentialism, systems and transaction theory, "behavior therapy," etc. (f) Research and statistical techniques. (g) Practice teaching of aids and student nurses.

Cultural Supplementation: Lectures in anthropology, sociology, linguistics, semantics, and philosophy.

Rotating Clinical Services: (a) Senior residency at the Institute and/or: (b) The Institute for Juvenile Research (six months) (c) The County M. H. Clinic (one month) (d) Orientation Services at the Criminal court (three weeks) and the county jail (two weeks). (e) Other rotating assignments as approved by the Residency Board.

I shall welcome suggestions for revisions or supplementations of these tentative plans.

With the principal features of the program available for evaluation, application for official approval could be made.

March 20, 1959

Dr. Walter S. Wiggins
Secretary, Council on Medical Education
American Medical Association

Dear Dr. Wiggins:

Dr. Lester Rudy, superintendent of the new Illinois State Psychiatric Institute, and I as the director of education, respectfully request your approval of its Residency Training Program in Psychiatry as described in the attached brochure.

Please be assured that all of the faculty members listed therein have pledged their active participation, that the didactic and clinical teaching will be given substantially as outlined, and that the institute, due to be completed within a few weeks and occupied shortly thereafter, will furnish superb facilities for training and research programs.

Since we hope to recruit resident trainees of high calibre to begin their duties not later than September, 1959, we would appreciate your tentative approval of this program—subject, of course, to later inspection and review—as early as convenient to you.

The program was promptly inspected and approved by the Council, the American Medical Association and the American Board of Neurology and Psychiatry. ISPI developed so rapidly that within another eleven months I could submit to the Advisory Board a rather lengthy and detailed report of progress. Excerpts:

Recruitment; the preparation and nationwide distribution of the new Residency Training Brochure, supplemented by personal efforts at recruitment by members of the ISPI staff, elicited about 150 written inquiries, each of which was given my individual attention. Fourteen first-year, six second-year, and five third-year residents have been enrolled and thirty more have accepted for 1960. Additional residents from the associated university and other training centers will rotate through their respective services at ISPI and also participate in the training program.

First Year at ISPI to consist of *(a)* fundamental didactic training in psychiatry and neurology and *(b)* intensively supervised clinical inpatient and OPD experiences. Schedules of lectures, instructors and supervisory clinical consultants include: *Neurology:* anatomy, chemistry and pharmacology, physiology, neurobiology, pathology, EEG and roentgenology, diagnosis, clinical neurology. *Psychiatry:* history, techniques of examination, clinical syndromes, child development, integrative psychiatry and psychotherapy, family dynamics, psychosomatics, social and forensic psychiatry, administrative procedures, techniques of psychotherapy, and hospital therapies. *Social Service:* History, Community Resources, and Techniques. *Psychology:* Diagnostic tests, Interpretations and Research techniques. *Ancillary Procedures* and *Activities:* Psychodrama, and recreational, music, and occupational therapies. *Other Didactic Teaching:* Daily ward conferences, biweekly seminars on group therapy, bimonthly intercom programs, weekly literature seminars, and approximately monthly lectures by visiting authorities in special fields. *Clinical Supervision:* Inpatient: four half-day consultants per week for direct supervision of the residents' diagnostic and therapeutic procedures. *Outpatient*: the OPD provides supervised intake conferences twice weekly and three additional hours of consultation per week for all residents. *Teaching Aides:* Each resident is furnished with a handbook of hospital procedures (assembled for ISPI in collaboration with Dr. Jackson Smith, Clinical Director, and for Chicago State with Directors H. Maltz and M. Gross) history-taking forms, medication guides, a classified list of required and other recommended readings, and other teaching aides. Library facilities and services have been expanded. *Films* (as film editor for the JAMA, I have arranged to have all new releases reviewed at ISPI), tapes and one-way screens will be used as indicated.

Second Year to be devoted to advanced training in clinical and administrative skills at one of the State Hospitals. By arrangements with the superintendents and staffs, Chicago State, Elgin, and Galesburg have been utilized to date, and other hospitals will be included as their personnel and facilities are developed. *Second Year State Hospital Training:* The principal center will continue to be Chicago State where most second-year residents will be assigned for didactic instruction and clinical supervision in modern methods of individual and group therapy, with interdisciplinary collaboration, ward management and administration responsibility. Arrangements have also been made to continue approved training at Galesburg where two residents are assigned, and to begin reinstituting it at Elgin by an initial six-month rotation of one resident.

Third Year: All residents in this category are now assigned to the Institute for Juvenile Research, ISPI-OPD, or in special classes and court services as indicated above. *Teaching Records:* Outlines or more detailed contents of all lecture courses as provided by each lecturer are kept on file in the education office. *Grading and Promotion:* A system with appropriate forms and procedures had been instituted for securing reports on each resident's progress in education and service as judged weekly by his teachers and clinical supervisors. These reports are co-ordinated in my office, relayed to the Department of Public Welfare, and made the basis for promotion or other action by the Residency Committee. To date, only one resident has been dropped, and only one other has not been granted a scheduled promotion. Group collaboration and morale are maintained by weekly group meetings and individual conferences.

Recruitment of Teachers: These fall into the following categories: (1) *Members of the ISPI Council:* The chairmen of all associated departments of psychiatry at each of the collaborating medical schools and institutes have given their time and effort gratis in direct teaching of residents and staff and in other invaluable contributions to the program. Monthly reports of plans and progress are given to the Council for their official advice, amendment or approval. (2) *ISPI Staff:* Many members of the technical as well as the medical staff have added highly effective teaching and supervision of residents to their other duties. (3) *Consultants:* After canvassing all the highly trained and experienced psychiatrists in Illinois who would be qualified as teachers and supervisors, the Director of Education submitted successive lists for approval by the ISPI Council. Attached is the current roster of seventy-six exceptionally well trained and able Consultants so appointed for service as needed; of these, more than half have actively participated, and the others have signified their willingness to serve at ISPI or at other state hospital programs to be described below. Monthly meetings are held with the consultants to foster their continued interest and collaboration, and they have accepted a fair fee schedule for time and travel as recommended by the council and approved by the DPW.

Service to Patients: Throughout his training each resident spends at least two thirds of his time in direct or indirect care of patients, and this service is supervised with sufficient frequency by highly trained and experienced men to ensure its high calibre. To this may be added the following advantages: (1) Direct therapy of patients by the teaching consultants. (2) Improved morale and therapeutic efficiency of nursing, social service, and other staff personnel. (3) Teaching services by advanced residents for nurses, aides, and ancillary employees. (4) Collaboration of residents in important research programs conducted by the Department of Public Welfare and associated medical schools and institutes. (5) Provision to these schools, institutes, and other agencies (e.g., the Institute for Juvenile Research, the Courts, the Cook County Mental Hygiene Clinic) of collateral teaching personnel and facilities, thereby further interesting them in DPW functions, training, and research. (6) Recruiting psychiatric trainees for permanent service to the DPW; in fact, candidates are now selected in large part because of a sincere intent to remain in academic and institutional work in this State. (7) Concurrently attracting trained and experienced psychiatrists, neurologists, and experts in related behavioral sciences to serve as clinicians, teachers, and research supervisors at ISPI and other DPW institutions.

Training of State Hospital Personnel

In further fulfillment of the purposes of ISPI as a training and research Institute to serve the entire State, a second general plan was developed to improve patient care in all Department of Public Welfare institutions by direct training and continuous expert supervision of their medical and associated personnel. Under the auspices of one of the participating schools and institutes, members and consultants on the ISPI staff were to provide one full day each week for nine months per year at each hospital. Their duties would be not only to give formal courses, but to make ward rounds, and provide individual and group supervision for all categories of professional personnel as particularly suited to the needs of each hospital. Annual or biannual intensive courses in psychiatric theory, diagnosis, and therapy are to be held at ISPI for State Hospital physicians.

Briefly, these plans have been put into effect as follows: (1) *Local Training at State Hospitals:* Individualized programs for each hospital are herewith listed alphabetically (and given in detail for six State Hospitals throughout Illinois). (2) *Training Courses at ISPI for State Hospital Personnel:* In accordance with plans developed in collaboration with the staff and consultants of ISPI and with individual State Hospital superintendents, one or two staff members from each state hospital will be sent to ISPI in October, 1960, for four weeks of review lectures in basic neurologic and psychiatric theory, and intensive clinical supervision in diagnostic, therapeutic, and administrative procedures; arrangements are being made by the DPW to cover their travel, living arrangements, and per diem expenses. It is hoped that when these physicians return to their respective hospitals they will impart some of their instruction to other members of the hospital staff, and thus multiply the effects of this section of the program. (3) *Other Methods of Staff Instruction:* The above arrangements are intended to fulfill the individual needs of each state hospital's staff by direct, on-the-scene, and competent instruction and supervision. Supplementary methods also currently employed are: Lectures, case discussions, seminars, etc. by telecommunication to DPW institutions twice monthly; Circulation of scientific films, tapes, books and periodicals from a central repository at ISPI; Regular visits to all DPW training institutions by Dr. Rudy, Dr. Smith, the Director of Education, and it is hoped, an assistant yet to be appointed.

Instruction of Non-Medical Personnel

Nursing Education: Nursing instructors attend designated lectures and seminars at ISPI, and all nurses participate in daily ward conferences. Instruction of nurse trainees at Chicago State and elsewhere is furnished by ISPI consultants and residents. *Social Service:* Similar arrangements have been worked out for teaching social service trainees and utilizing S.S. staff in turn in the instruction of residents at ISPI and the staffs of the various state hospitals. *Psychology:* This program includes conjoint seminars with staff psychologists and lectures in psychology by them to psychiatric residents.

Aides and Other Personnel: Clinical instruction has been furnished by service chiefs at ISPI and by consultants and residents at other state institutions.

Medical students: the facilities of ISPI are already being utilized for teaching psychiatry to undergraduates by Northwestern, Loyola, the University of Illinois, and plans for this liaison are being considered by the other medical schools. At no budgetary expense, this provides added service to patients, and further interests the faculties and residents of the schools in DPW activities.

Characteristically, Dr. Rudy wrote:

January 22, 1960

Dear Dr. Masserman:

Receipt of the year-end report of the Director of Education of the Illinois State Psychiatric Institute is hereby acknowledged.

You are to be commended for accomplishing the transition of the Illinois State Psychopathic program to the Illinois State

Psychiatric Institute with minimum friction and an improvement in the relationships with the state hospitals.

The ready acceptance of the program by the Council as well as the evolution of an outstanding Department of Education, has been due to your fine organization, devotion, and industriousness.

Please accept my sincere thanks and appreciation for all that you have done and what we may accomplish in the future.

Very sincerely yours,
Lester H. Rudy, M.D.
Director
Illinois State Psychiatric Institute

January 27, 1960

Dear Les:

Many thanks for your note. I doubt I would—or could—have done much if any one else had been director of ISPI.

Trainees from the staffs of the various state hospitals added:

October 26, 1960

Dear Dr. Masserman:

We wish to express our appreciation and gratefulness for being given the chance to acquire further experience in psychiatry. The series of scheduled lectures and case presentations will serve us enormously when we go back to our hospitals. For us this has been a new experience or one we have been away from for a long time, but in either case it has helped to clear up to a great extent many facets of development of our knowledge of psychiatry.

Multiple signatures

With ISPI well established and its training program accepted as an asset rather than a rival to the others in Chicago, I resigned my directorship of education to a full-time successor, Dr. Robert Drye, and continued as senior consultant. A bronze plaque commemorating the change in 1963 read as follows: "To Jules H. Masserman, M.D./In appreciation and Gratitude for his Contributions as an Outstanding Teacher/-Residents and Graduates of the Illinois State Psychiatric Institute."

Eleven years later, I submitted my farewell to the members of the Psychiatric Training and Research Authority:

June 1, 1968

Gentlemen:

As you may know, I am due to take my first sabbatical after 35 years of perhaps a not altogether wasted academic life. Beginning in October, 1968, I shall be lecturing at Australian and New Zealand universities as Invitational Professor, after which I shall be a Resident Fellow at the Center for Advanced Behavioral Studies in Palo Alto through June, 1969. During this period I plan to be in Chicago for about a week each month, timed insofar as possible so that I can attend the monthly meetings of the Authority (only one of which, as member and chairman I have missed since it was founded), continue to evaluate and report on grant applications assigned to my subcommittee in education and research, and perform all other services delegated to me by the Authority. However, I believe it to the best interests of the Authority to request relief from my duties as chairman, since (a) conducting the detailed and now often heavy duties of the office by mail to Palo Alto three weeks out of every four would not be practical, (b) we have a highly competent vice chairman and secretary who can efficiently conduct Authority affairs, and (c) their task will in turn be greatly lightened by our newly appointed and salaried executive secretary.

I therefore request leave to suspend my duties as Chairman of the Training and Research Authority from October 1,

1968, through June 30, 1969, after which I would be able to resume them until the expiration of my term in December, 1969.

Respectfully,

However, in the interim the Authority was dissolved by Richard B. Ogilvie, the newly elected Republican governor of Illinois.

Later, when called upon to help plan the reorganization of the Illinois Department of Mental Health:

August 29, 1969

John F. Briggs
Acting Director
Department of Mental Health
State of Illinois

Dear Mr. Briggs:

In response to your request, herewith a summary, with some additions, of our discussion of your thoughtfully prepared proposed reorganization of the Department of Mental Health. I shall review my suggestions as to your chart of July 1, 1969, very briefly, but shall be glad to elaborate them or propose alternatives as you may wish.

Levels of Organization

1. *Mental Health Director:* The qualifications for the post are not only a deep sensitivity to human medical and psychiatric needs and an awareness of modern modes of providing effective physical and mental care, but even more importantly, the foresight to envisage and the ability to manage realistically the highly complex financial, personnel, administrative, and political problems of the Department of Mental Health of a major state. Frankly, I know of only three or four psychiatrists in the entire country with this combined medical and executive ability.

2. *Director's Panels of "Blue Sky" Planning and Program:*

Advisory: I presume these would be analogous to a cabinet of medical, legal, sociologic, architectural, and other specialists directly advisory to the director and, therefore, properly his personal choice; if suggestions as to nominees in Illinois or elsewhere are desired, I shall be glad to furnish a roster of such consultants from the files of the American Psychiatric Association.

Director: This appointee had best be a psychiatrist with special training and experience in the social and community aspects of psychiatry, sufficient interpersonal charisma and skill to attract and retain professional and ancillary staff at all levels, and a greater interest in planning and supervising psychiatric services, training, and research in Illinois than in attaining personal prestige or power. Such men are available within the present department as well as elsewhere, and should be glad to leave the business details of the department to financial experts while working closely with them on matters of professional policies, planning, training and service.

Deputy Director of Research, Development and Training: I suggest that, since few men are equally interested or qualified in all three fields, this position be eliminated. Instead a better distribution of responsibilities would be to distribute these duties among three separate individuals on the level of management, namely: a divisional (or other appropriate title) supervisor of clinical services, a divisional supervisor of training, and a supervisor of research and development, with responsibilities as follows:

3. *Distribution of Divisional Responsibilities:*

Supervisor of Clinical Services: To help coordinate, under the Director and Deputy Director, the geographic, general catchment and special services of all Departmental hospitals, day care centers, halfway houses, OPD clinics, zones, etc. as listed in the fifth and bottom rows of the organization chart.

Supervisor of Research: A similar function for the laboratories and research programs at Illinois State Psychiatric Institute, the Pediatric Institute, Institute for Juvenile Research, Elgin, Galesburg, Anna, and elsewhere.

Supervisor of Training: To integrate and develop the training not only of psychiatric residents but also of psychologists, social workers, nurses, aides and other personnel as currently enrolled at Illinois State Psychiatric Institute, the Pediatric Institute, Institute for Juvenile Research and Galesburg to develop their simultaneous experience and service throughout all suitable Departmental facilities, and to coordinate such training wherever mutually advantageous with related programs at the several universities and institutes.

Advisory Panels: Even though (apart from management) each of the other supervisors (respectively of clinical services, training, and research) should be highly competent, they would want, for the advantage of their separate divisions, the benefit of advice from experts both within and out of the department, and in Illinois or elsewhere. Most of this aid could be obtained without departmental expense through the professional literature, association meetings, etc., but if special Advisory panels of four or five consultants could be set up for each supervisory division to meet three to five times a year, their members would soon learn the special problems of that division and be more helpful in their investigation and solution.

Recommendations as to Personnel:

Since you requested this also, permit me to submit names in confidence of persons not only well qualified by training, experience and personal dedication but also probably available.

1. *Departmental:*

Dr. Lester Rudy, Director of ISPI alternatively, Dr. Al Glass of Oklahoma;

2. *Divisional:* Supervisor of Clinical Services: Dr. Jack Weinberg, clinical director of ISPI. Supervisor of Training: Dr. Patrick Staunton of your department. Supervisor of Research: Dr. Peter Levison.

As you may know, when the Illinois State Psychiatric Institute was founded I organized its training programs, secured their approval by the AMA and APA, directed them for three years until a full-time director could be found, and since then have been senior consultant for Training until the present. During that time I had excellent opportunities to appraise the abilities of Drs. Rudy, Weinberg and Staunton, and can recommend them highly.

Again as you are aware, I was appointed a member of the Research and Training Authority when it was first instituted under the preceding Republican Administration, wrote its Code of Procedures, and served as its chairman until I left for my Fellowship year at the Behavioral Center in 1968-69. I can therefore certify that Dr. Levison, as secretary of the Authority, became well acquainted with research programs in Illinois and elsewhere, has good coordinating and administrative abilities, and is personally cooperative.

3. *Advisory Panels:* Under the present law, as I understand it, there is provision for only one panel of seven members, three from outside Illinois, to advise the department on all aspects of development, research, and training. To avoid any appearance of personal bias, I shall refrain from commenting on possible appointees from Illinois, who may have been members of the late Authority, and shall recommend only non-Illinoisian psychiatrists of national prominence in various fields to serve either on the seven-member Departmental Panel or as specialized consultants to the respective Divisions of service, training, and research. They are as follows: Dr. Milton Greenblatt, director, Massachusetts Department of Mental Health: Community Psychiatry; Dr. George Tarjan, professor, University of California in Los Angeles: Mental Retardation; Dr. Joel Elkes, chairman, Department of Psychiatry, Johns Hopkins University: Psychopharmacology; Dr. Jonathan Cole, National Institute of Mental Health: Research in Schizophrenia and Other Psychoses, Dr. Lewis R. Wolberg, director, Psychiatric Institute, New York: Psychiatric Therapies; Dr. James G. Miller, dean, University of Cleveland: Psychological Training and Services. In addition, I can recommend one local non-psychiatrist of national stature to serve as a valuable consultant on a training advisory panel: Dr. George Miller, head, Department of Research in Medical Education, University of Illinois School of Medicine.

The International Association of Social Psychiatry: Finally, as President of this Association, I am happy to formalize my invitation to the Illinois Department of Mental Health to join with Northwestern University and the Forest Hospital Foundation in sponsoring the next meeting of the International Association in Chicago sometime during the late autumn of 1970, with Governor Ogilvie and yourself among the official hosts.

To repeat, I shall be happy to elaborate or extend these suggestions as you wish and as circumstances warrant in further meetings or correspondence.

Sincerely,

Many of these recommendations were implemented.

15. EMPATHETIC DIAGNOSIS

Teaching and the writing of books have ever been fascinating indoor sports; fortunately, however, most psychiatrists cannot live merely by lectures or afterhours scribblings alone —a circumstance which, considering the quality of many of their didactic and literary efforts, is as it should be. So too, my own main interests have at all times been in clinical work: *i.e.,* in the dia-gnosis (Greek: thorough understanding) and therapy (Greek: *therapeuein,* to serve and cure) of my patients. As to the first category of practice, perhaps the most concise statements of my own approach are marshalled in the following *Suggestions for the Psychiatric and Psychosomatic Supplementation of the Medical Examination** I proposed for the use of trainees in *all* medical specialities:

Introductory Principles

Every medical disorder alters the personal and social behavior of a patient, and this in turn affects the symptomatology, course, and therapy of his illness. Similarly, environmental stresses, in persons born or made susceptible to them, may cause physiologic dysfunctions which, if severe and prolonged, may also lead to organic disease. Therefore no

*Modified from *Diseases of the Nervous System,* vol. 13, pp. 1-8, Aug. 1952.

medical diagnosis, prognosis, or therapy is complete unless it includes an evaluation of (1) the patient's deviations in *total* behavior as well as in organic function (present illness), (2) his constitutional and characterologic development (personality tendencies), and (3) the prospects of his responding favorably or unfavorably not only to medical and surgical treatment but to interpersonal and environmental readaptations (prognosis and psychotherapy).

Attitude of the psychiatrically trained medical examiner: The physician will remember, from his personal experiences, that under special life stresses he himself had occasionally reacted with excessive anxieties, unfounded fears or suspicions, minor depressions, and other deviations in thinking and mood with their accompanying physiologic expressions. Empathy so engendered will contribute to professional tact and understanding, sharpen the examiner's sensitivity to important psychiatric data, foster better relationships with the patient, and thus, even in the first interview, lay the groundwork for effective therapy.

Objectives

As indicated, it is the purpose of the psychiatric examination first, to establish rapport with the patient through sincere manifestations of concern as to his welfare, and then to elicit the following data:

The present illness, comprising the patient's complaints and the settings which precipitate, exacerbate, or relieve his accompanying symptomatology.

The personality evaluation, as derived from an anamnestic survey of the patient's *characteristic patterns* of behavior during his early childhood, in his schooling, and in his sexual, social, occupational, and other relationships. The nature of previous maladaptations to environmental stress and frustration or to bodily disease are to be noted, especially with regard to the circumstances that precipitated and complicated the present illness.

The mental status, deduced from the patient's spontaneous speech and conduct as directly observed, and his reactions under psychological and physical examination.

Dynamic formulation: Valid deductions from the data so secured as to (a) the patient's physical and intellectual endowment, (b) his acquired motivations, values, and tendencies of response, including his capacities and vulnerabilities and (c) the weight of other factors relevant to prognosis and therapy.

The transactional methods to be employed in securing this information must be varied to suit each patient, but the following general procedure will be found applicable to the great majority of patients.

The Present Illness

It must be remembered that in many instances the patient believes himself to be physically ill and may initially resent any implications that his symptoms have other than a purely organic causation. It is often advisable, therefore, to complete the usual systemic history and physical and laboratory procedures not only as an essential differential diagnostic step, but as an indispensable basis for the further investigation of psychiatric parameters. However, since a diagnosis of neurosis or psychosis *can never be made by exclusion* but must be based on positive data, it is well to look for such evidence fairly early in the diagnostic survey. Thus, with the medical findings reasonably complete, the patient may be tactfully but objectively informed that, whereas there is as yet little or no indication of bodily disease, his symptoms could also spring from other causes that require equally thorough consideration. Relatively neutral and acceptable terms suitable to the individual case (e.g., "overwork," "prolonged worry," or "emotional strain,") may be employed in these introductory explanations, but it is best to avoid confusing or pejorative pseudo-diagnostic phrases such as "neurasthenia," "exhaustion," "psychosomatic disorder," "nervous breakdown," or "mental illness." Most patients, if they are thus made to feel that the physician is understanding and sympathetic, will more readily accept the possibility of so-called "functional" or "emotional" elements in their illness, after which their examination may be conducted as here outlined to elicit *positive* evidence of such factors:

Review of the presenting complaints: Often these will in themselves be so characteristic of various psychiatric syndromes that a presumptive diagnosis can be made on this basis alone. The following are especially frequent and significant:

1. *Anxiety reactions:* recurrent episodes of precordial palpitation, shallow or catchy respiration, pounding pulse, sweating, tremulousness, and intense subjective apprehension, with or without a feeling of a lump or obstruction in the throat (globus hystericus), urinary urgency, splanchnic constriction ("butterflies in the stomach"), giddiness, or similar symptoms. Patients not infrequently complain of these as "heart attacks," "fainting spells," etc., but in most cases the symptoms are unrelated to exertion or other physical stress, and are so directly *precipitated or relieved by emotional circumstances* that the differential diagnosis need not be difficult.

2. *Depressive states:* with typical symptoms of insomnia, bowel irregularity, easy fatigability, anorexia alternating with occasional bulimia, impotence in males, dysmenorrhea and frigidity in women, and diurnally variable discouragement, hopelessness, hypochondriacal preoccupations, fixed melancholy, anaclitic demands for incessant attention and sympathy and, in severe cases, thoughts, gestures, or acts of suicide. Intercurrent periods of forced cheerfulness and distracting hyperactivity may supervene as "hypomanic" episodes; in most instances, however, there is little true euphoria, and such reactions merely represent attempts to deny and to overcompensate for the anxiety and depression.

3. *Phobic-obsessive-compulsive preoccupations:* characterized by fears partially recognized as irrational insistently recurrent thoughts or fantasies and ritualized behavior patterns, which, when prevented or frustrated, uncover an intense underlying anxiety.

4. *Epileptic equivalents:* even in the absence of *grand* or *petit mal* convulsions may be suspected on the basis of episodes of clouded thinking, momentary disorientations, and amnesias ("absences"), or transient fugue-like automatisms, with or without postdromal fatigue and headache.

5. *Toxic-delerious states:* due to drugs (including alcohol, tranquillizers, psychedelics, and narcotics) or intercurrent infections may be surmised from confusions, rapidly changing and often fearful hallucinatory experiences, distorted recall,

peripheral paresthesias, and variable sensory-motor disturbances.

6. *Psychotic admixtures:* revealed by bizarre ideation, gross illogicality, extreme and protracted deviations in mood or seriously altered rapport, or pathognomonic symptoms such as persistent hallucinations, grandiose and paranoid delusions and markedly impulsive behavior.

7. *Loss of cortical function:* indicated by variable loss of memory (especially recent integration and response), impairment of sensory perceptions, sensorial integrations, abstractive capacities, and communicative skills, diminished adaptability to unusual stresses or tasks, and progressive deterioration of personal and social habits.

Techniques of Inquiry

There are, of course, many other psychiatrically significant configurations; the above are reviewed only as a reminder of the fairly common syndromes that can be revealed by a direct inquiry as to the presenting semiology. In this exploration, however, the following precautions are advisable:

Specificity of description: Record the patient's complaint in his own terms, since his choice of language is always illuminating, even when ostensibly misleading. For instance, a patient may complain of "headache" to indicate feelings of inertia, emptiness, constriction, or other generalized discomforts vaguely referred to his "head". Other terms favored because of their ambiguity are "dizziness" (ranging from vertigo and slight faintness to syncope), "noises in the head" (tinnitus or obsessive sounds to auditory hallucinations), "nervousness" (meaning anything from mild restlessness and hypersensitivity to uncontrolled furors), "sleeplessness," "irritability," and "tension."

Sensitivities and resistances: However, it must be remembered that many neurotic patients cannot be pressed too intensely at their first interview without invoking further anxieties and resentments. In such cases, do not insist on an immediate inquisition into confidential or guarded material, such as secret drinking, sexual habits, marital infidelities, or parental failures. Indications of the importance of these may be evident, but their further exploration should be postponed until the patient's confidence, through the examiner's tact and skill, has been more securely won.

Circumstances that exacerbate or alleviate the presenting complaints: Information as to symptomatology can in most cases easily be obtained merely by a receptive attitude or a few evocative questions; in fact, the number and variety as well as the nature of the complaints poured forth under such circumstances may in itself be indicative of a neurotic admixture. When, however, it is necessary to make further inquiry as to the relationships of the patient's symptoms to inner emotional stresses, the following data should, with proper circumspection, be obtained:

1. Typical settings in which anxiety, phobias, obsessions, etc., are evoked: e.g., when the patient is called upon to perform an unwanted task, when he is reprimanded by some authority, or when he otherwise feels inadequate, threatened, or hostile.

2. Other circumstantial correlations, e.g., a wife's migraine headaches which appear only on weekends when she must contend with the continous presence of her in-laws as well as her spouse and children, or recurrent sexual impotence in a husband who unconsciously wishes to avoid impregnating his wife during her presumably fertile sexual cycle.

3. The nature of the symptoms may likewise by symbolically revealing, e.g., nutritive or gastrointestinal dysfunctions in immature "orally dependent" patients under circumstances in which they feel deprived or rejected, or urinary urgency and diarrhea in "anally aggressive" individuals who feel suddenly frustrated and angry. However, in the absence of recurrent and significant evidence, care must be taken not to make *a priori* presumptions about the so-called specificity of such "psychosomatic relationships."

4. The conditions under which symptoms are *relieved* may also be psychologically significant, e.g., change of work, vacations, moving the home, alterations in the family or social constellation, or hospitalizations. Particularly significant is an account that the patient had felt initially benefited by a wide variety of treatments administered by diverse therapists, but

that in each case the "illness" returned as joint enthusiasm flagged, after which the patient would seek another physician with renewed complaints. This, of course, also has an important bearing on current prognosis and plans of therapy.

5. Preliminary information may likewise be gathered about the deliberate or unconscious advantages which the patient may be deriving from his illness. These may take the form not only of financial compensation and relief from responsibilities ("secondary gain") but may concurrently satisfy security-seeking, regressive dependencies, aggressive hostilities, or other "primary" neurotic purposes.

Precipitation of the present illness: Whenever possible the physician should determine what circumstances exacerbated the current symptoms. In the case of combat or postcatastrophic neuroses, the history may be fairly obvious. But in most other cases, though the stresses involved affect the patient just as seriously, they may be less evident to the observer. In such instances they can consist of more subtle but equally disruptive threats operating on a previously sensitized individual, such as, a dreaded demotion or promotion, guilt over the secretly desired travails of a rival, an impending engagement or marriage, or various social or religious transgressions of unique import to the patient. Inquiry into such causes must be especially gentle and judicious, but is often highly revealing.

The Personal History

Since psychiatric disorders are accentuations of previously latent behavior tendencies, it follows that every neurotic or psychotic illness is an outgrowth of the patient's previous personality, and that the evolution of the latter must be traced as clearly as practicable from early familial influences through the vicissitudes of later life to the onset of his current disabilities. Training and practice in this task will make it far less formidable and time-consuming than it first appears, but here as elsewhere in the psychiatric examination the physician must remember that most patients will be ignorant of, and unconsciously resist recognizing, any connection between their behavior and engrained attitudes and responses derived from their past experiences. This may be particularly true when crude or even merely routine attempts are made to elicit the familial and personal history; under such circumstances the patient may well defend himself, verbally or covertly, with some rationalization such as: "I came here for relief from headaches and bowel trouble, and they send me to a mental clinic where the headshrinker asks me if my dear old grandmother was insane and whether I really like my wife. Do they think I'm crazy?" Such reactions may be avoided only if the patient is given a preliminary understanding of the importance of a comprehensive history to better diagnoses and more effective therapy, and if the interview continues to be conducted with proper sympathy and adroitness. The following considerations are helpful:

Interview arrangements: Whenever practicable, choose a quiet, preferably soundproof office, free of distractions and interruptions. Reassure the patient that all data will be kept professionally confidential, and do not consult any manual during the examination; to do so implies incompetence and impairs the ease, rapport and effectiveness of the relationship. For the same reasons avoid voluminous writing during the interview, but note key facts and expressions for later elaboration.

Transitions in content: If the patient describes himself as "nervous," "emotional," "high-strung," etc., ask him if these or other characteristics were familial traits, thus leading him to give significant descriptions of his parents, antecedents, and siblings—e.g., the "family history." Similarly, make logical transitions from the present illness to various categories of the past history by inquiry as to whether current or other symptoms were present in childhood, whether they were influenced by excessive study in school, "overwork" or other maladjustments at early jobs, the stresses of various social adaptations and so on. Information on particularly guarded topics such as sexuality can be more readily secured by an indirect anamnestic approach: a complaint of dysmenorrhea may be used as a basis for asking the patient to describe the circumstances of her menarche; once the subject is broached, she may more easily be led to describe her sexual fears and fantasies and possible neurotic reactions to psychosexual traumata. Similarly, tracing a complaint of ejaculatio praecox may reveal familial prohibitions of erotic activity and later fears of masturbation or homosexuality directly related to present marital or other difficulties.

"Irrelevancy": On the other hand, the patient's tendencies to surface diffuseness when given an opportunity to talk spontaneously and freely—as should be done insofar as practicable—may in themselves be directly significant if basic associative themes are detected. For example, an emotionally immature wife may "wander" quite significantly from an account of her marital conflicts to a description of her idyllic childhood with her indulgent mother, or an aggressively competitive obsessive-compulsive individual may "parenthetically" talk about his own multiple superiorities to his siblings, his business rivals and others less "conscientious" than himself, including by implication the physician. With limited time, a completely undirected interview is rarely as informative as a skillful guided one, but both techniques may be combined as indicated by the experienced examiner.

Supplementation of the personal history: In general, the patient himself is the most fertile and significant source for the needed data, but wherever necessary or available, other resources may be used: interviews with family and friends, perusal of physicians', employers' or social service reports, school or military records, etc. It must be remembered, however, that all informants have various limitations and prejudices so that each may require individual evaluation and check against the others.

Significance of the data: It is now apparent that a psychiatric history is not merely a chronological account of "what happened" in the patient's life, but an inquiry designed to discern those *characteristic patterns of response* which constitute his "personality" and therefore possess diagnostic and prognostic value. Because of the patient's defenses and biases complete "accuracy" is unattainable, but even if his own accounts of past happenings are unconsciously distorted by symbolic ("screen") memories or even deliberately falsified, the nature of these misrepresentations will also be psychiatrically significant. In this sense, the proferred "history" is in itself an excellent index of the patient's mental status, in that it furnishes valuable data as to his motivations, self-concepts, symbol systems, values and current interpersonal relationships. With these qualifications, the information secured may be arranged as follows:

The family history: Although it is highly questionable whether there are genetic factors in neurotic (as well as in "sociopathic" and many psychotic) disorders, it is undeniable that the personality of every adult is greatly influenced by those with whom he comes into intimate contact in childhood. Therefore, even apart from its genetic significance, the patient's own description of the personal characteristics of his grandparents, parents, siblings or other relatives is often significant, particularly when special aspects of, or gross deviations in, their behavior (overindulgence, tyranny, unpredictability, tempestuousness, sexual seduction, etc.) directly affected the patient's formative experiences. Note also his subsequent allegiances or aversions to parent surrogates such as governesses or teachers, attachments to and rivalries with various siblings, and the adverse influence of familial discord, divorce or desertion.

Birth and early development: Accurate data may be difficult or impossible to obtain, but the patient's or other informants' impressions about the following are significant: prematurity; ease or difficulty in delivery (asphyxia, injuries); type of nursing and method of weaning; delays in early habit acquisitions such as sitting, walking, word or sentence formations, and toilet training; play interests; manifestations of early neurotic tendencies, such as feeding difficulties, excessive crying, night terrors, tics, spasms, phobias, persistent thumb-sucking, or enuresis.

Schooling and early socialization: Ages of enrollment and at various grades attained; adjustment to school routine and discipline; scholastic and extracurricular activities liked and disliked; development, nature, and depth of leadership or group loyalties at various ages; and unusual dependence upon or friction with teachers or other school authorities. Repeated disciplinary difficulties, social isolations, truancies, and delinquencies are especially meaningful.

Sexual development and attitudes: Tactful, objective inquiry—without undue emphasis may be made into early sex preoccupations (autoerotisms, curiosities, phantasies, fears, inhibitions, voyeurisms, displacements) as well as into the later development, nature, pace and intensity of homo- or heterosexual expressions, deviations in technique or unusual attachments or aversions to sex partners. Such inquiries may include previous and current marital adjustments comprising not only sexual compatibility but also relative fidelity or promiscuity, use and justification of contraceptive techniques, attitudes to in-laws and children, mutual interests and other interpersonal conflicts and satisfactions. In most cases, it will be found that the latter considerations *determine* sexual adjustments in marriage, rather than vice versa.

Other habit developments: Concerning food, sleep, dress, hobbies, recreations, etc. In later life the survey should include habitual overindulgence in tobacco, caffeine drinks, alcohol or sedatives, stimulant, psychedelic, narcotic, or other drugs.

Adult social adjustments: Type and constancies of friendships and group loyalties; submissiveness, passivity, or leadership in joint activities. Nature and intensity of significant social, ethical, and religious sentiments, with special relation to unusual rigidities or prejudices. Circumstances leading to compatibility and belongingness, or conversely, feelings of diffidence, embarrassment, resentment, and social failure.

Occupational history: Types of work sought or idealized; jobs secured and periods held; variability of effort and application; acceptance of duties, and cooperation or competitiveness with fellow workers; reactions to supposed injustice, idleness, and failures, or to promotions and successes; evaluation of employers, superiors or employees.

Military service: Record the branch and duration, the patient's reactions to training, discipline, and combat; his demotions and promotions; his attitudes at discharge; the pensions sought and retained; and his current evaluations of his experiences.

Effects of injuries and illnesses: Record the patient's previous organic illnesses, including a description of significant reactions to them, such as excessive invalidism, frequent hospitalizations, prolonged disability and dependency, or lack of cooperation with medical care. Accident proneness and consequent litigation may also be significant.

Transition to present illness: Under this heading the psychiatric anamnesis may be completed by a consideration of the circumstances that interacted singly or in combination (as outlined above) with the special sensitivities and vulnerabilities of the patient to precipitate his present illness and to induce him to seek (or be referred for) psychiatric help. However, a complete demarcation cannot always be made, and the "present illness" will be seen as merely a continuation, or at most an exacerbation, of the patient's previous life patterns and neurotic tendencies.

Current "Mental" Status

Direct observation: A great deal of emphasis was formerly placed on this as a separate portion of the psychiatric examination, intended to reveal gross deviations in motivation, affect, thinking, and behavior relevant to the differential diagnosis of various forms of "mental deficiency" and "major" or "organic" psychoses. The clinician must, of course, remain alert to these possibilities; however, a far larger number of patients will have only characterologic, neurotic or functional-somatic disturbances, and in such cases direct and crude tests of intellectual capacities or questions as to disorientations or hallucinatory experiences may be not only unnecessary but needlessly alienating. Actually, valid information as to most of the rubrics of the so-called mental status will already have been gathered during the course of the history and physical examination, as will be indicated by the following review:

General behavior: As manifested by appearance, gait, posture, demeanor, dress, and personal hygiene, mannerisms, tics, characteristic activity, obvious idiosyncracies or compulsions, cooperation with office or clinic procedures, and general response to the examiner and others.

Intellectual level: This may be deduced fairly accurately from the quickness and accuracy of the patient's preceptions, the range, versatility, and specificity of his vocabulary, the scope and accuracy of his general information, his capacities for the nuances and differentiations of both concrete and abstract thinking, the richness of his imagery, his forms of wit and humor, and the general levels of his cultural attainments. In estimating basic intellectual capacities, however, allowances must be made for the previous presence or absence of social and educational opportunities.

Sensorium: Memory, retention, associative and communicative capacities, orientation, etc., are not organically impaired in the neuroses. If, however, intellectual failures, possibly due to cerebral dysrhythmia, trauma, or disease are indicated by gross discrepancies in dates, places, and logical relationships in the history, the patient's sensorium may be further checked by indirect questions designed to reveal his awareness of identity, time, and locale, his capacity to remember his past accurately, to repeat forward or backward a series of from four to eight numbers given to him, to subtract 7 serially from 100 (ostensibly as a test of concentration), to retell an anecdote, or to act on a set of simple directions adequately. Even when necessary, this portion of the examination may be so conducted that the patient need not resent or hardly be aware of the fact that he is "being tested."

Mood and emotional state: The fixity or range of the patient's affects: e.g., anxiety, depression, indifference, euphoria, hostility, etc., will have been verbally indicated by him during the interview and examination; in addition, the examiner may have noted such physiologic and mimetic accompaniments as flushings, lachrymation, pupillary dilations, tremors, jaw-clenchings or other muscular tensions, startle reactions, and related visceral and motor expressions of emotion. The stooped posture, slow movements, low retarded speech, and dolorous facies of melancholia are especially noticeable; in such patients, the possibility of self-destructive preoccupations is better investigated gently and indirectly (e.g., "Are you sometimes so discouraged about your illness that you feel there is no hope in going on?") than by direct questions as to frank plans for suicide. With empathy and experience the examiner will also more readily sense the fragile apprehensiveness of the anxiety neurotic, the bland pseudo-serenity (*"la belle indifference"*) of the relatively content "conversion hysteric," the strained, restless, false euphoria of the hypomanic, the demanding, self-pitying, preemptive depressive, or the dereistic thinking, distorted affects and deviant rapport of the schizoid or schizophrenic.

Preoccupations and special symptoms: When indicated, further inquiry may reveal persistent fantasies, significant dreams or nightmares, obsessive phobias and compulsions, hypochondriacal tendencies or fixations, diurnal or other variations in energy-level or temperament, recurrent *déjà vu* experiences, feelings of depersonalization, confusion or panic, transient absences, or prolonged fugue states. Even more serious psychological deviations may incidentally be uncovered: for instance, hallucinations may be described in response to an inquiry about "very vivid daydreams or imaginations," whereas paranoid or other delusions may emerge clearly if they are detected and accepted as possibilities (though never expressly agreed to) during the interview.

Insight: This is always a complex, relative and variable aspect of the patient's past attitudes and current status, but from a clinical standpoint what is usually called "insight" may be estimated along the following dimensions: (a) the patient's own explanations of his illness, (b) his ideas as to prognosis and treatment, and (c) the sincerity of his desires for, and cooperation with, medical and psychiatric therapy. The superficially polite acceptance by the patient of the examiner's pet formulation should not *ipso facto* be termed "insight."

Psychiatric significance of the physical examination: The patient's conduct during this procedure often contributes evidence as to his mental status: excessive shyness, modesty, or exhibitionism; unusual passivity; suspiciousness, hypersensitiveness, or avidity with regard to abdominal, vaginal, or rectal examinations; irrational fear of transillumination or retinoscopy, and so on. Incidental observations should include the adequacy of oral, ungual, hirsute, and other personal hygiene, tattoo marks, drug rashes, bruises from injuries or repeated syncopes, or skin punctures indicating the intravenous use of narcotics.

Supplementary psychologic testing: Whenever there are difficuties in differential diagnoses or other special problems, the patient may be referred to a competent clinical psychologist for the following: (a) tests of intellectual functions, such as the Wechsler-Bellevue or modified Stanford, (b) tests of occupational preference or special abilities, such as the Strong Vocational Guidance or the Seashore scales of musical aptitude, (c) personality tests, of which the questionnaire techniques such as the Bernreuter or the Neymann-Kohlstedt are least reliable and the projective techniques such as the Rorschach and the Thematic Apperception are the most revealing—but only if skillfully conducted and evaluated.

Ancillary techniques in psychiatric diagnosis: These include polygraphic recordings during questioning or history taking ("lie detection"), hypnotic catharsis or regression, or the administration of drugs such as scopolamine ("truth serum") or intravenous sodium pentothal or sodium amytal. Such procedures are rarely required, reveal only the patient's less inhibited attitudes and images rather than objective "facts," carry definite physical and psychologic risks, and therefore had best be used only after special training and experience; here too, however, the physician should be acquainted with their general significance.

Psychiatric Formulation

When sufficient information as outlined above has been gathered to make possible a comprehensive formulation, this should be integrated and summarized according to the following outline:

1. Brief statement of the precipitating circumstances, nature, duration and course of the present illness.
2. Organic factors as revealed by the medical history and by the physical, neurologic, laboratory and other special examinations.
3. Constitutional and personality factors as indicated by the familial and personal history.
4. The current behavioral status as shown by direct psychiatric observation and supplementary psychologic or other tests.
5. An interim diagnostic summary based on the above, including (a) the presence and relative prominence of various psychiatric syndromes (anxiety, depression, psychosomatic

dysfunctions, schizoid tendencies, etc.), (b) the relationship of these reactions to specific external stresses (environmental maladaptations), and (c) their roots in inner motivations, formative experiences, and derived character patterns (psychodynamics).

6. Indications for further medical or psychiatric diagnostic procedures.

7. Preliminary plans for therapy, as recorded under the following rubrics: (a) Immediate symptomatic relief by medication, sedation, physiotherapy, or other medical or surgical procedures; (b) environmental alterations such as change of residence, work, or environment, or, if necessary, hospitalization for total care; (c) projected nature and techniques of the dyadic, family, group, or other psychotherapy to be employed; (d) methods of securing the cooperation of the patient's friends and family in his treatment, or when necessary, in his legal custodial care.

This formulation should be supplemented by progress notes as the patient is treated and followed up, and elaborated and amended as new facts become available.

The above represents a fairly extended but by no means all-inclusive review of modern approaches to a comprehensive and dynamically oriented clinical examination. As a summary, the following *Condensed Guide* may be employed for ready reference in actual clinical usage.

Brief Outline of the Psychiatric Anamnesis

Rationale: Since the symptomatology, course and therapy of every illness is influenced by the motivations, personality, and environment of the patient, no medical diagnosis or plan of therapy is complete without an adequate survey of these factors. With proper sympathy and tact therefore, the examining physician should obtain the following information:

I. Psychiatric Aspects of the Present Illness

1. *Neurotic symptomatology:* determine the intensity and frequency of anxiety reactions, obsessive-phobic-compulsive states, depressive or hypomanic mood swings, disturbances of consciousness or motor control, drug intake, and recent impair-

ments of intellectual functions and interpretations of reality.

2. *Relationships to environmental stresses:* survey the circumstances that precipitated, exacerbated or alleviated the above deviations in behavior and their accompanying organic (psychosomatic) dysfunctions, including the patient's reactions to previous examinations and therapy.

II. Personal History

Since normal and abnormal behavior can be best understood as an evolution of genetic, constitutional and adaptational patterns in relation to physical and emotional stresses, this section of the examination should comprise a pertinent review of the following data about the patient as a person:

The family history: brief descriptions of significant traits in parents, siblings or important relatives.

Birth and early development: data on infantile traumata or illnesses, feeding disturbances, spasms, terrors, or other childhood neurotic tendencies.

Schooling and early socialization: scholastic interests and performance, adjustments to discipline and group participations.

Sexual attitudes: including marked deviations, special fears, and marital and parental adjustments.

Habits: of food, sleep, recreation, and intake of alcohol, sedatives, or other drugs.

Social adjustments: friendships, social belongingness, recreations, religious activities.

Occupational adjustments: goals, level of initiative and performance, cooperation with employers, fellows, and subordinates.

Military service: motivations and reactions in training or combat.

Previous reactions to injuries or illnesses: including tendencies to emotional over-reactions, dependency and invalidism.

The personal history so obtained should be less a chronological account than a biographical review of the *origin and nature of the patient's characteristic patterns of conduct,* and as such will lead naturally into the precipitation of the present illness as in paragraph 1 above.

III. The Current "Mental" Status

This consists of a summary of the patient's behavior as either directly observed during historytaking and physical examination, or as elicited by further inquiry. The data may be organized under the following headings:

General behavior: appearance, posture, mannerisms, dress, personal hygiene, etc.

Intellectual level: as estimated from perceptive grasp, vocabulary, general information, logic and versatility of thought and cultural attainments.

Sensorium: orientations to time, space and identity, clarity of awareness and retention.

Mood and emotional state: excessive anxiety, euphoria, passivity, hostility, indifference. In melancholic patients the possibility of suicidal impulses is of immediate practical importance and requires the quick and effective instillation of hope or adequate protection in home or hospital.

Special symptoms: such as hypochondriacal preoccupations, panic or fugue states; déjà vu; clouded consciousness, etc.

Psychotic manifestations: affective distortions, hallucinations, grandiose or persecutory delusions and paranoid systematizations are seen relatively rarely in general clinical practice, but must be recognized when they occur.

Insight: the patient's own concepts as to the nature of his illness, his ideas as to treatment and prognosis, and his cooperation with examination and therapy.

IV. Formulation

The above information about the current illness may be integrated and appended to the medical summary under the following headings:

Organic factors: determined by the medical history and physical and laboratory findings.

Psychiatric and "psychosomatic" components: their predisposing and precipitating circumstances, as determined by the psychiatric and personal history and mental status.

Indications for further diagnostic procedures: medical, psychologic or special techniques.

Psychiatric diagnoses and prognosis, in a clear, condensed summary.

Projected Treatment: comprising methods of immediate systematic relief or environmental readjustments, need of hospitalization for special procedures, and plans for long-term medical and psychiatric treatment and eventual social rehabilitation.

With sufficient familiarity and skill eliciting these important psychiatric data need take relatively little time, and will add immeasurably to comprehensive diagnosis and effective therapy.

16. LAW, SEX, AND INDUSTRY—PROFESSIONAL COMMUNICATIONS

Law

Whether he admits it or not, the psychiatrist is an officer of his social order, duly commissioned and licensed to wield important powers over material possessions, personal freedoms, and even life itself.

A psychiatrist can declare a millionaire incompetent to manage his own estate, certify him as "psychotic" and thereby confine him possibly indefinitely to a "mental institution." Again, a psychiatrist can deny a "plea of insanity" and thus help send a convicted murderer to his execution. Obviously, a psychiatrist has very serious obligations to obtain all the relevant data available, conduct his own thorough examinations, reach unbiased and balanced conclusions, and then convey these in untechnical and unequivocal language calculated to bring about the best results for all concerned—yet without infringing upon the final prerogatives of the referring agencies. This is especially important when the psychiatrist's opinions are requested by judges and attorneys, with whom it may be well for the psychiatrist to reach one other basic understanding: that he will refuse to appear in court as a special pleader for either the "prosecution" or the "defense"; instead, he will submit a written report to the judge himself, with copies to be sent to the contending attorneys at the Court's discretion.

It was invariably under these conditions that I acted as *amicus curiae* to the Criminal Courts and to the Courts of Domestic Relations in Chicago for twenty years, and submitted scores of reports to judges, or in duplicate to the contending attorneys when both wished to avoid trial. A few examples, chosen almost at random, are here reproduced:

Psychiatric examination of a young man held on a criminal charge of armed robbery.

REPORT TO: THE HONORABLE ________
SUBJECT: N. U., AGE 20

Conditions of Report: On May 20, 1965, Mr. I. D. B., attorney, telephoned my office to request a psychiatric examination of his client, Mr. N. U. The preliminary information furnished by Atty. B. was that Mr. U. had been identified by two attendants at a gas station as the man who robbed them of $35.00 at about 11:30 p.m. on April 4, 19__, fired two pistol shots at one of them while escaping on foot, and was then seen driving a car through which he was traced and arrested at his home early in the morning of April 5th. I agreed to examine Mr. U. only if the following conditions were met: (1) That he would submit to every form of inquiry or investigation I thought necessary. (2) That my fee be paid in advance so as to eliminate any suspicion of bias through subsequent financial or other reward. (3) That I report my findings directly and exclusively to the presiding judge, who would then use his discretion as to the distribution of copies to the prosecution or defense, without further testimony on my part.

Mr. B. accepted these conditions, and Mr. U. was interviewed and examined in my office on May 25.

Preliminary Interviews with Family: The above conditions were explained to N. U's mother and father, and both seemed so genuinely convinced of his innocence that they agreed to any procedure that would confirm the truth. Mrs. U volunteered only two additional items of information which she apparently considered significant: namely, that her son N was home from work at about 11:15 p.m., the time when the robbery really occurred, and that he was "wearing his pajamas, not his underwear" when arrested in his bedroom at about 2:00 a.m. on April 5th.

Psychiatric Anamnesis of N. U.: A carefully conducted and detailed account of N. U.'s life, checked and rechecked in various ways for over an hour, may be briefly summarized as follows: He is the third born and second son in a family of seven children ranging in age from a sister of 28 to one age 12. He sincerely respects and admires his hard-working father, a mechanic, and is perhaps overly attached to his protective mother; however, all his familial and sibling relationships have been predominantly close and cordial. Recurrently severe childhood illnesses (pneumonia and asthma) with subsequent respiratory and skin allergies contributed to feelings of familial dependency in early life and to traits of social reserve and heterosexual shyness during boyhood and adolescence, but he maintained better than average scholastic adjustments, was active in ROTC (where he handled dummy rifles, but never smaller arms), has no disciplinary difficulties, and has worked steadily for the same employers evenings, weekends and vacations since the age of 15. After graduation from high school 18 months ago he has been steadily employed as a gas station attendant, without absenteeism or other work deficiencies or delinquencies. He belongs to no clubs or gangs, and confines his recreations to attending shows with one or two neighborhood friends his own age. He has been a regular attendant at Catholic mass and confessional, and was assured by Monsignor M. that the latter stands ready to give him an excellent character reference.

N. U.'s Account of Events on the Night of April 4, 1965: In brief, this is as follows: He finished his afternoon-to-night shift by closing the station at about 10:45 p.m., drove his partner home, arrived at his own house at about 11:05 p.m., met his family who were watching a late TV show, and washed in the bathroom where he was observed by his elder brother at about 11:15 p.m. Then, as was his custom after work, he drove to a hamburger stand, purchased a hamburger and potatoes, and returned home with them as usual for his midnight meal. (On specific inquiry, he states that the brother of the proprietor of the restaurant served him that night, did not know him, and would not testify as to his presence, but that the proprietor would vouch for his customary appearance at this time.) After the meal, N. donned pajamas and went calmly to bed, where he was arrested at 2:00 a.m. on complaint of one of the robbery victims who had allegedly seen him driving to the restaurant and had the police trace him through the license plates on his car.

Mental Status: N. U.'s intelligence, as manifested in his perceptive, mnemonic, abstractive, and integrative functions is high average and without special defects of awareness or judgment. In personality he is somewhat timid, self-effacing, and limited in ambition: in the latter respect, he hopes his prospective Army training will qualify him as a mechanic, but he prefers to "take orders, because I never feel like bossing other people." Repeated checks of his accounts of his life and the events of April 4-5 by various cross-validating techniques indicate this sincerity and veracity: for example, although consistent in essentials, he did not insist on precise timing-by-minutes as would be expected if his stories had been prepared and rehearsed; so also, he admits he cannot be certain of details that would be to his advantage, and he is eager to cooperate in every avenue of inquiry. Moreover, he bears almost no rancor even toward his accusers, since he is reasonably certain that they will recognize their mistake and that he will be judged innocent by the Court.

Sodium Amytal Interview: As a final check on the above observations, N. U., in the presence of his parents, was requested to submit to a further examination while under the effects of sodium amytal, with the understanding that his replies would be tape recorded and all findings as to guilt or innocence reported directly to the Court; significantly, all three again readily agreed. N. U. was then isolated and given 7½ grains of the drug intravenously, constituting an amount sufficient to induce a relatively communicative drowsiness, remove inhibitions and promote direct expressions of emotionally significant material. The events of April 4-5 were then once more gone over in fine detail, with the same result: an internally consistent and affectively appropriate repetition of his experiences as outlined above, despite many evocative and provocative interrogations that would have produced evasions, lapses, contradictions, and significant emotional reactions had he been guilty as charged.

Conclusions: In the highly complex field of human behavior there can be no absolutes, but only highly reasonable probabilities. However, on the basis of the numerous psychologic and psychiatric data elicited in my interviews, it is my objective and unbiased judgment that N. U's previous personality and character, his consistently validated accounts, and the results of the amytal examination render the probability of his innocence very close to certainty.

N. U. was acquitted.

Another rescue:

REPORT TO THE HONORABLE __________
SUBJECT: PSYCHIATRIC EXAMINATION OF MR. F.W., AGE 24

Presenting Problem: Mr. W. states that while driving a school bus at about 7:00 p.m. on a Monday evening a month ago (details as to time, place, and date are imprecise) he picked up a youth who requested a ride, and drove him along the bus route for about twenty minutes. During this time they "talked about girls" and both became sexually excited—whereupon Mr. W., allegedly encountering no resistance, palpated the younger boy's penis through the latter's clothes and caused him to have two ejaculations. After the second of these the youngster grew angry, left the bus, threw a stone at it, and ran off. Two days later Mr. W. was arrested, and then learned that the boy (who allegedly gave his age variously as between 13 and 16) had complained to his parents, after which the latter had sworn a formal complaint. Mr. W. was held on charges of disturbing the peace and contributing to the delinquency of a minor, during which time he freely admitted to police examiners the occurrence as described above. Four days after his arrest he was released on bond for a psychiatric examination to be used at the discretion of the court.

Family History: F. W. describes his father as a hard-working but remote, rather strict and arbitrary person who has evinced little warmth or understanding in his paternal relationships. The mother is more kindly, though she too is apparently temperamental, old-country in her prejudices and unreliable either as a confidante or an ally in the home. The older brother (now age 30) has, according to F.W., always been overbearing or tyrannical and since his return from service has also grown increasingly alcoholic and physically abusive to other members of the family.

Personal History: F. W. was born in Chicago to a family life handicapped by considerable financial privation and internal strife. Another important drawback has been his marked intellectual limitations, which contributed to retardation at school, social awkwardness, and feelings of general inadequacy and isolation. He quit school after the 10th grade, worked at a minor postal job for a year, and then, because of adverse home conditions, ran away at 17 in an attempt to join the army. One year later he succeeded in this, and rendered satisfactory service both in this country and overseas as a clerk and psychiatric hospital attendant with a rating of PFC for the entire three years of his enlistment. Significantly, he enjoyed the regularity, discipline and security of army life, and would have remained in it except for his mother's pleas that she was ill and needed him at home. Since his return, however, he has held a long succession of civilian jobs only briefly, generally quitting or being fired because the skills and proficiencies required at nearly every task quickly exceeded his limited capacities and resourcefulness. Similarly, he found it difficult to cultivate interests and friendships on his own initiative, and has remained isolated and lonesome. He has therefore wanted to return to the army as the only place where he ever felt needed and useful, but has been deterred by his mother's continued pleas to stay at home and protect her from her unpredicable husband and older son.

Sexual History: Mr. W.'s sexual development was similarly retarded in that, aside from occasional masturbation, he had had no sexual experiences until one or two contacts with prostitutes during his army service overseas. On two occasions, also, he submitted to mutual masturbation or fellatio with a "service buddy" when both were intoxicated, but never solicited or assumed the active role, and avoided all sex thoughts on duty. Mr. W. states in apparent sincerity that this is the first such difficulty he has had since leaving the army, that he would greatly prefer to associate with girls ("except I don't have any money, and they don't think I'm very smart"), but that nevertheless he hopes a 17-year-old girl he now knows will marry him when she comes of age "so we can settle down and have our own home."

Mental Status: Mr. W.'s language, forms of thought, and limited capacities for abstraction, logic, memory, and other intellectual functions indicate an only borderline normal intelligence; so also his social techniques and occupational motivations are relatively underdeveloped. However, he is sincere, frank, friendly, and devoid of deeply rooted antagonisms or aggressions that might make him in any way vicious or dangerous, even in circumstances of threat and anxiety.

Diagnosis: Immature personality. The homosexual tendencies are not of pathologic intensity, and should subside under favorable circumstances.

Interview with F. W.'s Mother: Confirms in general the above data and analysis. Mrs. W. states that she is now willing to let her son re-enlist if so advised.

Recommendations: From a psychiatric standpoint, F.W. may be considered an intellectually limited and emotionally underdeveloped person subject to minor deviations under adverse circumstances but nevertheless capable of conforming well to limited duties under proper supervision in an accustomed environment. Severe punishment or prolonged incarceration in his case, in all probability, would be psychologically devastating; on the other hand, at the discretion of the court, a directed re-enlistment may be in order as a general rehabilitative procedure.

Mr. W. was placed on six months' probation and then discharged from legal supervision.

Conversely, to counter an unjustified plea of "insanity":

REPORT TO: THE HONORABLE W.J.L.
SUBJECT: PSYCHIATRIC AND NEUROLOGIC EXAMINATION OF MR. F.H.

Preliminary Conference with Mr. H. and His Attorney, Mr. O.O.: Atty. O. stated that approximately 18 months ago Mr. H. was indicted under the Hobbes law for the alleged mishandling of some $80,000 of relief funds during his presidency of a local labor union, Atty. O. now requests a psychiatric examination because, in his opinion, Mr. H. has been so uncooperative in preparing a proper defense that a question has arisen in Mr. O.'s mind with regard to Mr. H.'s mental competence, or his capacity to withstand the rigors of a long trial. During this joint conference Mr. H. volunteered only the following information: that the amount in question "was only $65,000," and that he positively rejects and resents any implications that he is "insane" or mentally incompetent in any way.

Examination of Mr. H.: Personal History: When Mr. H. was twelve years old, his father died, leaving a wife and family of 14 children (of which Mr. H. was the third youngest) to fend for themselves. Mr. H.'s schooling and extrafamilial social opportunties were correspondingly limited, but he worked steadily and productively as a construction laborer under the mentorship of his employer, C.P., and soon advanced fairly rapidly as the business agent of the local union. An unfortunate marriage ended in divorce some 17 years ago, and under the attendant familial, social, and financial stresses Mr. H.'s previously moderate consumption of alcohol became excessive. A so-called nervous breakdown resulted which was apparently, from his own symptomatic description and according to supplementary reports from Dr. J.P.W., a period of emotional depression complicated by alcoholic delirium. Mr. H. was treated by eight or nine electroshocks at River Forest Sanitarium and six more elsewhere, and recovered sufficiently to return to work. He readily admits that he has since continued to drink heavily and that espidoes of special stress (such as that following his indictment) still lead to alcoholic excesses, with neglect of food and rest to the point where medical care becomes necessary.

Neurologic Examination: The only abnormalities found were blood pressure 140/96, slight retinal sclerosis, mild irregular alcoholiform intention tremor of the extended hands, and variable paresthesias and formications indicative of early peripheral polyneuritis. There were, however, no indications of grossly disabling lesions of the peripheral or central nervous system.

Psychiatric Examination: Mr. H. shows slight and transient amnesias for recent events, occasional failure to follow rapid changes of ideation, and some tendency to defensive repetitiveness of thought and action; however, these are not in excess of what is common at his age. On the contrary, despite his history of chronic alcoholism, his intelligence, as tested by orientation to time, space and person, general comprehension, logical differentiation, integrative grasp, and appropriateness of reaction, is remarkably well retained. In personality he is genial, frank, friendly and sincerely cooperative when his confidence has been won. He then shows normal parental concern about his son—a military academy graduate now in the Marines—and considerable pride in his devotion to his "boys" —the men in his labor union whose benefactor he believes himself to be. The only hints of paranoid thinking were his remarks implying (a) that just possibly, his indictment may have been engineered by lawyers for large insurance companies who disliked his free-handed financial largesse to his "union boys," (b) that he did not proceed to get affidavits as to his disbursements to them because he wished to protect them from possible tax embarrassments, and (c) that he suspects that some of his current legal advisers are postponing his trial for their own advantages, rather than his best interests. However, such thoughts are fairly common rationalizations in men of his background, education, and position, and certainly cannot be considered indicative of psychotic deviation. Justifiably or not, Mr. H. seems to have no consciousness of guilt over personal financial gain, and repeatedly professes his eagerness to undergo due process of law without special favor or delay on medical or psychiatric grounds.

Telephone Conference with Dr. J. P. W.: This confirmed the presence of some degree of alcoholic liver cirrhosis, but Dr. W. agreed that there were no disabling medical impediments to Mr. H.'s standing trial.

Psychologic Tests: The results were in line with the clinical findings.

Recommendations: The data summarized above furnish no adequate medical or psychiatric reason for modifying any legal procedures involving Mr. H. on grounds of physical or mental incompetence. In his own best interests, however, he should diminish his intake of alcohol, at least during his period of legal jeopardy.

When a judge requests professional support for his courtroom impression that one party in a neighborhood dispute is "mentally disturbed":

THE HONORABLE ____________
RE: PSYCHIATRIC REPORTS ON MR. I. L. AND MRS. V. B.

In view of the nature of the case, the following reports on Mr. I. L., the complainant, and Mrs. V.B., the defendant, are being sent directly to you, with copies for distribution to the attorneys involved only at your own discretion. As is my custom, I have confined my conclusions to the psychiatric evidence and have avoided implying opinion as to any legal questions involved.

Mr. I.L.

Complaints: Mr. L. states that he had lived for six years

happily and at peace with everyone until Mr. and Mrs. V. B. moved next door about 3 years ago. The new neighbors soon began arguing with him about trespassing on their property, and since then they have allegedly spied on him, vilified him, his family and his visitors, sprayed water through his windows, unleashed a vicious dog who bit members of his family, and even had him falsely arrested for assault. Mr. B. is fairly frequently intoxicated, but most of these nuisances are created by Mrs. B., who treats her other neighbors similarly though in less extreme form.

Personal History: A detailed anamnestic survey indicates that Mr. L. has on the whole led a stable, well-adjusted personal life. After a good preparatory educational record he graduated from Chicago Technical School, held progressively better positions with the Central Electric Company and served commendably in the army. He has remained happily married for ten years, and appears to be raising his three children and conducting his other personal and social affairs in a competent fashion.

Mental Status: Mr. L. has superior intelligence and shows consistent logical, controlled thinking. Despite his resentments he maintains a balanced, tolerant and occasionally even compassionate attitude to the B.'s, whom he suspects of being mentally aberrant and therefore not totally responsible for their acts.

Mrs. V. B.

Complaints: These are in part so incoherent or generalized that they are difficult to specify. In effect, Mrs. B. believes that the entire neighborhood has been bribed ("with hundreds of dollars") by Mr. and Mrs. L. to "torture" her, that the Sanitary Bureau and perhaps the police have also been suborned to persecute her and that "bad stories" about her nationality and sex life are being spread to break up her home and to cheat her of her property. In order to protect herself, she has had to lock all her doors and windows and hide from everyone; once, when she ventured forth, she and her niece were shot at by Mrs. L.'s little boy. She "thanks God Mrs. L.'s brother died," since this disposed of one of her enemies—and hopes that the others will also be adequately punished.

Personal History: Mrs. B. came from an exceedingly adverse familial background: her father was recurrently ill, her mother was and is "so nervous she is afraid to go to a doctor because they'll put her away," and her sister repeatedly has been committed as psychotic. Mrs. B. herself did poorly both socially and scholastically in parochial school, could not speak English well until adolescence, left the grammar grades at 16½ and, except for some menial work, remained almost isolated in her home until her marriage at 24. Marital life has been stormy because of her husband's drinking, irresponsibility and mutual accusations of infidelity.

Psychiatric Status: Mrs. B.'s intelligence is estimated as only borderline normal; however, her main deficiencies consist of severe emotional instability and a marked tendency to confused and paranoid thinking and action. Unfortunately, she has little insight into these handicaps, and may disregard or resist advice and direction. A neurological examination indicated that Mrs. B.'s psychiatric disorder was of psychological rather than organic nature.

N.B.: Since neither Mrs. L. nor Mr. B. appeared for examination, no psychiatric opinion can be rendered about them or their role in the present difficulties.

Conclusions: From the evidence at hand, Mr. L. appears to be an intelligent and relatively dependable individual, whereas Mrs. B. is a retarded, unstable and paranoid personality as described, and may therefore misunderstand or refuse to obey customs or orders. This, of course, is not to be interpreted as a judgment as to their conflicting claims, which is a matter of the Court's decision as to facts and justice.

A consultation requested by the Chicago Bar Association:

SUBJECT: PSYCHIATRIC EXAMINATION OF ATTY. D.L.
ISSUE FOR CONSULTATION: FITNESS OF MR. L. FOR THE PRACTICE OF LAW.
DOCUMENTS REVIEWED: COMMUNICATIONS OF COMMITTEE ON CHARACTER AND FITNESS AND LETTERS FROM DRS. A. C., D. B. AND B.T.

Personal History: Mr. L. was born in Chicago, as the middle of three siblings whose mother, after much family discord, separated from her husband and took D. to Poland when he was a child. After many vicissitudes, he returned to this country at the age of 20, served marginally well in the military, and completed evening law classes on the G. I. Bill in 1953. By that time, however, he was already having serious marital difficulties, and was changing industrial and government jobs (FBI, State Department, Library of Congress) with growing frequency because of increasingly fixed and bizarre ideas that he was being continually observed, persecuted and poisoned, and that his home was wired and his wife employed by FBI agents for nefarious purposes. In 1956 he was hospitalized in Washington for highly disturbed and possibly destructive behavior, and thereafter was kept on ataractic medication for several years by Dr. A. of that city. In 1962 he came to Chicago "to get away from the FBI," but has been unable to secure work and has had to live on his pension for total psychiatric disability. Dr. B., after a recent psychiatric examination of Mr. L. with psychologic consultation, submitted an equivocal report.

Current Mental Status: Mr. L.'s general intelligence is high normal, and there are no signs of organic defect or deterioration. However, beneath a thin facade of polite rationality he maintains a complex delusional system to the effect that, possibly because of his association with a homosexual friend, he not only was under incessant surveillance by the FBI and hounded from job to job, but that in addition numerous attempts were made to subvert his wife and friends and to harass and, if possible, kill him by poison or other means. He admits that "as a lawyer, I can't produce the evidence in court," but this in no way diminishes his convictions that he was thus persecuted—and, more importantly, may still be in great danger from unknown enemies here in Chicago.

Mr. L.'s relatively intact accessibility, physical orientations, and appropriate affectivity are not distinctively schizoid, but this renders his delusional system all the more rigid and stereotyped.

Diagnosis: Chronic paranoia, with acutely delusional exacerbations in episodes of confusion and excitement.

Recommendations: Regrettably, Mr. L.'s mental state seriously impairs his objectivity, judgment and interpersonal relationships, and renders him incapable of the ethical and effective practice of law. Therapy may possibly improve his capabilities, but the prognosis, unfortunately, is dubious at best.

Sex and Marriage

I took with equal seriousness referrals from the Chicago Court of Domestic Relations, or from lawyers who sent me their clients for advice as to whether reconciliation, separation, or divorce was the best solution, and what had best be done with regard to custody of the children. Here, too, I laid down conditions of professional confidentiality and, to retain a reputation for fairness and imparitality, refused to take any contending party as a patient, except when I was specifically requested by the Court to conduct follow-up interviews:

Again, a few examples:

Duplicate reports to opposing divorce attorneys who jointly requested advice as to what would be best for their respective clients:

TO: MR. Z. AND MR. A., ATTORNEYS
SUBJECT: MR. AND MRS. E.

As is ethical in such consultations, it is understood (a) that the following report of my examinations will omit all data that either Mr. or Mrs. E. wished to be kept confidential (b) that the conclusions reached will have relevance only to the problem of their marital compatibility, and (c) that no portion of this report be made available to any person other than the parties concerned and their counsellors.

Mr. S.F.E., age 34:

Mr. E. arrived nearly forty minutes late for his appointment, remarked casually that tardiness was one of his lifelong customs, and was thereafter quite vague, evasive or stereotyped in his communications. Nevertheless, enough data were gathered for the following psychiatric summary:

Personal History: Mr. E.'s father died when Mr. E. was only 10 years old, leaving nine children ranging in age from 19 to one year old to the care of Mr. E.'s mother. Under these adverse familial and economic conditions, Mr. E. developed a somewhat overcompensatory ambitiousness coupled with a lack of self-discipline and social coordination—a combination which resulted in marginal adjustments at school, in a long series of failures at various jobs, and recent difficulties in his religious affiliations. Corresponding tendencies to grandiosity, irresponsibility and escapism also affected his marital adjustments; for example, he quit his job just before his wedding in 1947 and lived 10 years in a 2½ room flat on his wife's income, because he refused to work steadily for a series of employers or in his own business ventures. He was away playing golf when his wife delivered their only daughter, now aged ten; he insisted on more children despite his wife's fears of repeated miscarriages and their continuous poverty and indebtedness; and he was home as little as possible, because, only two years after their marriage, he "could no longer stand her nagging and her tempers and her always diminishing me—and her damned interfering sister." When at his wife's insistence, they finally bought a home some 18 months ago he threatened that he "would burn it down around her ears if she didn't have more children"; however, when their conflicts increased instead of abated in the new environment, he left her and the child a year ago, and now wants a divorce.

Mental Status: Mr. E. has normal intelligence without signs of organic impairment; but he is emotionally unstable and deeply insecure in many ways. For example, he wavers between confessions of abject failure and overreactive self-importance, passive dependency *vs* blustering aggressivity; semi-fanatic religiosity *vs* cynical agnosticism, and pathetic indecision *vs* stubborn intransigence. The latter attitude currently is crystallized into a sullen rejection of his wife, but extends also into interpersonal remoteness and increasingly antisocial postures. These processes now constitute a serious character neurosis which may progressively handicap all of Mr. E.'s life adjustments; however, he has little insight into his own pecularities and almost no current desire to seek help for them.

Mrs. E.K.E., age 36

Personal History: Mrs. E.'s father died when she was five years old, and her mother a decade later, leaving her to be protected, perhaps excessively, by a sister nine years older than herself. Mrs. E.'s early scholastic, social, sexual and occupational adaptations, though not as marginal as those of her husband, also showed areas of maladjustment; and she entered marriage with almost as little clear forethought and realistic planning as did her husband. When the inevitable conflicts over money, family, sex, children, etc. occurred in rapid succession and increasing intensity, her reactions took the form of complaints, tempers and hysterics, setting up cycles of sulking, absences and periods of separation during the past six years. Since the last one three years ago she has returned to work and has acquired insistent suitors; however, she finds her "marriage failure" unpleasant and wants to "try him out again because my daughter still loves him, and we know he is emotionally sick."

Mental Status: Superficially, Mrs. E. is more warm, friendly, communicative, and receptive than her husband, though she soon reveals a quite similar tendency to headstrong self-righteousness and blames nearly all of her difficiltues on others. This stand includes the saving grace of (a) considering Mr. E. "sick" and (b) offering to undertake therapy for her own lesser "nervousness" if he would do the same in a joint effort to save their marriage. Unfortunately, this offer is also in part a covert bid for implicit victory in their many conflicts, though it may be more constructively employed by a skillful therapist.

Recommendations: Present indications are that unless

both Mr. and Mrs. E. undertake effective treatment for their respective personality difficulties, any rapprochement between them would be short-lived and would only add to their current conflicts and the emotional traumata imposed on their daughter. Mrs. E. professes to agree to such therapy but if, as is likely, Mr. E. refuses, renewed frictions, separations and an ultimate divorce seem inevitable. In that case Mrs. E. seems capable of caring for her daughter, whereas Mr. E.'s visitation rights should depend on the reliability and rationality of his future conduct.

When a marriage is primarily a contest for dominance between two weaklings:

TO: MR. Y. AND MR. J., ATTORNEYS
RE: MR. AND MRS. I.V.

The following summary of my examination of your clients must omit much confidential material, but may serve as a basis for objective recommendations.

Mr. I. V., age 38:

As the thirteenth of 15 children of an imperious Teutonic father and a subservient but indulgent mother, Mr. V. very early in life, adopted the paternal patterns of arrogant and aggressive behavior whenever given an opportunity to dominate or control others. During his brief education (he did not complete high school) these tendencies were channelized into athletic activities with some success, but since his marriage they have been directed mainly against his wife and children. The wedding was forced 19 years ago because Mrs. V.'s father thought her pregnant, but Mr. V. refused to let his wife adhere to her Catholic faith. Instead he made her live two years with his Jewish family, attempted to abort their first child and kept urging her to work to supplement his meager income and lack of social progress. When she began to make an independent career several years ago, by applying her literary and executive abilities, he turned his envy of her superior drive and intelligence into personal depreciations, jealousy, accusations of infidelity and threats that he would get her degraded and discharged by denouncing her to her bosses' wives "as a home-breaker." He regarded these actions as justified, and intended them to restore what he regarded as his rights and privileges in his home; Mrs. V., however, rebelled, and has left him repeatedly during the past 10 years. Mr. V.'s current attitude, predictably, is that he wants his wife back on the grounds of her duties to him and the children (boys aged 14 and 17), plus a renewal of the customary but exceedingly vague promises to "work things out for real family spirit like I've been brought up in."

Mrs. K. V.:

For her part Mrs. V., as the less favored of two sisters, was raised in an atmosphere of economic, religious and social conflict that inculcated deep feelings of inferiority and inadequacy. She permitted and perhaps sought early seduction and then, on religious grounds, immediately insisted on marriage to the first boy who she thought would be available; after this, to restore her self-respect in the face of many disappointments and rejections, she decided that she "would force I. to love her." By this she covertly meant eventual triumph over him and revenge for her mistreatment, since her familial, sexual, personal and parental relationships in her marriage have never been satisfactory by normal standards, and have deteriorated rapidly in the last few years. At present Mrs. V., like her husband, is still ambivalent about the impending divorce; on the plea of "pitying, not loving, him because he falls apart so," she keeps telephoning or seeing him, and thus re-opening old interpersonal contests.

Psychiatric Appraisal: As is evident even from these partial statements, the marriage of Mr. and Mrs. V. has been based up to now not on essential compatibilities but on mutually supplementary personal insecurities and neurotic needs. With Mrs. V.'s recent social and economic emancipation her need for dependence has vanished, leaving what is at present primarily a contest for marital dominance and control. Unfortunately, it is mainly on this inadequate basis that the two are currently dealing with each other at all.

Recommendations: In view of the above, it is also evident that sweeping personality changes in both Mr. and Mrs. V. are necessary before a healthy and lasting rapport between them could be established. Even though, under their current severe emotional distress, both may profess to desire such changes and even undertake intensive psychiatric counselling or therapy, this will not necessarily be successful in altering their deep-rooted characteristics and thereby making a happy marriage probable. Nevertheless, this is the only remaining possibility; without it, the unpleasant but almost certain reality must be faced that further relations between them will lead only to increasing recrimination, hostility, social conflict, or possibly even physical aggression.

Should they decide on psychiatric therapy—which must be intensive and will take months—I shall be glad to direct them to competent psychiatrists and help in any other way I can.

A report requested by the Presiding Judge of the Chicago Courts of Domestic Relations:

TO: THE HONORABLE ______
SUBJECT: MR. AND MRS. K.N.

Mrs. K.N., age 36

Presenting Problem: Mrs. N. states her position quite simply: This summer she was given unequivocal evidence that her husband had been robbing her, her children, and her family for years through forgery and embezzlement; following this, she lost all confidence in him, and now wants at least a separation and at best an early divorce.

Personal History: Mrs. N. considers her father "dynamic and very competent," her mother "altogether darling," and feels that both always and unremittingly have been interested in and protective of her personal welfare. Accordingly, she never considered it particularly important to plan for her own future, spent her adolescence mainly in recreational or ancillary interests, developed ulcers when subjected to even the minor stresses of college (these cleared when she discontinued her education and consulted a psychiatrist for a year), and then worked at various minor jobs. Her first marriage at the age of "about twenty-two" was to someone she describes as "a brilliant boy named Jerry, but his family thought I was dumb." Difficulties ensued almost immediately over her continued irresponsibilities and escapsims, her sexual inhibitions and recurrent miscarriages; consequently, the marriage soon broke up amid familial quarrels, despite the fact that the couple had adopted a boy, D., now 11½ years old. Mrs. N. returned to her own family haven for another three years until she "fell madly in love with K.N. because he was kind and thoughtful—just like my father." However, "K. never supported me," did not fulfill his promises to find steady work, and as she learned later, "cheated my family out of thousands of dollars," while her sister and father protected her from this knowledge by covering up most of his defalcations. During this time she kept blaming her own "stupidity" for her unbalanced accounts and vanishing resources until, in August of this year, she was confronted with certain evidence that allegedly he had been "lying, forging, and embezzling from me, the children, the neighbors, and everyone else ever since we got married." She then developed a recurrence of ulcers and migraine, enlisted her family in arranging a separation and, as she repeatedly insists, now wants a divorce.

Mental Status: Mrs. N. has average intelligence, but is currently operating at a far lower level of general competence because of her emotional immaturity, dependent irresponsibility and persistent naivete, as particularly evident in her vagueness and lack of insight into her own personality deficiencies. If she did not have available the ready refuge of her family, she might be driven, despite her marital disillusionments, to resume her previous childlike and unrealistic dependence upon her husband, but this would probably be at the cost of more ulcers, migraine, and recurrent anxiety or depression. Under the present circumstances she is quite resolute in her decision to discard him, but characteristically has no other plans than to have her father support her and the children until "maybe I can marry again."

Mr. K.N., age 34

Presenting Problem: Mr. N. eventually made his stand equally simple: "I love my wife and children, and I'm not going to divorce her no matter what I promise the judge, or her, or you . . . and I don't care if I make everybody suffer either." As was predictable, he could not define precisely what he meant by "love" or how he was going to have it reciprocated if he continued his past and current behavior. Mr. N.'s accounts of his life are so evasive and contradictory that the following must be recorded as only tentative and impressionistic.

Personal History: As did his wife, Mr. N. describes his own parents as wealthy, self-sacrificing and almost completely indulgent: "They treated all three of us brothers like only children." He also never considered it necessary to put forth consistent efforts toward independent scholastic, social, or occupational adjustments, but claims he studied moderately well in school, obtained a university degree in architecture, and was promoted to a captaincy in the army in this specialty, even though he had not previously troubled to take his exams and secure an architect's license. He vaguely admits that after marriage he "deceived" his wife about his prospects and jobs, told her "half-truths" about his income, "covered his dealings by signing her name on stocks" (he claims he had informed her so on one occasion), and "borrowed from her accounts." When she finally had him arrested for forgery, he avoided criminal prosecution by making a partial financial restitution, hence "she can't get me on a felony." He "can't explain" why he had neither succeeded as an independent architect, nor sought work during the past six years, except that he "didn't have contacts and took on too much," however, he claims he is now "chief architect for a $9,000,000 building at the city airport," is making "large fees," and "will soon be well off" even though he has had to "waste $15,000 in three months on my lawyers to fight the divorce and pay off my old debts." At this point Mr. N.'s statements become increasingly bizarre, to wit: "My wife is being hypnotized by her father, like Svengali . . . she is in a trance all the time . . . Dr. S. said she was in a trance too . . . but if I get rich and pay off her father—all he wants is money—he'll let her out of the trance. . . . I know she loves me but she is hypnotized and can't say so until I break the spell. . . ."

Mental Status: Mr. N.'s intelligence is adequate, but his motivations, values, and conduct disturbances are typically those of a person with only a marginal sense of social responsibility. Recently, his cumulative failures and the shock of his final rejections by his wife, in-laws, and parents seem to have impaired his grasp of realities and caused an increase of grandiosity, a recourse to irrational fantasies and self-deceptions, and rigid defiance of any advice or guidance. Since he has little insight into his own reactions and their effects on others, there is almost no likelihood of spontaneous improvement either in his values or his trustworthiness within the immediate future, and certainly none without prolonged guidance and therapy.

Conjoint Interview: When Mr. and Mrs. N. were interviewed together, she openly reiterated her complete rejection of him, whereas he insisted that he would not give her a divorce, because she really loved him and was only being forced against her will by her father. It was evident that this impasse would lead only to more quarrels and perhaps violence should a "reconciliation" be attempted without fundamental changes in the attitudes of both parties.

Consultation with Dr. S.:

My conversation with Dr. S., who had interviewed Mrs. N. and had treated Mr. N. for several months, confirmed the diagnostic surveys as outlined above.

Recommendations: There seems no present prospect that this marriage can be reconstituted to the benefit of anyone, including the litigants, their children, and respective families, unless Mr. and Mrs. N. separated and were sincerely motivated to undertake prolonged individual therapy—which neither is at present inclined to do; even then, in view of their longstanding personality deviations, the results would be dubious. The most reasonable course from a psychiatric standpoint would nevertheless be a prolonged separation while each undertakes such therapy, the outcome then to depend on their consistent conduct, rather than the opportunistic promises or temporary maneuvers of each. The eldest son D. is already receiving psychiatric care; the other children should also be placed in a receptive, non-contentious environment and watched and treated for behavior disorders. I shall be glad to refer any of the parties concerned for further counselling if the Court or they so desire.

A judicial consultation occasionally reveals a situation that involves not only the psychiatrist's professional but social responsibilities. A case in point is the following:

REPORT TO: THE HONORABLE ________
SUBJECT: MR. AND MRS. J. U. SUMMARY OF PSYCHIATRIC EXAMINATION

Mrs. U:

As will be seen under the description of her mental status, the information furnished by Mrs. U. is at best confused and at other times so fantastic and self-contradictory that it cannot be given direct credence. However, it is here summarized as typical of her attitudes and thinking:

Personal History: Mrs. U. idealized her father (to whose memory she is still exceedingly attached) as "perfect in every way, even though he had pernicious anemia," whereas her mother is described in highly adverse terms. She admitted that she herself was always "high strung," but managed to complete normal school and engage in substitute teaching. After "dating many men," she "fell in love with a man who I thought was much like my father; but when he propositioned me and didn't have father's perfect integrity, I decided to go to Nevada with Mr. U. instead. On the way he had a nervous breakdown, but I thought he had pernicious anemia like my father, so I married him. But for a long time my other boyfriends shadowed him and my brother threatened to kill him because they were so jealous."

Marital History: This portion of the anamnesis is even more fantastic. In effect, Mrs. U. relates vaguely that for the first month after marriage her relations with her husband consisted of his "putting smelly substances on her hair and rubbing his own stomach" while she rubbed his back, and that thereafter they practiced various perversions, particularly per anum. When her boys were born her husband switched to pederasty, and apparently has practiced it frequently on the younger son K., ever since the latter was four years old. She now remembers having heard the child screaming repeatedly while locked in the bathroom with his father, but she made no moves to investigate until the boy was thirteen. Then a Dr. O. reportedly confirmed the fact that the child had been sexually abused, after which she accused her husband of homosexuality *elsewhere* and separated from him. Scattered through her account were vague admissions that her son K. had been seen by a psychiatrist in early childhood, that she herself had been under psychiatric treatment, and that she had not followed recommendations to the effect that she should be divorced and that K. was seriously retarded and needed special care. Instead she had taken the boy for years to a so-called non-directive counselling center for his "speech disability"—even though the boy has made no discernible progress and is now mentally defective in many respects.

Mental Status: Mrs. U.'s ideation is diffuse, repetitious, illogical, and at times definitely delusional. For example, she is convinced that Judge P. has been victimized in a plot by four of her former lawyers whom she has dismissed, and that her present attorney also instructed her to deceive the examiner so that her husband would win the case. Her emotionality is correspondingly labile and excessive, making her interpersonal contacts precarious and unstable. Her only plans are (a) to secure a divorce and alimony, (b) to protect K. from further sexual seduction during his weekend meetings with his father, and, of all things, (c) to derive her livelihood by expanding her "school for children" from its present enrollment of four (aged 2 to 5) to an indefinitely larger number.

Mr. S. U.

Personal History: Mr. U.'s father was a minister who apparently dominated Mr. U. since an early age, especially after the latter's mother died when he was nine years old. A latent, highly ambivalent homosexually-tinged bond between the father and son became established, and continued to the elder U.'s death last autumn. Mr. U. grew to be a retiring, dependent, ineffectual person with relatively poor school, military, and occupational adjustments until late in life. He had almost no heterosexual interests, did not marry until he was "about 38," and almost immediately decided that he "did not love" his wife; thereafter he "retired from her into other interests." He accuses her of variously mistreating both children and of "beating K. with a strap to make him stop being dumb," but he seems never to have interfered with such abuse. He vociferously denies sexual relations with either boy, and offers "to take a lie test any time—providing my wife will pay for it"; however, such denials are accompanied by manifest anxiety and discomfort and either a resigned apathy or overreactive anger. He admits that when she accused him of homosexuality a year ago, he quite specifically threatened to kill her and then "gladly left." His preferences now would be to divorce his wife and place his son, K. (whose exact age he could not recall) in a foster home five days a week "if I can see him weekends"; otherwise, he has no special plans.

Mental Status: Mr. U. is somewhat more intelligent and superficially better integrated than his wife, but at deeper levels he is as irrational, disturbed, and deviant as she. My examination could not determine whether he had actually committed pederasty, but did reveal strong indications of homosexual patterns of thought and action. In any case, Mr. U.'s insight and judgment are inadequate to look after his own, let alone his children's, interest.

Impression of K. U., age 15:

In the absence of a request to do so, the boy was not examined formally. However, judging from his speech and behavior in my office and samples of his writing, he seemed seriously retarded and in manifest need of prolonged and expert care.

Recommendations: In view of the above, separation or divorce between Mr. and Mrs. U. seem inevitable and probably desirable. However, neither parent at present is sufficiently stable, emotionally mature, or intellectually competent to be entrusted with the care of their child, K. On the contrary, the boy is urgently in need of psychiatric examination and diagnosis at the Institute for Juvenile Research or a similarly competent institution, to be followed by proper foster home placement and expert supervision. It is even more alarming that Mrs. U. seems to be running some sort of children's "day school"—a trust for which she is eminently ill-suited, and in which she might do considerable harm to impressionable children. I earnestly request the Court to take this under advisement or refer it to the proper jurisdiction.

The marital problems of later life.

REPORT TO: THE HON. S.J.
SUBJECT: MR. AND MRS. I.C.

Mrs. M.C, aged 56

Mrs. C. admits that her emotional insecurities and hypersensitivities date to her childhood, when she was raised by an invalided mother who suffered from "hysterical fevers" during the father's prolonged absences from home. Nevertheless, she completed a fair education, worked steadily, maintained her marriage faithfully for 32 years, "raised and married off" her only daughter (who now has four children of her own) and even helped support her husband during long periods of his illness by piecework at home until a year ago. At that time, however, she discovered he was having occasional sexual relations with a neighbor's middle-aged wife, and in reaction developed a chronic depressive state characterized by fatigue, loss of appetite and weight (down to 100 lbs.), frequent crying spells, and a maintained mood of suspicion and recrimination. Last February, after many broken promises and ensuing quarrels, she sued for divorce "to see if the shock would change him"; since it did not, she now confides that without letting Mr. C. know, she has confronted her husband's paramour and plans to "sue her for alienation of affections just to see what he will do then."

Mental Status: Mrs. C is a cooperative and fairly intelligent woman who, unfortunately, seems to have been exceedingly disturbed by what she considers a recent and devastating assault on her fragile security system. In overreaction, she has harassed her husband excessively with suspicions and demands, and by her own retreat into a variably agitated and hostile melancholic state. Her present plans to "test" her husband by further new threats and suits are correspondingly unrealistic and confused, being compounded of motives of revenge and a contrary fear of being totally deserted and helpless at her present age unless she can frighten him into compliance. She has partly recognized this irrationality and has occasionally sought help from physicians and made single visits to two psychiatrists, but obviously needs more thorough and consistent guidance.

Mr. I.C., aged 62

Mr. C's personal history is here irrelevant other than that he apparently never developed truly deep and consistent feelings of responsibility and loyalty toward anyone, including his wife. His affair with a neighbor began casually as a reassertion of aging virility some 18 months ago, and was admittedly not occasioned by any actions or deficiencies on the part of his wife other than that she was not invariably sexually responsive. Since then, however, he feels very bitter about her "nagging and crying and calling me up all the time; if she'd just leave me alone things would probably work out by themselves." He intends neither to marry nor to leave his paramour, but at the same time wishes to retain his marriage—with just a "period of separation so I can have some time to myself." Naturally, he desires his wife to drop all accusations and suits immediately, and feels martyred that she does not do so.

Marital Status: Mr. C, too, has intellectual capacities within normal range, but his exercise of them, especially in the current situation, is handicapped by long-term personality characteristics of recalcitrance, thoughtless and sometimes arrogant self-seeking, insensitivity to the feelings of others, a tendency toward conscious hypocrisy, and resort to frank hostility when not given his own way in his interpersonal dealings.

He, too, regards a divorce as eventually inconvenient yet, despite half-hearted disclaimers, feels no real contrition about his past behavior or any sincere desire to alter it except under direct threat of punishment.

Recommendations: In view of the currently incompatible motivations and interactions of Mr. and Mrs. C., it is probable that a period of directed separation would do little toward really healing the breach, since after the usual mutual promises the same or similar conflicts would soon recur between them. Divorce and ensuing litigations would be no less futile in giving either of them stable satisfactions. One course would be to refer each for competent marital counselling with or without temporary separation; if they agree and the Court assents, I shall be happy to help them arrange it. In any case they will probably rejoin each other eventually, since neither has much of an alternative.

And another instance, in briefest summary:

TO THE HONORABLE L:

Herewith the reports on Mr. and Mrs. L.S., both aged 55. From a psychological standpoint neither really wants a divorce, since each basically needs the other. Unfortunately, however, with each the conflict has now become a matter of personal prestige and dominance: Mrs. S., consciously or not, has the attitude that if she acceded to her husband's sexual and other demands before he gave up drinking she would lose status and control, whereas Mr. S. feels that drinking and sex are indispensable trappings to mask his fears of inferiority. The solution would be to make each feel personal satisfaction rather than supposed defeat in a reconciliation—a task in which you have had long experience. As to Mr. S.'s drinking, I can help him control that, if he so desires, with Antabuse and other modern methods.

When an attorney requests an unauthorized Court report:

TO THE HONORABLE PRESIDING JUDGE J.C.,

I am in receipt of a request from Attorney M for a copy of my report on Mr. F.G., whose examination by me was directed by Judge M.M.

If Your Honor please, it has been my custom in the past to observe both medical and legal ethics by sending all reports in duplicate only to the referring judge, and then leaving it to the discretion of the Court as to who should have access to this confidential material. For the sake of the efficiency and validity of the psychiatric examination, I would prefer to have this practice continue, but if you order otherwise, I shall of course comply.

The Court authorized me to keep my reports confidential.

Myself as Judge

Considered with equal seriousness were requests from seminaries and religious societies to assay the qualifications and handicaps of candidates for ministerial or missionary training, since such evaluations might determine the future not only of the candidate, but the myriads of people he would influence during his career:

YE SHALL NOT ANOINT THEM

REPORT TO: THE X BIBLICAL INSTITUTE
SUBJECT: THE QUALIFICATIONS OF MR. I.T.C. AS A CANDIDATE FOR THE MINISTRY

Mr. C. himself disclaims knowing any reasons for the referral.

Personal History: Mr. C. grudgingly describes his father as an active, outgoing, energetic, relatively successful businessman with a deep interest in his church and so great an urge to preach that he acquired a "preacher's license." His mother is described in somewhat similar terms with an addendum—obviously depreciatory toward his father—that "she makes snap judgments much easier than he does." Mr. C.'s attitudes, as further revealed in the tenor of his descriptions of others who influenced his early life, indicate similar feelings of remoteness, resentment, and interpersonal estrangement. In childhood, these early attitudes became manifest in dislike of elementary school, playmates, and most of his teachers, frequent truancy, and a general sense of rebellion and isolation. He felt less restricted in high school, cultivated some interest in abstract subjects such as mathematics, and planned to become an accountant; nevertheless, he continued to be shy, socially backward, and highly limited in his extracurricular activities. During this period he sought guidance from a local pastor, who apparently believed that entry into religious work would solve the youth's problems and urged him to consider the ministry; indeed, Mr. C.'s later choice of your seminary may have been strongly conditioned by the fact that he followed this pastor to his assignment in your city. After a term in military service to which he adjusted only minimally well, Mr. C. entered T____ College on his veteran's allowances as a means of "marking time while studying" until he "could find himself between accounting and the ministry." Once again, whereas he developed few friendships and social interests, his one "love affair" became so intense and conflictual that when the girl informed him that she was tired of his idiosyncracies and self-centeredness and wished to terminate their relationship, he reacted with deep depression and thoughts of suicide. This episode seemed to swing the balance toward an attempt to find solace in the ministry, and he enrolled in your seminary.

Unfortunately, his course since then has again been scholastically and personally unsatisfactory. Torn by conflicting goals and preoccupations, he does not enjoy or concentrate upon his studies; instead, he rationalizes his failures with statements that the requirements are unjustly high, the teachers dull, the work mostly uninteresting and much of the teaching unacceptable. The latter statement leads to a revelation of even deeper motivational and intellectual turmoil to the effect that, since his very faith in the existence of God has been shaken by his readings, he would be unable to expound His existence in a way that would be acceptable to future congregations.

Symptomatology: On further discussion, Mr. C. fitted a varied but generally ominous list of symptoms in reaction to recurrent situations of stress. For instance, periods of doubt and indecision had always resulted in severe headaches; and, if there was much concurrent frustration (as in military service, after his love affair, etc.), periods of depression supervened and would lead to an occasional agitated melancholia. Special or acute stresses would also precipitate episodes of trance-like day-dreaming, with or without actual feelings of stupor or faintness.

Current Mental Status: Mr. C.'s general intelligence is relatively high and shows a fair distribution of special abilities in grasp, comprehension, abstract reasoning and communication. Unfortunately, these capacities are considerably vitiated by deep internal conflicts which also impair his social, sexual, and current occupational adjustments. The origin of these conflicts may tentatively be traced to intensely ambivalent dependencies on his parents and autistic withdrawals from extrafamilial discipline in early youth; but, whatever their precise nature and origin, these conflicts pervade most of Mr. C.'s behavior and render his reality adjustments tenuous and difficult.

Diagnosis: Schizoid personality.

Recommendations: Mr. C. will require intensive psychotherapy in order to be able to continue at the seminary, but even then his prognosis is uncertain and guarded. On the other hand, an abrupt dismissal would be highly traumatic to him and might induce a serious depressive reaction. Therefore, if he does not undertake intensive treatment, his separation from school should be arranged tactfully and every effort be made to orient his immediate future favorably. In either case, I would be glad to render any further assistance which may be needed.

REPORT TO: THE BIBLICAL INSTITUTE
SUBJECT: MR. X. A. AS A CANDIDATE FOR THE MINISTRY

Reasons for Referral: Mr. A. professes not to know any reason for his being referred for examinations.

Personal History: Mr. A. is exceedingly defensive about his familial background and only under the most tactful questioning can be led to "confess" that his father "died insane in a Colorado State mental hospital," allegedly of an "accident." This occurred when Mr. A. was seven years old, after which he was moved by his restless and emotionally unstable mother among various branches of the family in New York, Kansas, and finally back to his home near Denver, Colorado; consequently, his adolescent schooling was sketchy and his social and occupational adjustments transitory and inadequate. After variable periods as a domestic servant, a farm hand, a restaurant worker, and a trucker, he was drafted in 1943 and sent to serve with the Seabees in and about Saipan, at which time, as will be noted, his previously minimal personality difficulties and neurotic tendencies became exacerbated.

Marital and Sexual History: Mr. A. remained almost childishly naive about sexual matters until adulthood and shy and awkward in his relationships with women, until, at 22, he "took pity on a physically very attractive girl whose father had been a wastrel who abused her" (here Mr. A. stopped and quite audibly smacked his lips and sucked his tongue). After an acquaintance of only a few months he married her, as he put it, "to raise her up among living and decent people," but soon afterwards had to depart for military service. Upon his return in 1945, he found that "she had been unfaithful and extravagant, and so I permitted her to divorce me and keep the children." Asked to elaborate upon this, Mr. A. becomes confused and contradictory; e.g. he states that his two daughters aged nine and eleven "adored him" yet chose to go with their mother, that his wife was "sorry that she had lost me" and yet had been obviously enthusiastic about securing her divorce, etc. Since then, Mr. A. has "avoided women and all thoughts of them," yet "some day when I meet one really worthy maybe I will marry again."

Mr. A. states as his immediate reason for coming to the seminary that he wished to prepare himself for the task of "teaching religion in some great university." Asked why he had chosen his goal so relatively late in life, his answers once again become characteristically defensive and evasive: He had "terminated his pastorate in Colorado," because he had felt that his "abilities could be better utilized in the field of pedagogy," and also because "I have been divorced—and nobody trusts a divorced pastor." When requested to elaborate further, he launched upon a somewhat incoherent exposition to the effect that he was "a prophet rather than a preacher" and followed this by a depreciation of a pastor as being "just an administrator and an organizer who has to deal with church boards who don't know anything about religion." When his attitude on this too was mildly questioned, Mr. A. became quite overtly antagonistic and threatened to expound to the seminary administration the unwisdom of having ministers examined by people who, "like the great majority of all Americans, are never conscious of God. You can't expect me to explain my philosophy to anybody who can't understand such things." The tactful diversion of the examination to other topics, however, restored Mr. A.'s professed but essentially brittle and precarious cooperation.

Symptomatology: As may be inferred from the above account, Mr. A. began suffering from episodes of anxiety, various compulsions and phobias, and recurrent depressive episodes during adolescence, and has manifested those reactions to stress in increasing degrees ever since. There seems to have been a serious neurotic breakdown requiring temporary hospitalization during his military service, but Mr. A. is so evasive about this episode that no precise data are available. His divorce and his recent personal frictions and failures in the ministry have likewise precipitated episodes of anxiety and melancholia; moreover, since his resignation and his enrollment at the Seminary, his suspiciousness, hostility and covert feelings of being misunderstood and persecuted have reached almost paranoid levels.

Diagnosis: Depressive personality with compulsive and paranoid tendencies.

Recommendations: I regret to report that Mr. A. is suited

neither intellectually nor temperamentally for the ministry, and that his adjustments to an academic post would be rendered highly problematical by his personality difficulties. It is doubtful whether he would cooperate with psychotherapy, and even if he did so and could secure a highly skilled therapist, the prognosis would still be uncertain. I therefore cannot recommend his further training at present.

REPORT TO: THE BIBLICAL INSTITUTE
SUBJECT: MR. S. T. AS A CANDIDATE FOR THE MINISTRY

Reasons for Referral: Possible homosexuality. Mr. T.'s version is that he himself wishes psychiatric or psychologic consultation, but mainly for the reason that he is finding it "increasingly difficult to concentrate" on his studies.

Significant Aspects of Personal History: Mr. T. regards his father, who dicd four years ago, as having always been a distant, shadowy figure whom he "didn't know very well." In contrast, his mother is described as a driving, nagging, "nervous" woman who has controlled his life since childhood, usually managed to have her own way and even now participates in many of his activities and interests. Many of Mr. T.'s comments on this score imply covert incestuous guilts and conflicts involving his maternal relationships, and indicate attempts to escape from these through a diffusion of interests, shallowness of interpersonal bonds outside the family, derisive attitudes toward women in general, and, finally, compensatory homosexual preoccupations. These reactions seem also to have extended to education and social maladaptations since an early age so that, for the most part, Mr. T. has been a restless, emotionally unstable, and frequently anxiety-ridden individual.

Presenting Situation: Mr. T.'s own account of his current difficulties may be summarized as follows: Eight or nine months ago one of his roommates, a Greek student named "something like Goromykalas" (characteristically, Mr. T. was uncertain of the name) allegedly made "an attempt to pinch my shoulder or maybe to kiss me." Mr. T. says he resisted these advances and was "popped a couple of times for my pains." He became greatly excited and preoccupied with a fear that "he might lay his hands on me when I am asleep," and therefore reported this incident to the school authorities. Asked why, by his own description, he had been so disturbed at the time, Mr. T. launched into a glib harangue about "being caught in the specific culture of our civilization, with its senseless opposition and indoctrination about homosexuality..." Finally, with many circumlocutions, he conveyed that whereas he "understood homosexuality," he "could not countenance it culturally." But from this, and with hardly any transition, he shifted to an attack on "the ministry not being up to moral standards," whereas he himself "preferred to be interested in the phenomena of morality and emotion in terms of man's effects on his culture—in a word cultural psychiatry." These thoughts, again with almost no hiatus, led to a supposedly sophisticated but almost incoherent attack on Dr. B., a previous examiner who, according to Mr. T., had "so structured his interviews" that "when I asked him about religion, he said that he could discuss it only in terms of my neurosis." This indicated, according to Mr. T., that "Dr. B. planned to impose his philosophy on me and thus deprive me of my individuality." As to the present interview, Mr. T. also wished it clearly understood that he would "resist any similar maneuver" on my part and would, indeed, have to be "persuaded" that he needed any sort of therapy. At this point only with difficulty was he reassured that no one concerned had any intention of imposing any course of action on him whatsoever.

Mental Status: Mr. T. is oriented for time and place, conversant with sensorial reality, and is as yet unimpaired in the usual intellectual functions. Nevertheless, his stereotyped mannerisms, evasively confused elocutions, emotional overreactions and blockings and unmistakable paranoid tendencies indicate a markedly disturbed personality, only precariously adjusted at present and highly vulnerable even to minor social stress. More specifically, latent but explosive homosexual tendencies are clearly present and likely to erupt into direct activity or aggressive countermeasures under unfavorable circumstances.

Recommendations: Regrettably, S. T. is unsuited for the

ministry. It is, in fact, problematic whether Mr. T. desires or can be benefited by brief therapy.

A difficult choice between Jove and Jesus—misinterpreted as between Vice and Virtue—was involved in this referral from a missionary board.

REPORT TO: THE MISSIONARY BOARD
SUBJECT: MISS K.G., AGE 27

Presenting Problem: Miss G. is struggling with a decision as to whether to continue her career as a singing actress, or whether to surrender this in favor of marrying her fiancé and joining him in the missionary career for which he is training.

Relevant Personal History: A highly important influence in Miss G.'s life has been her intensely ambivalent and unresolved attachment to her alcoholic father. She describes this somewhat as follows: When he was sober she idealized him as a devoted and fun-loving companion who was proud of her accomplishments; when he was intoxicated, she spent hours in silent prayer that he would overcome his "faults of blasphemy and irresponsibility." When Miss G. was thirteen years of age her parents were divorced, leaving her with conflictful drives toward active self-sufficiency and independence *vs.* a yearning for passive security and belongingness. Both were reflected throughout her schooling by a need for status and popularity in various extracurricular activities, such as concerts and class plays; in her church work she was simultaneously troubled by religious doubts and excessive concern with service or choir; so also, her social and heterosexual development was marked by a series of intensive attachments either to men she described as "domineering and masculine like my father" (she was "engaged" to one for six years), or to weakly effeminate ones "like my mother" (she nearly married one three years ago), or to the "moral, dedicated Christian type like my stepfather" as exemplified by her current fiancé. Significantly, during most of these intensely ambivalent relationships she was travelling from Korea to England with dance bands, USO troupes or musical shows, and in each case except the last finally decided that her devotion had been misplaced. Now also, despite her current idealization of Mr. F. and her self-styled "burning of bridges behind me, so maybe I can marry him in December"—she has, as an instance of this "resolution," declined some tentative offers of musical comedy contracts—her inner indecision and turmoil are still manifest in episodes of tension, anxiety, depression, and ruminative obsessions as to whether she "really made the proper choice."

Psychological Examination: Miss G. has superior general intelligence and considerable talent in imagery and both verbal and kinesic communication; in this connection her somewhat exaggerated gestures and mannered speech seem more a part of ingrained stage and TV training than marks of insincerity. As indicated, she has deep longings for status and companionship, but is at the same time fearful of being unappreciated, disappointed, mistreated, and deserted, as she had been in childhood. In the latter regard, she confesses to persistent resentments of her fiancé's self-righteousness, religious unctuousness, and preachy prejudices against what he terms "frivolous theatrical people." His main attraction is his presumed altruism, reliability, and the offer of the "true Christian missionary life"; but unfortunately her concepts of being a missionary wife are rather unrealistically roseate with regard to adventure, travel, and rewards. Toward the end of the interview she became more conscious of her inner conflicts not only about her marriage but about other goals and values, and recognized that she needed help to work out a stable decision that would be lastingly satisfactory to her fiance, herself, and the missionary board.

Impression: An intelligent, talented girl deeply conflictful over unconscious fears and yearnings which cannot be resolved by immediate, arbitrary, or impulsive action. If Miss G. chose the role of missionary wife and then became seriously regretful of her choice, she would almost certainly become subject to severe and disabling depressive reactions.

Recommendations: Miss G. will need a period of expert counselling to help her resolve her conflicts; until then, it would be best to postpone all irreversible decisions. If the Society so directs, I shall be glad to recommend a competent psychiatrist wherever she may be during the next several months.

Follow-up "Social Call" Four Years Later: Miss G. is now the better half of an apparently happily married and jovial musical comedy team occasionally to be seen on national television.

About a woman who wished to become a missionary at the age of nearly sixty:

REPORT TO THE Z MISSIONARY SOCIETY
SUBJECT: MRS. E. E. AS A MISSIONARY

Presenting Problem: In essence whether Mrs. E, after an early orphaning followed by a relatively sheltered and protected life, can at the age of 59 function as a missionary teacher in a foreign field.

Relevant Personal History: This revealed that, after the early parental deaths and resultant familial separations, Mrs. E achieved excellent individual, sexual, and social adaptations throughout her school and college years despite problems arising from foster-family care and economic limitations. She performed well as a primary grades teacher, and concurrently was a competent and beloved mother while she and her husband cooperated well in dedicated and fruitful church service. They served as missionaries in the Congo after their marriage in 1930—he as a dental surgeon and she as a teacher—but he later assumed university and clinical duties in this country until his death from cancer three years ago. It is particularly significant that she rebounded well even from this loss, returning to teaching within a week "as the best thing I could do for everybody," and has continued to readapt well individually and socially in nearly all respects. However, after three years of reorientation she now feels ready to give what she hopes, despite her late years, will be greater Christian service than she can render in her present limited position.

Mental Status: Mrs. E. has a well-maintained general intelligence, with no clinical evidence of definitive senile or other significant impairments in perceptive, abstractive, phasic, and related capacities other than a bit of slowing commensurate with her age. In personality she is gentle, soft-spoken, interested, fairly well balanced emotionally, and modest—particularly with regard to her capacities to learn a new language. Nevertheless, she has derived additional motivation and confidence from the approval of her three children for her plans, from a recent European trip during which she "proved I can take care of myself where I am," and from the fact that, even so, she hopes to live and teach in Asuncion, Paraguay, where she will be with familiar friends at the Friendship Mission.

Recommendations: With medical clearance and with no mnemonic or phasic handicaps revealed by special tests, I am happy to recommend Mrs. E. for a few more years of foreign service as a missionary teacher—preferably, however, in initially partly familiar, nonstressful, and friendly surroundings.

When the executive secretary of a missionary society sought advice as to how to respond to outraged complaints from candidates that they had been inadequately examined when they were informed of their rejection—sometimes, unfortunately, not by the society, but directly by the psychologic or psychiatric consultants who had interviewed them:

June 8, 1962

Dear Mr. ________:

Imparting unwelcome information to anyone is a difficult task, and when that results in serious disillusionment and disappointment, it is almost sure to elicit disbelief, resentment, and hostility—particularly in the types of persons whose inner weaknesses, marginal interpersonal skills, and deficient insight necessitated their rejection in the first place. Some clinical psychologists have the tact and skill to handle such situations; others, (including some psychiatrists) do not—and finally, some people cannot be reassured and pacified by the most skillful examiners, again confirming the wisdom of the original decision. As to the actual length of my own interviews: I generally spend about sixty minutes reviewing the records and psychological reports, a minimum of forty-five minutes and longer as necessary with each candidate, and up to two hours formulating the reports.

All in all, I suggest that you really need not invariably assume the obligation to explain, let alone apologize, for the rejection of candidates; in most cases, a kind, tactful, and considerate letter advising the candidate that he is best qualified for other fields should suffice. On receipt of such a letter, the reactions of rejected candidates would range from regarding it as God's directive toward domestic service, to its being a sign of Satanic subservience or hopeless idiocy on the part of the Society and its consultants—and proceed from there toward more comfortable rationalizations. In instances where candidates demand an explanation, some could be told, again with firm kindliness, that all decisions were made on the basis of *many* data from many sources, all of which must be kept confidential, and only in special instances where the interview would not be misused would referral to a psychologist or psychiatrist be advisable. This would save not only the Society's finances, but many a needless headache or heartache for all concerned. However, I'll continue to help in individual instances in every way I can.

Industrial: The fear of employees' litigious cupidity has become so general among some employers that occasionally a reassuring report may encourage the rehiring of an injured workman:

REPORT TO: THE COMPANY, INC.
SUBJECT: MR. C.A.'S SUITABILITY FOR RE-EMPLOYMENT

Presenting Symptoms: Mr. C. A. states that six months ago he inadvertently pushed his right hand and forearm too deeply into a mechanical grinder and suffered a mangling injury which necessitated amputation. He makes no claims about lack of safety devices or other company liability, and voluntarily informs the examiner that he has considered himself well treated surgically, orthopedically, and personally. His only request at present is that he be rehired at some job suited to his limited physical capacities.

Personal History: Mr. A. was born in Chicago into a family environment rendered unstable and contentious by almost continuous parental disagreements. However, there is no history of serious nervous or mental disorders in his heredity, and other members of his family are normal; e.g., his only other sibling—an older sister—is at present making adequate adjustments as a university student. Mr. A.'s own schooling was irregular and did not progress after a third year of high school; however, he has held various jobs since an early age after school and during the summers, and was apparently a consistent and reliable worker. He spent two years in military service; during this time, although he was disciplined twice for minor infractions, his record on the whole was satisfactory and he received an honorable discharge. Mr. A. claims, apparently truthfully that he has had no significant occupational, social, or personal maladjustments prior to the onset of his disability.

Neurological Examination: Essentially normal neurological findings. There is no evidence of peripheral neuritis in the stump, and Mr. A. is learning to use his prosthesis fairly effectively.

Mental Examination: Mr. A. was at first curious and somewhat suspicious as to why he had been sent to a "mind doctor" for his examination, but his confidence and cooperation were secured relatively easily. His intelligence is within normal limits, and in personality he is relatively frank, pleasant, and extroverted. His ambitions sometimes exceed his apparent capacities; for instance, he plans, if possible, to attend trade school and learn "radio or radar." On the other hand, he is realistic in that he expects to support himself by working and makes no present claims for extra compensations, special grants for his disabilities, or other demands. His current job expectations are likewise reasonable: He is willing to accept any sort of routine work which he feels capable of handling with the limited use of one arm.

Recommendations: There are adequate indications that Mr. A, far from being litigious or "accident-prone," is a capable and reliable individual who earnestly desires to return to work and deserves consideration in this regard. If treated fairly, he will very likely again prove to be a grateful and productive worker.

Confidential reports to medical colleagues could be made more explicit—provided they were to your friends. Plain talk to a physician about an adolescent sent for consultation:

Dear Dr. ____:

Your 17-year-old nephew K.N. can be characterized briefly: about as badly spoiled, self-willed, and undisciplined a perennial pubescent as I've had in the office lately. Unfortunately, he has learned all the standard techniques of seducing and controlling his parents—particularly his wishfully gullible mother—and is firmly convinced that these will serve him indefinitely everywhere. Some of his misinterpretations of reality border on the schizoid, but his main patterns of escapism, indulgence, bravado, and explosive aggression when frustrated are sociopathic and still possibly reversible.

His treatment, of course, will have to be directed as much to his family as himself, along the following lines:

1. Simple explanations, avoiding all technical terms and medical implications, of his need to learn different character patterns and external adjustments.
2. Insistence on regular hours, a job, social decency, etc., to be encouraged by set predictable rewards or enforced by inevitable punishments.
3. Failing adequate control at home, an adequate boarding school with psychiatric help or trial of military service.
4. Failing that, legal commitment for therapy before, rather than after, he develops more serious delinquencies.

I made this as plain as I could to all concerned within the limitations of time and tact, and referred them back to you. But without the cooperation of all concerned, I doubt I can be of further help.

To Dr. Raymond Headler, who referred a patient almost ruined by a prolonged, poorly conducted "classical analysis":

Dear Ray:

Mr. T. presents a case history instructive enough for a book: a preemptively demanding and covertly hostile dependent who perverted the "classical analytic technique" of one of our own colleagues to his own neurotic advantage for many years, leading to the inevitably bitter and possibly tragic pay-off. I am not sure he can be rehabilitated at this late date; but, if therapy is at all possible, it would now have to take the following lines:

Interviews with his wife, brother, and associates to lessen their victimization and diminish the important—and quite conscious—dependency and aggressive gains he is now deriving from his "illness," and its consequent need for interminable "analysis."

A radical change in technique away from "dream analysis," "symbolic interpretations," and escapist regression to a quite literal and practical concern with present activities and tenable future goals. Should he temporarily revert to a dramatic and invaliding "psychosis," a small sanitarium with no EST but with no privileges or visitors either would be indicated.

These and other considerations speak against his coming from Milwaukee to Chicago for therapy, since he would use the three days a week "off" as another officially sponsored escape into irresponsibility, fogged by "free-associative" double-talk. I have therefore recommended that he return to you, and that I discuss his progress with you and see him only occasionally as you direct. I have had fairly extensive and successful experience with many such cases that have come to me after years of such misguided "therapy," and perhaps I can, on your occasional visits to Chicago, help you a bit with this one.

Your letters still indicate a peculiar ambivalence toward analysis, which can spring only from still being *either* "for" or "against" it as a cult or dogma. Eventually, I hope you can become whimsically sophisticated about the behavior of some "psychoanalysts," but accept the field itself as another moderately interesting and informative dialectic excursion in our search for interpersonal understandings and skills. But I trust you are on the way to such eventually satisfying integrations.

17. HUMANITARIAN THERAPY

In Chapter 15 I outlined the principal objectives and techniques of the psychiatric interview, namely: (a) to establish initial rapport, (b) to survey the patient's current difficulties and dangers in the light of (c) his previous personality so as (d) to lay the ground work for (e) his intermediate partial relief and (f) for his extended therapy. In effect, the examination should never lead merely to the affixing of some single diagnostic label to a patient, but instead to these more comprehensive concepts:

1. That the nosologic terms still used in psychiatry refer roughly to predominant modes of behavior rather than to definitive disease entities.

2. That every diagnostic designation can be only relatively "differential" and never exclusive, since nearly every known pattern of "normal" or "abnormal" propensity is operative to a greater or lesser degree in every subject. Rather, psychiatric diagnosis consists in identifying and weighing the predominant aberrations and deviations of behavior from the current "norms" of time, place and culture, with full recognition that all other reactions are also present to a lesser degree. In this sense, all "neuroses" and "psychoses" are "mixed," although the relative prominence of a few patterns

may justify a currently meaningful emphasis.

3. Correspondingly, prognosis is not an inevitable consequence of any descriptive diagnosis, since nearly all behavior tendencies are reversible to a greater or lesser extent contingent on the origin, tenacity, and influenceability of the patient's patterns of conduct, and on the possibility of channeling them into new and more favorable adaptations by available therapeutic means. Indeed, many acute psychotic reactions have a better prospect of recovery than others labeled merely "chronic neurotic," or "sociopathic," which are far more resistant to therapy.

But to describe briefly a matrix of therapeutic techniques that I am still trying to refine after some forty years in the field would be analogous to writing a short dissertation on how to play the organ with artistic finesse without years of self-critical practice. On the other hand, I cannot plead, as do other writers on the subject that the "art" of therapy, as distinguished from the "science" involved, is too esoteric and ephemeral for exposition; indeed, *Webster's Dictionary* defines art simply as "skill derived from training and experience." Seemingly more directive aphorisms are equally difficult to apply. For example, it is true that all therapy can be summarized in a dual sentence: Help the patient recognize and abandon his deviant patterns as no longer either necessary or satisfying—and since such insight, if merely verbalized, would still leave him anxious and bewildered—concurrently guide him by word, deed, and example to adopt new patterns of conduct that he will eventually find more personally and socially rewarding. This is excellent advice, but it requires a dedicated acceptance of iatric responsibility and the development and application, through years of training and experience, of a great variety of technical and transactional skills.

I have elsewhere attempted to describe my own medical, dyadic, familial, social, and other therapeutic techniques in a number of texts: *Behavior and Neurosis* (1943), *Principles of Dynamic Psychiatry* (1946), *Practice of Dynamic Psychiatry* (1955), *Modern Therapy of Behavior Disorders* (1967), and in some scores of specific articles published in the annual issues of *Current Psychiatric Therapies* and elsewhere. Here, however, I propose to recall a lecture on "Brief Psychiatric Therapies," which I presented at the New York Postgraduate Center some five years ago, in the hope that the historical perspectives of various "modern" modes of therapy and the spontaneity of my answers to subsequent questions would be in greater accord with the style and spirit of this book than would a more pedantic exposition. The transcript of that discussion, edited only to eliminate the occasional halts and redundancies of casual verbal interchange, reads as follows:

Once upon a time (said I), Arthur Mirsky, in a complimentary introduction to a talk I gave at the University of Pittsburgh, mentioned that some of my books had been translated into German, Japanese and other languages—but then turned to me to say, "and, Jules, if you'll give me the right, I'll also translate them into English!" Which brings up a trenchant point: namely, that in psychiatry we too often attempt to conceal ignorance by mythical allusions and pretentious jargon rather poorly designed to gloss over gaps in our data and conceptualizations. One example is the use of the root term *psyche,* as in psychology, psychopathology or psychotherapy. In the classical Greek myth, Psyche herself was a beauteous mortal maiden who enjoyed a mysterious lover until one night, contrary to their initial agreement, she lit a candle and discovered that he was none other than the Olympian Eros—for which transgression she was condemned by gods and men alike. In this symbolic fable, the intellect or *psyche,* deriving its inspiration from hidden lust, could remain happy were it not for its nagging spirit of research—something about which Eve could have warned Psyche.

But in modern science we must deal with processes and transactions rather than myths called "psyche" or "mind"—let alone "psychopathology," a philologic miscegnation literally translatable as "the science of diseased abstractions." Instead, let us simply convert the term "mind" from a protean noun to the verb in a series of operational phrases—and lo, Anglo-Saxon pragmatism makes sense of Greek Platonism. Thus, if we "put our mind" to something, we're referring to the processes of perception and attention; if we "keep a thought in mind," we mean the unique property that living beings have of processing, storing and cross-indexing information at a level of complexity (though not of speed) far greater than any calculating machine; and if we "mind our parents . . . manners . . . customs . . . laws," we recognize social education and the transmission and acceptance of mores and culture. The concept of "mind" thus becomes a study of verbal and other motor *behavior:* i.e., we know someone's "mind" only by the way he adapts by voice and action to his physical and cultural milieu. In this connection, "therapy" is another highly significant word which, in its Greek origin, simply means *service;* ergo, what we really mean by psychotherapy is the service which one human being can render another in whatever modality, by whatever techniques, and in whatever culture the two happen to coexist. In this sense the parameters—"brief" or "long," as misapplied to "superficial" or "deep" therapy—may have little relationship to the effectiveness of the service actually rendered. As a parallel example, the more training and experience one acquires as a surgeon, the more rapid as well as effective his operations. In fact, psychotherapy and surgery can well be compared further; in both, the physician first establishes confidence and then uses appropriate measures to reach a comprehensive diagnosis without unnecessary elaborations or delay. The patient's trouble may have been a congenital defect, an early injury, or the more recent residues of stress or trauma. In any case the physician, without unnecessary dissection and as rapidly and as skillfully as possible, corrects what he can and then reapproximates the tissues so that there will be no wound difficult to heal or which may leave a disfiguring scar. Both the surgeon and the psychotherapist thereby gently help nature's reparative powers and expedite the recovery and social rehabilitation of the patient. As to the current fad of "nondirectiveness": Once in a talk to a group of Rogerians, I made a mildly regrettable slip of the tongue by referring to Carl Roger's system as "non-*cor*rective therapy"; actually good psychiatric therapy is about as non-directive as good surgery.

But are there no ways to bring some degree of clarity and consistency out of our present theoretic confusions and disparate practices? I submit that there are indeed three modes of inquiry and integration as applicable in our field as elsewhere in science, to wit: the historical, the comparative, and the experimental. Let us here examine the first of these heuristic sources.

An Historical Review of Psychiatric Therapy:

In essence, man throughout history has tried to ensure his existence and expand his powers in three fundamental ways: first, by asserting technical mastery over the physical universe; second, by cooperating with his fellows in this endeavor; and third, by postulating transcendental systems of beliefs (whether designated as science, philosophy, metaphysics, or theology) designed to find order and predictability in an otherwise chaotic universe. H. J. Muller has perhaps expressed most trenchantly our temporal parochialism in his aphorism that our historical perspectives seem to be confined to the minutes of the last board meeting; ergo, we neglect the precious lessons not only of half a million years of human development, but of three billion years of biological evolution.

In contrast, may I point out that in the primal Algonkian slime where life was created, it almost immediately showed the first two vital principles that I mentioned: a capacity to maintain itself by manipulating the inorganic elements of the universe, and soon thereafter, a tendency toward collaborative effort to preserve the species. Even now, so relatively simple a creature as the primitive myxamoeba remains a rugged individualist as long as all within and about it is going well; however, should food and water become scarce, some cells may deliberately form themselves into a stalk upon which the others can feed, sporulate, and survive. Even in later stages of evolution, it remains difficult for an ethologist to tell whether organisms such as the Portuguese man-of-war are merely collections of individuals, or cooperating transpecific colonies, or integrated, functioning animals adapting to their external milieu, their fellows, and their universe.

If we now jump countless aeons to the earliest records of humanity, all three principles remain operative. Let us take the indications of early human behavior, say artifacts from the Mousterian era fifty thousand years old. The paleolithic people who bequeathed them to us were equipped with the brain potential and the physical endowments we possess today, and had already invented stone axes, scrapers, darts, needles, and other tools with which to control their environment. They had also reached a high level of social development: They lived not only as familial groups, but also in clans and tribes which joined in common endeavors with apportioned roles and hierarchies of command. They apparently took care of their aged; they certainly took care of their children, or we would not be here to philosophize about them. But in addition to their technology and social organization, they had evolved a third technique: a system of magical beliefs and practices designed to influence their fate not only on earth but also in some imagined hereafter. How do we know all this? We have, for example, the little stone statuettes (by our standards, unlovely but unforgettable), "paleolithic Venuses," whose physical features of unmistakably exaggerated womanhood antedate the worship of the beneficent goddesses Ishtar, Isis, and other ancient mothers of men. We find other works of art that express not only man's creative strivings, but also a trust in his capacity to determine his own future. Witness the superb drawings and paintings in the caves of Altamira in Spain and Lascaux in France, in which the tribal hunt was represented. There is no deliberate cruelty in these pictographs; they simply show human beings in a common endeavor for the good of the clan. These pictographs were placed in alcoves in the remote regions of the common cave, as in primitive chapels where they were surrounded by other articles of magic and worship. Thus, through form and ritual, they represented man's dreams and hopes in a sense that, if he depicted time and place in the poetry of his own imagination, he could thereby control the universe. L. S. B. Leakey, curator of the Coryndon Memorial Museum in Nairobi, describes similar paintings possibly a quarter of a million years old in the Olduvai Gorge of Africa.

In effect, the basic principles by which men always sought equanimity, and which we now employ in what we call psychotherapy, had already governed the behavior of our Stone Age ancestors. We can very well imagine a Neanderthal man, troubled or lost, coming home to the cave, being accepted into a society of his fellowmen, being reassigned a role and feeling once again secure—provided, of course, that he fitted into the technological and cultural requirements of his society, participated in its philosophy and, if you will, in its primitive theological-religious system.

By the time of ancient Egypt many of these practices had achieved a high degree of elaboration. Men who were ill or frightened came to the temples of the local gods. There they found a haven of refuge and healing and performed rituals which gave them a sense of magical mastery, reinforced by the concordant actions of others with similar fears and faiths. Individually or in groups, the temple supplicants were also given drugs that "tranquillized" them or induced a gentle sleep, during which they had dreams which the priest interpreted. He then revealed to them who and what had troubled their spirits and intoned directives which, if properly interpreted and followed, would not only solve their problems on earth but in life thereafter. And so the Egyptians were a happy people insofar as they had evolved not only an enduring earthly civilization but also, through the revealed authority of their sacred Book of the Dead, a promise of serene immortality in Ra's eternal Land of the Setting Sun.

Continuing in the Nilotic tradition, there is hardly a method of individual or social psychotherapy employed today that was not also practiced in the Asklepiad Sanatoria of classical Greece and Rome, during what might be called the Golden Era of Hellenic Humanism.*

When these parameters became obscured during the Middle Ages, the Catholic Church offered a religious haven of refuge that much of Western humanity sorely needed as a retreat from the difficulties of a hazardous and conflictful world. True, the Church was sometimes ruthless in also preempting worldly prerogatives, but churches of various categories and denominations have always been materially supported because they fulfilled this third human need for the securities of unquestioning faiths.

One of the first Western therapists to claim that he could cure human ills without the aid of divine intervention was

*For a development of this theme, see Chapter 21.

Greatstrakes the Stroaker, who asserted that he could massage people in such a way that the evil humors they had accumulated from unwholesome foods and other noxious sources would be forced out of their extremities. Three centuries ago, he had thousands of people flocking to his clinic because, in the post-Cromwellian era when many encounters were murderous rather than gentle, they found a healer who, with reassuring self-confidence, would feed them special diets and pat and comfort them much as though they were children. And so do thousands of people today who believe in chiropractic, or Swedish massage, or "sensitivity groups," or Yogic exercises—with or without yogurt cheese—find comfort in strange dietary regimes and their favorite brands of "stroking." Not because the massage, the rotting proteins, the "spinal adjustments," the baths, or the calisthenics are essential to the cure, but because the faithful are like troubled children who are reassured, petted, fed, and played with until they feel better.

A century and a quarter later there lived the founder of a great many more of our "modern" therapeutic techniques—another pseudoscientific charlatan by the name of Anton Mesmer. (Incidentally, I wonder, what will people think of our current psychotherapeutic "science" a hundred years from now?) Mesmer observed that when he made certain intentionally meaningful movements with his hands, he could influence others not only by touching them but also at a distance. Since at that time the only known forces that acted at a distance were gravity and magnetism, Mesmer inferred that he exerted a form of "animal magnetism" that could produce remote physiologic effects. Inasmuch as the same forces also governed the stars and planets, Mesmer included astrology in his rationale and wrote a doctoral thesis on the topic. (For that matter, Kepler and Copernicus, two of the greatest astronomers of all time, were also astrologers, who reassured their patrons with vaguely comforting zodiacal predictions.) Thus did Mesmer, employing what he thought were the human embodiments of cosmic forces, induce "Mesmeric spells" from which a compliant subject would wake claiming to feel rested, reinvigorated, and exhilarated.

Mesmer literally entranced a great many influential people, and was therefore, for a time, highly successful and fashionable. In view of certain highly organized cults of our present day, it is disconcerting to recall that then also there were official and officious Mesmeric societies, with local and international journals of Mesmerism. Any candidate for membership in these societies had to be himself Mesmerized by a properly Mesmerized person, and have a prescribed number of controlled Mesmeric sessions before he could be certified as an accredited Mesmerist who operated according to the Rules; however, if he proposed new and better methods, his loyalty and professional qualifications were criticized and he became subject to disqualification and expulsion. Mesmerists, as did the later Freudians, quite sincerely believed in their theories and felt themselves misunderstood and martyred by the medical men of the day. And they had indeed discovered a universal System of Healing in that they had tapped a basic human yearning for encounter and relationship: not "animal magnetism" (later renamed hypnotism by Braid, Esdaille, *et al.*) but a form of reassuring and suggestive communication that had been practiced in the temples of Akkad and Egypt. There, too, in a setting of diminished light, the priests had intoned repetitious, monotonous, rhythmic lullabies known to all mothers of troubled children who seek comfort and rest in a trusting security.

Predictably, Mesmer's own practice grew to such proportions that he could no longer give individual attention to every patient; ergo, he began to deal with them in groups. Mesmer's patients would form a circle, hold hands, feel overpowered by the "magnetic spell," have erotic, hallucinatory, and other sensations that might now be termed "psychedelic" or "sensitivity" experiences, and leave praising the system and spreading the Mesmeric gospel. Mesmer himself was eventually investigated by Benjamin Franklin and others in a French Royal Commission, which concluded that he was a deluded charlatan; he ultimately died in poverty, though still convinced that he was a scientific martyr.

From Mesmerism there arose many therapeutic cults that we can now call by their modern mames. One is a belief in the efficacy of "magnetic belts," hundreds of thousands of which people still wear in the hope that these surcharged diapers will "revitalize the iron in the blood" and so alleviate frigidity or restore potency. Also derivatively, we have current schools of hypnotists who, in their theorizing if not in their practice, ignore the simple fact that people like to be treated by supposedly wise and magically powerful persons; consequently, some professional hypnotists themselves seem to forget Bernheim's caution to Freud that "a wise hypnotist must always know who is hypnotizing whom."

Another interesting derivative of Mesmerism is the Christian Science Church, which invokes all of the powerfully therapeutic modalities we have already reviewed. These comprise first, a system of transcendent beliefs, not only religious but purportedly "scientific." Second, over three thousand Churches of Christ Scientist nearly everywhere in the world provide opportunities for an almost universal kinship; so that a Christian Scientist can hardly feel alone anywhere. Third, the Church offers a very simple, repetitious, and assertive dogma, which resembles some aspects of analytic therapy in being confidently serene in its semantic obscurity. Church services consist of repetitious readings from Mary Baker Eddy, so that if one learns a few key phrases, he knows all the essential passwords. Thus armed, Christian Science healers, outdoing Mesmer, are confident that they possess mystic powers by which they can conduct "absent healing" at any distance. Consequently, a great many troubled, lonesome human beings join Christian Scientist churches or other organizations with similar beliefs and practices that afford comfort and companionship. No one can deny the tragedies that can result from the misapplication of such doctrines, yet as humanitarian psychiatrists, we can neither neglect nor deny any modality that may help our patients.

But there is another derivative of Mesmerism that seems at first sight almost completely unrelated; to wit, latter-day psychoanalysis. Its derivation, though a long story and a somewhat discursive one (i.e., Mary Baker Eddy learned her craft from Phineas Quimby, a disciple of Mesmer), can be summarized for our present purposes in the light of the therapeutic transactions we have traced. Freud began by using hypnotism much as a directed confessional—to command his patients to tell him what was troubling them. But since many subjects resented this, Freud later instructed his patients simply to say anything and everything that they thought without fear of condemnation or judgment. So invited, they would confess, often with emotional histrionics, recent sexual episodes which Freud seemed to think had precipitated their difficulties. This process was labelled "catharsis" in the sense of ridding "the psyche" of something noxious, accompanied by "abreaction" when the emotionality was intense and thereby presumed to be corrective. And, of course, some patients felt better in the thought that they had found a friendly physician who was interested and understanding rather than judgmental or punitive, and who ardently believed in his mode of therapy. But Freud went on to a deeper recognition: namely, that his patients must have been chronically troubled long before the relatively trivial "sexual traumata," which he had at first considered significant; instead, they must have been sensitized by earlier adverse experiences. Indeed, most patients began to recall familial insecurities, jealousies and conflicts during their adolescence and eventually in their childhood that had rendered them particularly sensitive to similar hurts, rejections, and sorrows in later life. Thus, for a time psychoanalytic therapy consisted of an attempt to reconstruct "primal sexual traumata," particularly in relation to a so-called family romance between child and mother, constituting a universal "Oedipus complex" with its attendant "castration fear" of paternal punishment.

However, Freud also began to recognize something that every minister, physician, or other adviser had implicitly observed: that the patient inevitably placed the therapist in the role of a parent, sibling, or other surrogate. The patient thus attributed to the therapist various characteristics that he did not necessarily possess, and then treated him as a mother, a rival, an erotic object, a persecutor, a protector who must look after the patient indefinitely, or in various other roles revelatory of the patient's pre-Oedipal "anal aggressions," "oral fixations," or "primal narcissistic" patterns as derived from varied extra-therapeutic relationships. Freud thought that once the patient, through "transference analysis," was helped to recognize the artificial positions into which he forced not only the therapist but various other people in his life, he would alter these interpersonal transactions to everyone's advantage. This is about where Freud stopped, but by this time he had already rediscovered and reformulated (sometimes unnecessarily fancifully or obscurely) various basic principles of human behavior and clinical therapy that have been operative throughout the ages—and, of course, need still be applied if any form of treatment is to be effective.

Since then, of course, psychiatrists have employed a great many other approaches, none of them new. We have rediscovered the efficacy of reestablishing control of the material universe through "occupational" therapy, job training and creativity. We have rediscovered the necessity of progressive social rehabilitations through making our offices, clinics, and hospitals not places divorced from reality, but integral parts of their community. And, finally, we have rediscovered the intimate relationships between psychiatry and the various religious systems. As is our American custom, we have departmentalized the latter in various Institutes of Pastoral Counselling, some of which, unfortunately, are in their turn becoming doctrinaire and stereotyped, thereby vitiating principles on which they were professedly founded.

These, then, are the leads culled from our historical perspectives, rich in their implications for current psychiatric theory and practice. In essence, therapeutic methods, whatever their supposed rationale, have been effective through the ages primarily as they strengthened three of man's essential beliefs, precepts, categorical imperatives, or ultimate (Ur-) defenses—call them what you will. These can be summarized as follows:

1. *A presumption of personal invulnerability, power, and vicarious immortality,* rooted in primary narcissism and never completely surrendered.

2. *A hopeful "faith in humanity,"* derived from the almost equally illogical assumption that because each child's mother presumably at one time loved and cherished him, the rest of mankind is assumed to be almost equally provident and indulgent. This expectation of survival through dependence, when

combined with ancillary erotic yearnings tinctured with rivalries and mistrusts, determines many of our interpersonal relationships, including those in psychotherapy.

3. *A wishful postulate of a Transcendent Order and Perfect Servant* within mortal ken and control, expressed consciously in the belief that one can impose order and security on a universe of chaos and danger by the invention of necessarily "anthropocentric" scientific or philosophic systems, which somehow include the intercession of omnipotent and omniscient Beings, who can be influenced by wheedling, bribery, or command, much as one once controlled one's subservient parents.

These, of course, are but bare statements that, taken alone, may sound pretentious and oracular, yet strangely disturbing. However, reflection will reveal how many physical, verbal, and other therapeutic maneuvers resonate with these mystic, irrational, but ubiquitous beliefs, and consequently how futile or explosive are the results of any attempt to traduce or abolish them either in an individual or in a society. While it may be too cynical to propose outright that therapy consists in reestablishing these and other of man's essential *Ur*-delusions in proper working order, wise psychiatrists eventually learn—along with wise teachers and ministers—that truly to aid a man, one must help him rebuild his own universe of *useful* fact and fancy, and largely on his own terms, his faith in himself, in his fellowman, and in his personally conceived social and cosmic systems.

Thus ended my talk. Wisely, Dr. Lewis Wolberg, director of the Center for Postgraduate Studies, had limited me to these sixty minutes of didactic abstractions, to be followed by more precise answers to questions from the mixed audience of psychiatrists and other professionals about specific details and contingencies of comprehensive biodynamic (or, as preferably designated at his Center, "short-term") therapy. These were now invited, and my replies recorded as follows:

Question: Are there any special kinds of symptoms or syndromes that respond better to your short-term than to long-term methods?

The true measure of therapy is not its length, but its effectiveness, and the issues involved are rendered even more confused by the fact that we classify "syndromes" in large part by their supposed amenability to treatment. In effect, I accept all patients that come to me, never consider any two-word diagnoses worth even a file card, avoid "long" therapy because I'm not interested in being a subsidized, tax-deductible baby sitter, and treat everyone as effectively—and therefore, as briefly—as possible.

Question: Since it is manifestly impossible within the confines of a short-term psychotherapy program to arrive at the definitive psychodynamics in many cases, is it possible to present a general formulation of dynamics that may be meaningful to the average patient?

What I'm interested in—and what I try to help the patient achieve—is for him to become a relatively happy and useful member of society. This may take only one interview for an acute anxiety state over a resolvable stress, a week to a month for a "depression," six months to a year for many a person discarded by others as "schizophrenic," or a bit more time for the social parasites, dilettantes, or escapists who had almost learned how to get away with it. Perhaps the greatest shortener of therapy is one bit of essential "insight," namely that whether the patient admits it or not, he *is* responsible for what he does—and that whether they say so or not, other people will hold him to that fact. Under proper guidance, he can also learn that the vicarious gains of neurotic behavior are evanescent, and socially adaptive patterns eventually prove to be more fun and, therefore, preferable. This is most of the "dynamics" he needs.

Question: Are goals in short-term therapy limited to symptom relief, or are reconstructive personality changes possible?

The term "personality" is derived from the Greek *persona,* a facade or mask; in the classical Greek plays of Aeschylus or Euripides the actors wore masks to conceal their "true" identities. However, whatever the patient's preferred "inner identity" or "self-image" the favorable changes in his behavior are the only true indices of good therapy regardless of its duration. These improvements can be limited and transient or sweeping and enduring—but they alone are the measure of the effectiveness of any mode of therapy. Operationally, "personality" is not what a person says nearly as much as what he does.

Question: Are there qualitative differences in techniques in short-term as compared to long-term treatment?

Lucy Ozarin once defined long-term psychosis as the permanent deviation in behavior *produced by* hospitalization in a long-term hospital. So also, overprolonged therapy can complicate the very difficulty we are supposed to be treating.

Question: Psychotropic drugs deal with target symptoms. Are there any special psychotherapeutic techniques that can also deal with target symptoms?

Again, much of the internal logic of science consists of examining the questions asked. Is there any internist or surgeon in this audience who can tell me of any single drug or operation that treats only a symptom? Even Ehrlich's "magic bullet" was aimed not at the symptoms, but at the infectious agent (itself only a *partial* cause) of syphilis. So also, diphtheria antitoxin is "aimed" not at the rash or the fever, but at the general toxicity that causes both. All good psychotherapy resolves underlying conflicts and promotes healthier adaptations; it is, therefore, always more than merely "symptomatic."

Question: Is a transference neurosis desirable in therapy? How may it be managed most constructively, if it does develop?

Once more the crucial term is "transference neurosis." Freud, who was never an orthodox Freudian, implied in his autobiography that a "transference neurosis," when it was *not simply a neurotic transference being analyzed,* was really "an artifact of poor therapeutic technique!" A "transference neurosis" is thus to distinguished from a "neurotic transference," which comprises the relationship that the patient plays out with his therapist as well as with everyone else, as derived from the patient's transactions with previous important persons in his life. But if, instead of revealing and correcting these patterns, the therapist enhances them by cooingly inviting the patient to regress into an analytic crib *sans* sidebars, or by fostering an escape into fantasies of dreamy omnipotence, or by providing another set of temporarily shared delusions called "insights"—then the therapist is creating *a transference neurosis in the sense that he is transferring his own neurosis to his patient.* In the Middle Ages surgeons insisted that they had to operate so that the wound would inevitably develop a discharge called "laudable pus," thought to be essential to the cure. It was not until the thirteenth century that Master Chirurgeon Teodorico Borgognoni cautioned his fellows that: "It is not necessary, though modern surgeons teach it, that pus be generated in wounds! No error can be greater than this. Such a practice is indeed to hinder nature, to prolong the disease, and to prevent the conglutination of the wound." If we can't help a patient, let's not, in any form of therapy, complicate his life with an *induced* neurosis, "transference" or otherwise.

Question: Are there ways of managing dependency in short-term therapy that differ from the methods used in long-term therapy?

We have already touched on one referent of this question in our discussion of the artificial complication and prolongation of therapeutic dependency through the induction of a "transference neurosis." On the other hand, one can't live *without* many normal dependencies. I'm very dependent on my secretaries, my patients, my publishers, my bankers, my students, my university, and many other relationships—and so are all of us; indeed civilization is a maze of interdependencies, which imply mutual service and profit, not as "cooperation" spelled out in the terms of you coo, while I operate. If the therapist himself has this understanding, he can impart it to his patients.

Question: Do you ever supplement psychotherapy with physical therapy?

If you mean drugs, I avoid most so-called tranquillizers because of the escapist-addictive tendencies of patients avid of them, but I have no hesitation in prescribing Dilantin or Phenurone for epileptic seizures or equivalents, the new l-dopa for Parkinsonian complications, or occasionally allowing a patient a barbiturate to abort needlessly restless nights until we can trace and alleviate the sources of his despair. If you refer to the induction of Metrazol or Indoklon convulsions, decerebrating electroshocks or other such drastic and destructive measures—I put these in the same class as supposedly curative medieval tortures for witchcraft; however, about once a year I may hospitalize a suicidal depressive for two or three —not more—mild ESTs that may haze over some of his troubles and, when combined with intensive individualized and group psychotherapy, help him realize that a reorganized and reevaluated life may be preferable to the near-experiences of death after all. With this qualification, permit me the *hubris*—which the gods may have me regret tomorrow—of stating that I have never had a suicide in thirty years of a highly diverse practice. But the contention that there can be far less dynamic distinction than is usually thought between "physical" and "psychological" therapy may be illustrated by the following example:

A 47-year-old woman, after seven years of therapy by three successive psychoanalysts, was referred to me for continued alcoholism and recurrent depressive episodes; characteristically, she made an immediate dive for my office couch in the middle of our first interview. To establish what rapport I could through the only channel thus offered, I permitted her for several more sessions to ramble on supinely about her dreams, her early childhood, her intricate "object cathexes," "introjections," "transference distortions," and various other periphrastic vacuities, by which she and her former analysts had long tried to avoid dealing with the realities of her life. One day, however, she walked in with an obvious limp, and when I responded to this overture by asking why, she told me that, while gardening that morning, she had stepped on a rake, one prong of which had penetrated the sole of her foot. Having gone only this far, she tried to preclude further intrusions by informing me that she herself knew that her adventure in the garden was a form of acting-out designed to cause a symbolic erection of the rake handle, and that she freely wished to admit unconscious erotic satisfaction in the penetration of the phallic prong into her downwardly displaced vaginal instep—with the ensuing bleeding of course, representing a regression to, and a reenactment of, her fantasied adolescent defloration by a "brother-father surrogate," who, because of his erotic activities, had been called "a rake" by her "castrative mother" . . . At this point I interrupted her harangue (which only a somewhat retarded first-year analytic trainee could regard as anything but evasive and derisive) with the statement that, whether or not she regarded it as neurotic voyeurism on my part, I wished to examine the wound in her foot. In shocked amazement, she complied and showed me a puncture lesion on her heel still surrounded by specks of imbedded dirt. I promptly sent my secretary for a vial of tetanus antitoxin, and after proper inquiry as to the patient's serum sensitivity, asked her to bare one buttock while informing her that, whether or not she interpreted the syringe and injection as a sexual intromission and ejaculation, no patient of mine was going to develop tetanus convulsions if I could prevent it.

That "physical" treatment, taken by the patient as evidence of my realistic and competent concern, proved to be a crucial point in her therapy and in her life. In later interviews she abandoned her covert methods of using pseudo-analytic persiflage to frustrate analysts at their favorite one-upmanship games; instead, we both began to deal with her specific concerns about children who had grown, married, and left her, a husband who seemed only occasionally successful either in his business or in concealing his extramarital adventures, her failures to find security in a minor political career seasoned with a sexual liaison, her dread of losing the rest of her fading attractiveness, and other such actual or fancied stresses. Within three months she found new satisfactions in greatly improved relations with her children, husband, and lover, in being elected president of her state PTA, and in other achievements which rendered her alcoholism or punitive depressions no longer necessary.

Question: How does one utilize dreams in therapy?

In line with the old song, "Did You Ever See a Dream Walking?" no one has ever really analyzed a dream *per se.* What one deals with is a patient's *communications* the day or the week after he had a "dream." These are contingent upon his particular situation at the moment, his motivation, his "transference relationship," and what he's working through: hence, such communications are no more or less the "royal road to the Unconscious" than if he fantasied that he had won a Nobel prize or married Brigit Bardot, or saw me sinking in Lake Michigan. As do the patient's dreams, these would represent wishes expressive of *the patient's ever-changing situa-*

tional and transactional attitudes and responses. The more experience I accumulate the fewer become *my* free associations to dreams, and the less I explore their "symbolic significance in the roots of infantile neurosis"; instead, I regard them as but another of many equally significant modes of communication. Nor do I as readily fall for the patient's ploy: "Let me take this hour to tell you what I dreamt last night . . . Isn't that fascinating? Now *you* interpret it [(in *sotto voce*) because I want to deal with *your* fantasies rather than my realities]."

Question: What supportive approaches are helpful in short-term therapy?

I have a couch and a chair, with a good solid floor beneath to support the patient, and I pay rent on all of them. But the support that remains useful outside the office occurs when the therapist has opened a bridge to a physical and social reality in which the patient can continue to live.

Question: Is it helpful to see related family members in short-term therapy? If so, for what purpose?

Of course it is helpful; especially if they are invited to become aware of their own roles in the patient's problems—though that very often takes therapeutic tact and courage. However, at a recent international peace conference in Athens a member of the British Cabinet half-seriously proposed that the heads of various states, who were putting the world in chaos, should be induced to seek my professional help. When the chairman, President Robert Hutchins of the Center for Democratic Studies, asked my opinion on this technical point, I told the apocryphal story of the patient who came into a psychiatrist's office dressed in a tiger skin with spinach hanging from his ears and a fried egg on his head, and said, "Doctor, I would like to consult you about my brother." Members of patients' families will come to you in the same spirit, unmindful of the fried eggs on their own heads.

Question: Do you use psychological testing and other psychological approaches in short-term treatment?

Infrequently, except when the employer, the court, or other referring agency, with the patient's consent, want such supplementary reports. This is not because of lack of confidence in the tests; on the contrary, I once used them extensively and still have a long chapter on them in my *Practice of Dynamic Psychiatry.* It is merely that I have developed more confidence in a thorough direct examination than in one done through pictures, paper, and pencil, and have validated this by decades of collaboration with competent clinical psychologists.

Question: Is it very dangerous for a patient to be treated by a neurotic therapist?

Let us once again focus on the two key terms in the question. "Treatment," as we have seen, has very broad connotations, whereas "neurotic" often means only "somebody I don't like." For example, some observers might regard the Negro mystic who called himself Father Divine as a "paranoid psychotic." Should we have committed him? So also, Father Divine had a group of ardent followers who actually believed he was God, had cured their ills, and saved their souls by divine power, and had constituted them a heavenly host of angels on earth. Many of these people were good providers and useful citizens; should we have committed them also? At any Holy Roller meeting, the preacher may go off into trances, and the congregation may shout and roll in the aisles, crying out, weeping, singing, dancing, sometimes tearing off some of their clothes and acting in a way that in the back wards of a state hospital would be diagnosed as a schizoaffective furor. Yet at the end of the service, preacher and congregation get up, dust themselves off, straighten up their neckties, and blouses, put on their hats and coats, go back home, have a good night's sleep, and go to work the next morning. Is the preacher subverting his congregation or is he operating on a significant *folie* desired by all concerned in this supposedly post-Dionysian era? With reference to the possibility that interminable psychoanalysis may, in act, prove to be but a quieter *folie,* I may relate another anecdote:

I once gave a relatively innocuous lecture on *The Biodynamic Roots of Analysis* to the British Psychoanalytic Society which, like most British societies, is divided neatly down the middle by an aisle. To the right sat the conservative Anna Freud and her disciples; to the left, Melanie Klein and her cohorts. At the end of my lecture there was a question period during which people would get up from the right side of the aisle and say: "Dr. Masserman, what you are presenting, of course, is a searching confirmation of the tenets of our great leader Anna Freud, and I am happy that the data you furnish are so compatible with her teachings." Whereupon others would get up from the opposite side of the aisle to counter with: "On the contrary! on the contrary! What Dr. Masserman has told us, with regard to his research and his inferences, supports without any reservations the basic understandings of our great leader Melanie Klein." Finally, somebody asked me a question that I felt I could answer, to wit: "Dr. Masserman, in your country, we understand that psychoanalysis lasts only two or three years, whereas here in Britain, we think that a proper psychoanalysis should persist at least for seven, eight, or nine years. How do you explain this difference?" My reply, recorded in the annals of the British Psychoanalytic Society, was simply that I had heard somewhere that it took the British a little longer to see a joke. Nevertheless, I had a pleasant visit that evening in Anna Freud's home.

Question: Are there any special considerations and techniques in the treatment of the aged?

In the United States we seem to shuttle dizzily between extremes of antipathy and anticipation about aging. On the one hand, *sen*ility has become a term of opprobrium, often implying the need for permanent confinement in a mental hospital, yet *sen*iority (up to a point) is an occupational privilege, and the *Sen*ate is our highest deliberative body. We deplore the prospect of twenty million ailing aged on public relief, yet our advertising folders picture tanned septuagenarian playboys with alluringly well-preserved wives cavorting about the country in boats and trailers on permanent vacations subsidized by Eternal Life Insurance Companies. If I recollect the statistics accurately—a bare possibility—in 1910, not one man in ten retired from work until terminal illness; now one in four does so, often while he still has much to contribute. What, then, as a background to the therapy of those baffled by this double bind, should be the Golden Mean for the Golden Age?

Obviously, since every individual is unique and his situation different, here we can deal only briefly with the general physical, psychologic, and social rationale of geriatric therapy. However, let's again review the *Ur*-strivings of all human beings at all ages, and see how they apply particularly to those of us in our middle and later years.

First, we seek continued strength and power through maintained health, expanding knowledge, and adequate skills. Threats in the first category become more disturbing with advancing age, yet L. Z. Cosin, the British geriatrician, reported that he could reduce by 85% the permanent hospitalization rate for "senile psychosis" merely by correcting metabolic errors or curing intercurrent infections which caused temporary confusion or panic in his elderly patients. As to the importance of preserving self-reliance, in my own practice I have often restored a crotchety, troublesome, "mentally deteriorated" old man to a moderately happy life and the good graces of his previously exasperated family mainly by arranging for his return from "retirement" to resume at least part time a trade, art, or profession in which he had found erstwhile pride and status.

Second, every human needs an array of reciprocated loves and loyalties. As our families, children, and friends depart over the years, we either concentrate our demands on those that are left, or else must establish new and satisfying relationships. Unfortunately, our former Homes for the Aged at best furnished reluctant baby-sitters for our second childhood; at worst, they were tragic concentration camps for the discarded and isolated. We must instead provide facilities in every community where the elderly finally deprived of all other relationships can find new friendships and join in what they themselves feel are useful pursuits.

Third, every intelligent human yearns to reach beyond the confines of his earthly existence and escape an intolerable sense of cosmic weightlessness. As the ever-denied shadow of death approaches, each of us, peon or philosopher, seeks comfort through various beliefs in eternity and universal purposes. For that matter, scratch any self-styled agnostic or materialist hard enough to hurt, and you will find a mystic, though each will rationalize his faith in his own way. To the sociologist

Auguste Comte, God was the Great Humanitarian; to the mathematician Arthur Eddington, God was the Perfect Computer; to Sigmund Freud, God was a Psychoanalyst.

What, then, can we do to alleviate the problems of aging? As to prevention, each of us can in part mitigate the empty futility and loneliness of old age by developing, while yet young, a range and versatility of interests, skills, and satisfactions that we can utilize throughout life. Literature, art, science, music, philosophy—these are deathless, and unimpaired by the inevitable hardening of joints, arteries, and habits. Any enthusiasms permanently shared with others can help: The ancient mariner with a love of the sea and a knowledge of the proper rig and trim of a boat will be welcomed among ship lovers at any time. Yet an essential bit of wisdom of another sort must also be acquired, long before the senium: Namely, that in this less than perfect world, a modicum of personal dignity, resilience, and self-sufficiency in the face of inevitable disappointment and even injustice is an invaluable asset. But when prevention fails, therapy must again accord with our aging patient's basic (*Ur-*) needs as follows:

First, and most urgently, we must improve his physical health and energy by every means at the command of modern medicine.

Second, we must restore insofar as possible satisfying familial and group relationships or, when necessary, help the patient cultivate new friendships through retained social skills. Whereas the *speed* of many responses inevitably declines after early middle age, their versatility and effectiveness can be retained until actual organic deterioration sets in; ergo, relatively old dogs can learn relatively new tricks (e.g., flying a plane or learning Swahili) whenever they really wish to do so. And as to sexual activity, Newman and Nichols, in a recent survey published in the *Journal of the American Medical Association,* reported that in both sexes "physically healthy, elderly persons [with capable partners] continue to be sexually active into their seventh, eighth, and ninth decades"; Masters and Johnson now agree.

Question: Can you cite a case illustration?

I accepted on referral a 65-year-old ex-president of a cigar company, who had been retired with his firm's gratitude, a gold watch, and half a million dollars. For four years he had had little to do except try to reassert his authority over his sons and daughters and grandchildren and everyone else within his crotchety, ill-tempered reach. Obviously what this old gentleman needed was to recover his status and self-importance, and so my therapy once consisted of accompanying him on some pretext down to the cigar counter in my office building, and waiting five minutes while he got increasingly angry about the poor merchandise and the poorer service. The next time he came in, he said: "You know, Doc, I think I've been wasting a lot of time plaguing my poor family. They think I'm a has-been, but I'm going to show them that I can set up a chain of cigar counters that will really give service with a smile and not charge high prices for poor merchandise." This he proceeded to do, and got so busy, successful and happy at it, that all talk of appointing a conservator for this putative "presbyophrenic" ceased. This nice old gentleman and I are still friends, though he slyly sends me a box of fine cigars every Christmas, knowing I don't smoke.

Question: When do you discontinue therapy?

At a time corresponding to when any competent internist or surgeon discharges his patient as adequately recovered. Psychiatrically, when the patient is sufficiently equipped with broader understanding and restored skills to function well enough in his society so that he no longer needs continuous guidance. This may occur after one interview or may not occur after two or three years. Again, the only measure of treatment is whether it has been skillful and effective.

Question: Should hypnotism be used by the general practitioner?

I have written much about hypnotism in my textbooks and elsewhere, and have lectured about it and demonstrated it to students for a quarter century. And yet, after the usual novitiate enthusiasm, during the past two decades I have used it in my extensive neuropsychiatric and psychoanalytic practice perhaps in only one patient every two or three years. The reasons are simple: Experience has shown that there is nothing that can be done by hypnosis that cannot be done better by other means—with fewer misunderstandings and complications for both the patient and physician.

Question: Isn't psychoanalysis the only "true" cure for neurosis?

The term "psychoanalysis" has three somewhat disparate meanings:

First, it is a mode of research into human behavior through purportedly "free" associations, the reporting of dreams, fantasied recollections of childhood, etc. There can be no objection to any ethical methods of clinical investigation, though the inferences drawn from such data are always subject to critical reexamination. Second, psychoanalysis is also a theory of behavior which includes various constructs such as "libido," "the unconscious," "the death instinct," "transference," etc. These and many other of Freud's original formulations are being abandoned in favor of more fruitful biodynamic concepts and behavioral equations. Third, "classical" psychoanalysis also connotes an expensive and somewhat ritualized mode of therapy which requires almost daily hours on a couch over a period of years. However, there has never been any proof that this mode of therapy has produced better results in the common disorders of behavior than briefer and more practicable forms. Accordingly, the "classical" techniques are being greatly modified by progressive psychoanalysts, so that eventually psychoanalysis will become identical with more dynamic and comprehensive modes of therapy for all forms of behavior disorders including what, two centuries after William Cullen, we still miscall "the neuroses."

Questions: Don't you think accurate psychiatric diagnosis is essential to effective therapy?

As I have tried to make clear in my textbooks,* much psychiatric diagnosis is intuitively obvious. For example, there is no cardiac, thyroid, or gastrointestinal syndrome that can match the symptoms of severe anxiety. I sometimes make this clear to medical students by saying, "If you can't remember what the anxiety syndrome is, just imagine you have been asked this in a final examination, and your whole career depends on your answer, and if you fail this question you are

*See Chapter 15 on empathetic diagnosis.

going to be expelled from medical school. Now, describe what you feel."

Or we may try to protect ourselves from unformulated apprehension by regulating our lives and being meticulous in our habits; on the other hand, if our patients become overly elaborate in trying to order their universe to the point of tolerable predictability, we say they have obsessive-compulsive or phobic neuroses.

Or have any of us *not* felt depressed—that is, literally pressed down by what seems to be a weight that cannot be borne? Feeling threatened, we do not sleep very soundly or eat well, are preoccupied and apprehensive, and buttonhole our friends, whining and crying a bit to get some succor and comfort. We think that because the world has mistreated us, we are justified in making everybody around us uncomfortable too.

And who has not felt the desire to escape from his underlying melancholy by drinking too much, or by vacillating from one to another empty diversion in a vain attempt to escape from restless anxiety through what we call hypomania?

Or, instead of admitting our own failures, we may prefer to think we have made powerful enemies who are organized to keep an important man down; ergo, we can understand why a paranoid functions as he does.

Finally, if the world seems too inimical, we tend to revert to our private worlds of wishful fantasy and unique symbolism. If such reactions are more intense and persistent in our patients, we call them "schizoid" or "schizophrenic."

All of these "psychiatric syndromes" may, of course, be accompanied by somatic resonances, such as feelings of weakness, cardiac disturbance, or various expressions of "psychosomatic" disorders. And if we take a few drinks and perhaps a sleeping pill too many, and experience a diminution of external perception and an impairment of reality testing and concept formation, illusions may build up into hallucinations and delusions to the intensity of delirium. In essence, then, we have all sensed the larval "neurotic" or "psychotic" phenomena that our patients experience. So I tell my residents, as I am sure all good teachers do, that there isn't anything you can see on the ward that you have not experienced, and therefore can't empathize with and understand; it is only a question of degree, intractability and severity.

Question: Are then, the modes of therapy you would recommend correspondingly eclectic?

I prefer the terms comprehensive, versatile and integrative to the designation "eclectic." To retain his patients, every physician must practice psychotherapy every medical moment. Fortunately, most do it intuitively well unless they involve their patients in their personal troubles. I used the phrase "do it intuitively well" to mean what it says: a skill inwardly taught. By the age of adolescence, everyone learns how to deal with those who appeal to him for comfort and solace, else he soon becomes a social outcast. To this inner knowledge, the future physician's education is more specifically designed to *lead out* (L., *e-duco)* and develop his capacities to serve his fellow man. Indeed, I have insistently defined psychotherapy as *any* form of help *any* practitioner can offer to make the patient healthier, happier, and more creative and to please the patient's family, his associates, and society in general with the change. With these broad orientations, it becomes evident that all medical procedures are effective in curing (L., caring for) disease (i.e., un-easiness) *only insofar as they ease the three fundamental anxieties of man.* To repeat, our basic therapeutic methods therefore always have been—and will probably always continue to be—these three:

First, to alleviate our patients' fears of pain, disability and death.

Second, to rebuild his confidence in, and his capacities to deal with, other human beings and thereby resume his desired role in the social order.

And third, to restore his faith in the comprehensibility and benignity of some universal system in which he has a place, a value, and a dignity, whether he calls that order scientific, philosophic, or for that matter religious.

How does the practitioner do this? By employing his generalship in reenacting his traditional roles of friend, expert, and mentor as follows: *As a physician* able to apply the best of medical and surgical skills, as outlined below. *As an ally in need.* Whether they admit it consciously or not, patients come to us much as hurt, frightened, and dubious children appealing to their parents for instant, individualized, devoted and seemingly unselfish care. Ergo:

Make it known that you wish to be always available to them, and to be informed immediately if they require your services. From a practical standpoint, if your patients believe you are sincere in this, your necessary leisure is *less* likely to be troubled by frantic calls from patients who want to make formal reservations in advance for your attention.

Place as few intermediates between you and your patient as is consistent with rounded service. Do not direct your secretary to enter a frequently misleading "systems-review" on a stereotyped form; do *not* assign the patient to a serial number in a crowded waiting room; do *not* shuffle referral laboratory reports between glances at the office clock while the patient, perhaps by now feeling thoroughly dehumanized and rejected, finally tries to get you to take an interest in *him.*

Supplement the "medical history" in every case with an equally important inquiry as to whether familial, economic, social, or other life stresses may have preceded and presumably contributed to, the patient's symptoms. This can be done briefly and tactfully by using common but easily understood euphemisms, such as inquiries about "overwork," "worry about the family," "business troubles," or other such inviting allusions that will be accepted by the patient as evidence of proper medical concern rather than unwarranted invasions of privacy. The argument sometimes heard that "no one but a psychiatrist has time for this" is particularly weak in this context, since a few minutes spent in such a survey will often reveal direct etiologic relationships between intercurrent life stresses and subsequent anxiety states, obsessive-compulsive-phobic reactions, psychosomatic dysfunctions, prolonged depressions, and other easily recognizable psychiatric syndromes—and thereby spare both the doctor and the patient from weeks to years of fruitless diagnostic searching and misdirected therapy.

Unless absolutely *contra*-indicated (e.g., in homosexual, seductive, paranoiac, or delusional patients), further signify your medical concern by doing at least a partial physical examination, if for no other reason than that the mother's pat, the king's touch, and the prophet's laying on of hands have always been touchingly effective in promoting good feeling.

Once begun, you must continue this personalized care of the patient—without ever delegating it wholly to others—until he no longer needs you in this central role. All laboratory reports and consultations must be mediated through you, and you must be his special friend and protector during subsequent hospitalizations, operations, and convalescence.

In essence, the doctor has an opportunity and privilege granted no other mortal: the use of his knowledge and skill in healing physical disease—a birthright some breeds of psychotherapists seem to have surrendered for some rather messy pottage. I myself am a psychoanalyst—yet in addition to my couch and easychair, I have an examining room fully equipped for physical and neurological examinations, a prescription pad, and a syringe for parenteral use as needed. The following measures may also be essential to comprehensive therapy:

The prescription of *specific medications* for the removal or relief of symptoms; in this sense, *every illness* is "functional" in that the patient is disturbed only insofar as his current or potential functions are threatened. The best way to treat the desuetude that may accompany some forms of anemia is to administer the indicated iron, copper, liver extract, B_{12}, or other antianemics; the most effective available relief for the sword-of-Damocles anxiety and over-reactive assertiveness which characterize an epileptic, or the regressive dependency of Parkinsonism, is to prescribe the proper anti-epileptic or extrapyramidomimetic drugs. As another example, I never treat a gastric or duodenal ulcer by "verbal psychotherapy" alone, since the antacids and antispasmodics are equally necessary to break the neurotic-psychosomatic cycle.

Nonspecific drugs may be correspondingly useful, if judiciously employed. An agitated, distracted melancholic may much more readily listen to reason after a night or two of restful sleep induced by simple barbiturates, bromides, or chloral hydrate; a patient in a state of exhausted lethargy may be helped back to activity by an amphetamine or some of the newer—though as yet insufficiently tested—stimulants. Again, however, my own experience has been that very few of the horde of ataractics, tranquillizers, or energizers now flooding the market have much advantage over the standbys mentioned above, and many have adverse effects. But whatever drugs one chooses, one must again observe two all-important cautions: First, sedative (sitting) or hypnotic (sleeping) medications must be used only for temporary relief while more basic life readjustments are achieved; and second, all drugs must be prescribed *with proper safeguards* when the patient is inclined to escape realities by cultivating addictions to the drug employed, by using it for suicidal gestures, or as leading to a facile substitute almost everywhere available, alcohol.

In verbal communications, avoid labelling your patients with a one-or-two-word "psychiatric diagnosis"; such nosology is no longer taken as adequately meaningful by experienced psychiatrists. Try instead to understand the nature of the patient's desires and tribulations; the effective (normal), deviant (neurotic), or unrealistic (psychotic) way he tries to deal with them; and the relative accessibility of these patterns of behavior to therapeutic influences. By the same token, avoid pseudo-analytic cliches, such as "oral fixations," "Oedipus complex" or "latent homosexuality." These obsolescing epithets may vent your concealed dislike of the patient, but they reveal little insight and furnish no leads to dynamic therapy.

Whether or not your patient's disabilities are the salient aspects of his illness, your personal relationship to him may be the most important single instrument in restoring his trust in humanity, and your wise guidance may indicate how he can cultivate other interests, companions and friends. Or, if you feel that he will need more specialized therapy, only through you can he be led to such referral—after which once again you may be one of the most important links in his physical and social rehabilitation. I need not here develop in detail the principle cautions necessary in this aspect of psychotherapy, since no sensible practitioner will permit the patients' dependencies upon him to become mutually paralyzing, and no ethical physician would ever exploit them for his personal, as opposed to his professional satisfactions.

In helping the patient deal with his problems, concentrate on the *real* and the *present.* It is true that the patient's conduct evolved from his previous life experiences, but the latter cannot be relived and changed, whereas the best way to alter the patient's reactions to his past is to have him reexplore and reevaluate his *current* misconceptions of physical and social realities, and thereby readjust his total behavior.

Never violate your patient's trust; however, this does not mean that you must exclude conferences with—or even the concurrent psychotherapy of—his friends, family, employer, or other persons in your practice who may be contributing to, or sharing in, his neurosis.

In no case should you furnish arbitrary directions as to major changes, such as the selection of a career, conception or adoption of a child, initiating or stopping a divorce action. If the patient is helped to see clearly the alternatives and consequences of his behavior, he will not need your advice; if he follows it blindly, dubiously, or resentfully, his actions are quite likely to circumvent your intent and backfire on you both—after which you will, quite justifiably, be blamed for the results. Nevertheless, if after using all your common sense and educated skill for a few weeks or months you are not witnessing satisfactory improvement, or if the patient seems too difficult or inaccessible in the first place, refer him to a psychiatrist—preferably one who, being broadly trained, avoids cults and doctrines, and can be as eclectic and versatile in his therapy as each patient requires.

Finally, we must acknowledge and respect the yearning for existential absolutes in each of us, whether we call our faiths science, humanitarianism, or religion. In effect, each man, as he ages, must preserve in adequate measures—or restore if they are impaired—his trust in himself, in his fellowman, and in his individually conceived God.

But perhaps I should here recall a third anecdote that affirms everyone's right of immunity to any challenging or disturbing statements I may have made. One of the delights of travelling round the world is having various people you have met repay visits to you when they in turn come to the crossroads of Chicago. Not long ago a likeable English psychiatrist came to dinner. Over liqueurs, I asked him if that talk I had recently given to the British Psychoanalytic Society had had any discernible effect. To which he replied: "Well really, old chap, in England we're getting away from this talkie-talk back to scientific psychiatry; I mean, making really definitive diagnoses preparatory to specific therapy. Then, if the patient has simple schizophrenia, we prescribe Largactil; if paranoid schizophrenia, why the thing to do is to give him insulin; and if he has a psychotic depression, we use electroshock, and so on. So instead of useless conversation we're returning to medicine, biology, physiology, and specific therapy. And how are things in the States?"

I know I should have refused the gambit, but instead I countered with: "Well, we're a young country, and haven't as yet developed such firm convictions. For one, we're not as adept at diagnosis; in fact, we're not very happy with the whole current system of classification in psychiatry. Instead, we try to understand each patient in a more holistic way: his genetic predisposition, his early environment, his crucial experiences, his current physical and emotional stresses, and so on. Therefore, we use not only drugs and EST, but individual therapy, social readjustment, group techniques, and many other therapeutic modalities." I went on this way for fifteen or twenty minutes as he kept stroking his chin and listening quite politely. Then, when I was through he said reflectively: "Dr. Masserman, you have given me a bit to think about. What I propose to do is to go home, sleep on it, and I'll warrant that by tomorrow morning, I shall have forgotten all about it. We are all entitled to our own opinions you know."

Fortunately, in a wondrously diverse world, this is still everyone's privilege. My own more extended views on clinical psychiatry are further expounded in Chapters 20 and 21 of this volume.

18. EPISTLES TO THE GENTILES

In this chapter also, I shall keep explanations and interpretations to a minimum, and let events, long ago and recent, be inferred from their context of correspondence. Perhaps the following array, selected in barely chronological order, bespeaks what in retrospect may seem an equally random life.

Early correspondence with a distinguished colleague in a twin discipline:

April 4, 1945

Dr. Livingston Welch
Director
Institute for Research in Child Psychology

Dear Dr. Welch:

Your research indicating that anxiety *expedites* rather than retards learning isn't "lucky"; that term I reserve for my winning opponents at tennis or bridge. It is turning out consistently because one manifestation of anxiety is an apprehensive hyper-reactivity to external threats (including psychotherapists) and an overmobilization, aberrant or not, of defensive "learning" adaptations. At least I think so, and therefore hope you will prove it.

That Puss in Purgatory article (about my work on alcoholic cats published in *Time* Magazine) was a bombshell. One letter from a nice old lady expressed the following intriguing sentiments: (a) I "must be a fiend whose family trembles at my approach;" (b) my "research is useless, since all alcoholics should be shot anyhow;" (c) I should see that a law is passed making this solution to the alcoholic program legal; (d) then my tortured body should be found in the gutter so that kind-hearted old ladies could feel safe about their cats. *Sic transit gloria mei.*

To a pioneer in psychosomatic medicine who wanted me to revise an article for a chapter in her new text:

October 1, 1953

Flanders Dunbar, M.D.
Editor
Psychosomatic Medicine

Dear Flanders:

I solved the problem of revising my old writings long ago: I never re-read them and so save my self-respect and peace of mind. Right now I'm finishing the long-delayed *Practice of Dynamic Therapy* which has been lying dormant in my drawers (no pun) for some seven years, but if you want me to mobilize more energy I'll see what I can do about the chapter you request.

One gratifying feedback:

World Health Organization
Interim Commission
Office of Director-General

350 Fifth Avenue, New York 1
Palais des Nations, Geneve
Telegr, Unsante, Geneve

Geneva, 22nd September 1948.

Dear Dr. Masserman,

Please accept my sincere thanks for your courtesy in sending us a reprint of your paper "Mental Hygiene in a World Crisis". It is indeed a very clear, concise and convincing statement.

I should like to see that copies of it are put in the hands of the Delegates to the General Assembly of the United Nations and to the World Health Assembly.

I am asking our New York Office to obtain some two hundred copies for this purpose.

May I congratulate you on adding another to the many useful contributions you have made to the cause of human understanding.

With kindest personal regards,

Sincerely yours,
Brock Chisholm, M.D.
Director-General.

In reply to an editorial request that I respond to Dr. Joseph Wolpe, who in an article in the *British Journal of Psychology* questioned the significance of my experiments on the ground that all my neurotic animals (cf. Chapter 21) simply "feared electric shock," and claimed complete originality for his methods of behavior therapy:

April 6, 1954

D. W. Harding
Editor
The British Journal of Psychology

Dear Dr. Harding:

The publications listed below* will show that during the past fifteen years my colleagues and I have noted and specifically countered the criticisms raised by Dr. Wolpe; I shall, therefore, not further dilute the literature by replying in detail to his interpretations of our data, except to point to our quite relevant experiments on the production of "masochistic" cats that avidly *seek* electroshocks when these *resolve* their adaptational conflicts. Instead, it may be of greater interest to comment on a general tendency among some psychologists (and, alas, not a few psychiatrists) to preempt a few words in the English language, take out a special patent as to their meaning, and then attempt to live off the royalties. One example is Erik Erikson's preemption of the term "identity," which apparently can now cover (in the sense of conceal) any aspect of human conduct. Another is Dr. Wolpe's solipsistic use of "motivational conflict," an expression which he apparently wishes to restrict to a clash between "learned feeding responses" and "grid shocks." Actually, rational reflection must expand "conflict" to encompass (a) *any* disruptive impasse among accustomed adaptive patterns (including, in a cat's universe, the opportunity simply to explore an experimental cage without being rudely electro-shocked), and (*b*) any new set of experiences that runs counter to such expectations—and is thereby rendered operationally "noxious" or "traumatic." Were this not true, human neuroses would quite literally be confined to people who had either been caught in an electrical short circuit or struck by lightning at the moment they were pushing a button to secure food from an Automat.

*Cf. research reports in Bibliography

As to Dr. Wolpe's therapeutic inferences from his own work: I regret that the "recent publications and manuscripts" he refers to are not as yet available here, so that I must be content to await patiently if not breathlessly for further information from him. However, I do not quite understand what he means by "treatment procedures . . . very different from those generated by Masserman's theory," since, in my *Principles of Dynamic Psychiatry,* based in part on our research, I tried to encompass all principal therapeutic methods from Ra to Rank. However, if Dr. Wolpe will accept an exchange of stakes he may consider not in his favor, I shall wager a set of autographed copies of my texts on therapy against correspondingly incribed reprints of his forthcoming papers (a) that the therapeutic principles he derives from his studies were already in use in the Asklepiad Sanatoria of classical Hellas and, (b) that they have been applied in infinitely variable forms with names other than "behavior therapy" ever since. And as a further instance of my trust in Dr. Wolpe's probity: if he will but consult the appropriate historical experimental and clinical sources I quote, he can be the sole judge of the matter.

Dr. Wolpe remained unmollified and continued the epistolary polemics, which I tried to terminate as follows:

May 6, 1954

Dear Dr. Harding:

The primary issue seems to be either that Dr. Wolpe thinks it unnecessary to read more than the titles of the publications I sent him, or else refuses to comprehend their contents. A simple instance is his reiteration that my "production of so-called 'masochistic' cats is easily explained on conditioning principles"—which is precisely what I tried to demonstrate (cf. my film "Experiemental Masochism," distributed by the Psychological Cinema Register of the State University of Pennsylvania)—although, I hope, without such simplistic concepts as "negative conditioning." Unfortunately, to deal adequately with Dr. Wolpe's other misconceptions of my work would require a specially annotated reproduction of a score or so of my papers in your columns—an eventuality that we would both deplore as a possible strain on Anglo-American friendship. The publication of Dr. Wolpe's second set of strictures and this reply is, of course, up to your editorial judgement; if it were my own, I would devote the space to material of greater scientific import.

The exchange ended.
A request from Karl Menninger:

April 7, 1954

Dear Jules:

I have picked out ten men in the American Psychiatric Association whose thinking and judgment I deeply respect, among them, of course, you. I have selected them for the purpose of imposing upon them a rough draft of a line of thought with which I have been preoccupied recently relative to some theories about conceptualizing ego regulatory functions. I present this humbly, so humbly in fact that my secretary wouldn't even put my name on it. But I did write it (with Dr. Mayman's help). I have thought about it and talked about it so much here that I am in a rut until I get some other reactions.

Read it, please, with a pencil in your hand. Scribble your comments in the margins or on the back of a page with an indicative asterisk. Then mail it back to me (stamped envelope enclosed). I shall take your comments most seriously, and when I have revamped it in the light of all the ideas I get, I will send you another copy for your memory book!

And I shall be grateful.

Sincerely yours,
Karl A. Menninger, M.D.

April 17, 1954

Dear Karl:

Flattery will get you nothing but instant service.

I went through your Chapter V, admiring your clarity and consistency, and here and there pencilling a self-explanatory comment. But about Freud's instinct-dichotomy theory—once again picturing eager Eros hopelessly against terrible Thanatos —I prefer Occam's razor-sharp *Entia non sunt multiplicanda praeter necessitatem,* to Tertullian's *Certum est quia impossibile est.* Actually if, as you say, neuroses are considered not as "sicknesses" but as deviant adaptations, "recovery" implies not a "realignment of instincts," but both more simply and complexly, *re*learning and *re*adaptation. One other comment: the book begins with a fine phillipic against sterile descriptions and questionable taxonomies, but lets these creep in again toward the end in its divisions of the personality and its categorizations of various "types" of "egos." We may need such transitional expositions—but I hope it will not be long until we can transcend them.

I shall look forward to the publication, and to seeing you soon.

To Manfred Bleuler, illustrious son of the famous Eugen:

May 11, 1954

Professor M. Bleuler, Director
Psychiatriche Universitatsklinik
Zurich, Switzerland

Dear Dr. Bleuler:

I have been a careful student of your illustrious father's writings, and am flattered indeed that you compare my modest contributions to his. While I cannot accept completely some of his theses—for instance, the inheritance of acquired characteristics—I follow his insights in many others: *i.e.,* the biologic nature of memory and the definition of "psyche" as behavior.

I greatly appreciate your gracious letter, and hope to renew our discussion personally some time either in Zurich or here.

A requested commentary on a Conference on the Mathematics of Behavior:

M. Ralph Kaufman, M.D.

Dear Moe:

As I wrote Iago Galdston about some of the presentations, there was one mathematical formula I was tempted to put on the board at our meeting in Chicago: $C_t\ C_s\ L_n$, or, the total Confusion equals the Confusion of the Speakers multiplied by the Number of Listeners. But I refrained.

In support of a friend being considered for academic promotion:

August 19, 1955

Karl M. Bowman, M.D.
Chairman and Professor of Psychiatry
University of California

Dear Dr. Bowman:

Dr. Jurgen Ruesch's contributions to our understanding of the modes of human communication, to the nature of interpersonal and social relationships, and to the derived dynamics of psychotherapy have been invaluable to a modern and integrative approach to the science of behavior. I specifically included such favorable evaluations of his work in my recently published *Practice of Dynamic Psychiatry* and am happy to reaffirm them here. Perhaps the only deterrent to the more rapid and general acceptance of his writings has been Dr. Ruesch's tendency to be outspokenly impatient with traditional theoretical vacuities and illogical practices in our field, but this also has been an understandable expression of his scientific consistency and honesty. I am therefore thoroughly in accord with your recommendations for his promotion to a full professorship, and hope that the trustees of the university will agree to give him greater opportunities for service to the university and to psychiatry in general.

Or for a chairmanship of a new Department of Behavioral Sciences:

April 9, 1955

Dr. Raymond Waggoner
Chairman, Dept. of Psychiatry

Dear Dr. Waggoner:

In pursuit of negotiations between Dr. James G. Miller and the University of Michigan, he has informed me of your request that I write you a letter of evaluation of his scientific and personal status. You will recall that at our Detroit meeting on March 17th, we discussed Dr. Miller, his associates and his plans in some detail, so perhaps it is necessary here to review only briefly and explicitly the opinions I then expressed. They are these:

1. Dr. Miller is a highly intelligent, broadly informed, sincere behavioral scientist dedicated to perhaps the most important task in our field: its reformulation in valid, operational terms and its systematic reintegration with the other disciplines of the biologic and humanistic sciences.

2. From my frequent contacts with Dr. Miller and from my fairly intimate knowledge of the academic milieu at the University of Chicago during the past fifteen years, I can say that the recent regrettable disintegration of the Department of Psychology at that institution is the result of deplorable university policies, and can in no sense be attributed to Dr. Miller. On the contrary, to my knowledge he inspires friendship and loyalty in his associates, and in a favorable atmosphere will serve the best interests of your own department and and of the University of Michigan.

Or for the directorship of a hospital:

December 23, 1955
Re: Dr. Anthony E. Maniscalco

Sister Loretto Bernard
St. Vincents' Hospital
New York, New York

Dear Sister Bernard:

In the six years in which I have known Dr. Maniscalco as an administrator, academic colleague, collaborator, and friend, I have found him to be invariably well informed, intelligent, high-principled, conscientious, and exceedingly effective in both his professional and personal relationships. I am not accustomed to superlatives, but in the case of Dr. Maniscalco I am certain that you will find him, as we have, a major asset to your institution.

To Percival Bailey who, at my recommendation, was designated by President Karl Bowman to present the academic address to the 1957 annual meeting of the American Psychiatric Association, and who sent me a preliminary draft of his manuscript:

January 31, 1956

Dear Percival:

Because I feel I can talk freely to a friend, let me do so. I like the typical Bailey directness and unequivocation, but there is not yet in this preliminary draft the measure of incisive logical organization, critique, and inescapable conclusions I have grown to expect in your publications and which will undoubedly appear in later versions of this one. You have the knowledge and ability to render American psychiatry a great service by doing what I have also tried to do in writing which analysts won't read: *i.e.,* put "psychoanalysis" in its proper context and perspective and so help get psychiatrists back to their senses, patients, and laboratories. Also, many of us would like to hear some positive directives in your peroration: possibly that analysts leave their monkish institutes and rejoin their colleagues in the academic and scientific settings of universities, where serious students also belong. Parenthetically, some of us this year are launching a new American Academy of Psychoanalysis with this as one of its major objectives.

I'll look forward to these future versions, and to talking them over—if you still want me to.

Sincerely,
Jules

Dr. Bailey made few revisions, and left a lasting impression of castigated shock on the APA.

A letter of indignation about a published calumny of a friend and colleague honored elsewhere in this volume:

May 4, 1956

Dr. John Frosch
Editor
Journal of the American Psychoanalytic Association

Dear Dr. Frosch:

In the interest of simple decency as well as professional dignity, I must protest Kurt Eissler's implication (your *Journal*, 4:315, 1956) that Dr. Frieda Fromm-Reichmann, one of the most respected analysts in America with whose opinions he does not happen to agree, is merely a "dynamic psychiatrist" allegedly lacking in "self-discipline and adequate training." I have been informed on excellent legal authority that such insinuations constitute actionable libel, but in any case they are unworthy of scientific discourse and are particularly out of place in our field. Since the respect with which all analysts are held may depend on the words and deeds of a few, I suggest that Eissler either retract this reprehensible form of *argumen-*

tum ad hominem or, if he prefers, maintain it and suffer the judgment of his colleagues.

Respectfully

Dr. Frosch published a dignified editorial regretting the incident.

The continuation of a personal friendship with a pioneer ethologist:

September 29, 1958

Konrad Z. Lorenz, M.D., Ph.D.
Departmental Director for Comparative Ethology
Max Planck Research Institute
Westphalia, Germany,

Dear Konrad:

Please do not trouble yourself further about our delayed correspondence; I am fully aware of how many unpredictable events can interfere with efficient long-distance communication. We have announced and look forward with renewed pleasure to your lectures at Northwestern, and we shall have facilities for projecting slides and motion pictures.

Also please let me know the time and mode of your arrival at our home, and Mrs. Masserman and I shall arrange everything for your comfort, including your room, your transportation, and a dinner party Monday evening. We hope that your wife is fully recovered and will accompany you.

Cordially,
Jules

To avoid joining a futile panel on Existentialism:

October 20, 1958

Jordan M. Scher, M.D.

Dear Jordan:

While Straus is a "phenomenologist" rather than a *Be*-mused or *Zen*-type "existentialist," he is still perhaps one of the most obscure speakers alive in a sphere highly competitive in that area. I admit myself outclassed and beg to beg off.

Reply to a temporarily tempting invitation to accept a professorship at the University of Southern California and an appointment as Chief of Psychiatry at the Cedars of Lebanon Hospital in Beverly Hills:

May 8, 1959

Harold Mazur, M.D.
Medical Director
Cedars of Lebanon Hospital

Dear Dr. Mazur:

Since our last correspondence I have discussed the Cedars situation with Drs. Alexander, Marmor, Ziskind, and others, and have thought long and seriously about your kind offer. My conclusions have been that the opportunities at the Cedars are gratifying, the anticipated personal and professional associations very pleasant, and the prospects of developing a Division of Psychiatry at the Cedars splendid; nevertheless, the position seems to call for a younger man with fewer requirements as to staff, finances, and facilities than I might perhaps expect. I also concluded that, since I have no immediate plans for a visit to Los Angeles, I should in all fairness apprise you of my present feelings on the matter so that you can proceed to process other desirable candidates.

I deeply appreciate your offer, and truly regret relinquishing the chance to join the Ziskinds and other current and potential friends on your staff. With personal thanks and regards.

Only once was I involved in evaluating the ethics of two

psychiatric colleagues, M.C. and V.F., and their "assistant psychologist" K.N. After the death of M.C., K.N. had traveled bimonthly from a city 1200 miles away to have me supervise the therapy of patients who continued to be referred to him by local physicians. At the request of the American Psychiatric Association, I reported as follows:

August 11, 1959

Dr. Francis J. Gerty
APA Committee on Ethics

Dear Dr. Gerty:

I knew the late Dr. M.C. personally, but regret that I can give you no direct information either on him or on his medical associate Dr. V.F. except whatever bearing my contacts with their psychological assistant, Mr. K. N., may have on Dr. V.F.'s current difficulties with your APA committee on ethics. Herewith:

Dr. M.C. was a fellow-trainee with me at the Chicago Psychoanalytic Institute, and to my knowledge graduated there, was recognized as an accredited psychoanalyst by the American Psychoanalytic Association and later as a training analyst by the Institute. He then returned to [a southwestern city], developed a highly lucrative analytic practice, and secured teaching appointments at the VA and the university. When I lectured at the VA hospital in [his city] a year or so before his death he introduced me to a "Dr. K.N., Ph.D." as an able psychologist whom he "had analyzed and further trained" and who was doing "analytically-oriented counselling" in Dr. C's office under his personal supervision. Later in 1951, when Dr. C's health was failing, he requested that I, as a friend who had helped him previously, take over this task for the sake of the patients he and other physicians "had referred to Dr. K.N.," and this I agreed to do. Following Dr. C's death, K.N. earnestly desired to continue this supervision, came to Chicago faithfully nearly every month, brought and took meticulous and accurate notes, and was receptive and intelligent in following therapeutic cautions and guidance, including referral of all medical problems to local physicians. Indeed, he successfully treated a number of physicians himself (including one psychiatrist), their families, and other locally prominent people. I regarded his conscientiousness, caution, and sincerity favorably, and acted in accordance with APA policies of supervising properly recommended psychologists in their clinical work just as we all do at our universities, VA hospitals, and elsewhere. It was therefore with deep personal regret that I learned early this year from the AMA that Dr. C had apparently deceived his psychoanalyst and the Chicago Psychoanalytic Institute as to his own qualifications for training, and that his assistant, K.N., was therefore similarly under a cloud. To the latter's further credit he told me this voluntarily, and accepted my advice that he cease all activities until he could associate himself with a university or an ethical, accredited clinic or psychiatrist and had full approval on his own merits from such constituted authorities. I advised him to refer his remaining patients, whatever their progress to date, to local psychiatrists, and left the matter there.

Now as to the late Dr. C's medical associate, Dr. V.F., currently under investigation by your committee for [seriously unethical conduct.] As far as I know, Mr. N took over only one patient on referral from Dr. F, brought her case record to me, at my advice changed her therapy, and incidentally effected her recovery despite alleged previous mishandling by Dr. F. Mr. N made no mention of supervision by Dr. F and was correctly guarded in his comments as to the latter's methods of treatment; further, since Dr. F. was listed as an APA member and a licensed board diplomate, and since I had none but hearsay data, I could not ethically criticize or report him in any case. Moreover, in view of Dr. C's original endorsements by the Chicago Psychoanalytic Institute, the American Psychoanalytic Association, and other official bodies, I saw no reason at the time personally to question his status or his recommendation of K. N. as a psychoanalytically trained and qualified psychologist with a doctoral degree who, unlike many who practiced independently, sought continued psychiatric supervision. I attach the only other correspondence I have in the matter and would be happy to help further in any way I can.

In reply to an understandably anxious inquiry from Dr. F:

August 12, 1959

Dear Dr. F.:

I can well appreciate your anxiety, and would naturally be glad to help any human being, let alone a troubled colleague, in any way I could. You must realize, however, that I had and have no knowledge of your situation except as given me by Dr. C and Mr. N, and more recently, the AMA, and that I have forwarded all I know to Dr. Francis Gerty at his request. To my knowledge Drs. Gerty and Tarumianz are eminently fair-minded people, and if your conduct has been well-intentioned and ethical I am certain you can feel confident of just treatment.

Dr. V. F. was reprimanded and retired from private practice; K.N. was absolved and has since functioned well on the staff of a state hospital.

When I was mistakenly listed in *Who's Who* as president of the American Psychiatric Association:

May 14, 1960

Editor
Marquis *Who's Who*

Dear Sir:

I hasten to be the first—I hope—to inform you that the honor of being listed in *Who's Who* does not entail my election to the presidency of the American Psychiatric Association. In future editions, please edit the entry to read, more truthfully, that I have admittedly (and simultaneously) been president of the American Academy of Psychoanalysis, the American Society of Biological Psychiatry, and the American Society of Group Therapy—which is a record of delinquency regrettable enough.

June 6, 1960

Martin Grotjahn, M.D.

Dear Martin:

Thanks for the copy of your most sensibly and engagingly written book *Beyond Laughter.* Like mine, it *may* conceivably sway future generations, the current one being manifestly hopeless. Your final chapter of dialectics is, curiously, also like the final one in my *Principles*—and will proably be similarly ignored in this decade.

Colleagues also submit their grant proposals, manuscripts, and miscellanea for comment and advice:

July 7, 1960

Raymond Headlee, M.D.

Dear Ray:

Thanks for your letter and your projected outline of a "Socio-clinical Study of Marriage Dynamics." With regard to the latter, as a recipient of now well over a million dollars in successful grant applications over the last quarter century, and as a member of various granting councils in the last decade, I can repeat almost verbatim the comments that would be made on your present grant application were it to be deliberated at NIMH.

"Headlee's research protocol is far too diffuse and intangible, and that Latin Square attempt just points it up all the more."

"Doesn't everyone examine the interpersonal dynamics of the marriage in all married patients"?

"How many times must it be shown that 'social work interviews' tell more about the worker than about the subject"?

"Since when is hospitalization an end-point, or even a definite turning point in interpersonal transactions"?

"To mean anything, this must really be a 20-year, not a two-year project—and we can't support these at NIMH."

"Headlee, like most of these recent trainees, starts with theoretical premises about fantasies and values that he apparently fully intends to prove. Why spend money in between"?

"Psychoanalytically-oriented interview techniques have invariably been shown by objective follow-up work to be grossly misleading, and psychoanalytic theory of negative heuristic value. Headlee seems to be getting to understand this, but we'll have to wait until he can formulate his research more scientifically."

"Where's his budget in dollars and sense"?

"He cites a few articles, but hasn't he heard of Ackerman, Laidlaw, Mudd, and all the others who have been studying this field for years"?

In weary days during many Advisory Council meetings, I've heard hundreds of comments like these from experienced and sophisticated psychiatrists and social scientists—and one or two really hep psychoanalysts—on scores of proposals like yours, with eventual rejection. I don't agree with all of these comments, but I long ago learned to avoid them with reference to my own applications, and I'll tell you how when I see you.

Meanwhile, I'm also glad to hear that you are recovering from the Procrustian wounds of the Chicago Institute and, though better for the experience, resuming normal functions in academic, familial and social affairs. Best of summers.

Appeal to an NIMH official in aid of a friend whose application for grants in aid of his research to find physio-anatomic factors in schizophrenia had been repeatedly, and without explanation, rejected by a governmental agency:

June 30, 1961

Dr. Ellis Kelsey
Washington, D.C.

Dear Ellis:

I am forwarding a letter from Dr. Robert Heath to you in confidence. It is my long-term judgment that Bob is among the very few psychiatrists who combines original and integrative thought with research skill and clarity of presentation. These qualities, inevitably in our field, have threatened a few hierarchs intrenched on committees, and these have treated him shamefully. As you know, I rarely ask much directly for myself, but am inclined to go pretty far for a friend and a cause. Could you, without prejudicing yourself or any NIH secrets, tell Bob or me what happened, why, and what might be done to save his program at Tulane before its unique research opportunities are lost?

I'm due East for some lectures next fall, and hope to see the new Kelsey Manor, on which congratulations and best of wishes. Until then, how about boarding the Naiad on her cruise anytime this summer if you are anywhere near her mooring?

June 30, 1961

Robert G. Heath, M.D., Chairman
Dept. of Psychiatry and Neurology
Tulane University

Dear Bob:

The attached letter to Kelsey is only one indication of my indignation. I'll try to find out what happened, and then do all I can. I can well understand that you might feel that the world isn't worth saving; however, as in my case, a few friends might help restore the precious illusion that it's worth another try.

You may know that, on request, the NIMH is obligated to inform you of the reasons given by various consultants (only their *names* are kept confidential) for rejecting any application. This is usually justified on the basis that future applications may be properly revised or amended.

Meanwhile, a vacation and some second thoughts about the remaining joys in life is an excellent idea.

Response to a research questionnaire as to "how it felt to be filmed in color and sound while demonstrating a clinical interview at the University of Pennsylvania":

December 5, 1961

Dear Dr. Scheflen:

My reactions to being filmed?

Simply those of an old pro. I have been doing demonstration interviews (i.e., interchanges of views with friends, students, and/or patients) for lo! these thirty years, nearly always without the interposition of a desk, notebook, tape-recorder, half-silvered mirror, movie camera, or videotape between the interviewee, myself, and an audience if present. Frankly, I regard all such devices, whether recognized as physically present or not, as handicaps to both therapy and teaching. Reasons? Even in a supposedly private dyadic interview the patient peoples the place with an infinity of presences from his past, whereas the interviewer does the same with a different but similarly imaginary claque, ranging from his clinical supervisor or his analyst through the hovering figures of Freud, Adler, Rogers, et al. to more ethereal divinities whom he must face on some Judgment Day. On the other hand, to record interviews without the patient's knowledge and consent is not only unethical, but what is worse, constitutes scientific hypocrisy. As to bequeathing my own acts in deathless hi-fi and technicolor to posterity: that has already been done, for good or ill, in the minds and attitudes of many patients and students, although with no more "consensual validation" than would be derived from viewing a film.

Parenthetically, after seeing scores of movies and videotapes of myself, I need no longer take the trouble to exhibit my "good" profile or try to use my "most expressive" voice; I am resigned to the sad circumstance that neither profile is very good, and that my voice occasionally sounds like a tyro practicing on an inferior viola. But the interview's the thing, and I shall be interested in reviewing my slips in technique.

December 15, 1961

Q and A Section,
Journal of the American Medical Association

Thank you for the copy of the letter by Dr. P.Q. about his "diagnostic use of physical features in detecting schizophrenia." Physicians at one time ardently diagnosed "amativeness" or "criminality" by bumps on the head or pointed ears—and were just as mistaken as to the value of these "physical aids to diagnosis."

To the Northwestern residents collaborating with me in writing the annual chapter on "The Neuroses" for Spiegel's *Progress in Neurology and Psychiatry:*

Pointers on How to Win Publishers and Influence People

Organization:

1. Make an outline of topics and subtopics in some logical, progressive sequence.
2. Put references together that belong together, either in confirmation or contradiction.
3. End each section with some comprehensive and *meaningful* summary.

Content: Condense. It's a delightful and profitable intellectual exercise to substitute a word for a sentence and a phrase for a paragraph.

Style: Avoid tautology. Don't begin "Blank studied ______"; your report will show he did. Never say "from his studies he concluded, etc;" how else could he? Avoid "he further states" and similar redundant expressions.

Tense: Put work done in the past tense, conclusions in the present. Observe rules of grammar: Don't split infinitives, end sentences with prepositions, etc.

Structure: Don't repeat words; English is 500,000 words rich! Don't leave out articles, e.g., "Author claims", or use telegraphic style.

Revisions: Can't it be said more briefly, clearly, elegantly? You can't know until you have carefully revised at least three times—and then reread it critically twice at least two weeks apart. But it pays.

Another typical response to more invitations to leave Northwestern, whenever the bids were ethical, dignified, and potentially interesting:

January 15, 1963

Dr. Alexander G. Karczmar
Chairman, ad hoc Search Committee
Loyola University

Dear Dr. Karczmar:

Since I long ago dedicated my life to research and teaching in psychiatry, your invitation to continue the work of my late friend John Madden and build a distinguished Department of Psychiatry at Loyola University deserves thorough and serious consideration. I am therefore enclosing a recent *curriculum vitae* and a copy of one of my textbooks. These will, I hope, well illustrate my agreement with you that the teaching of psychiatry should integrate not only the medical, neurological, pathological, and pharmacologic factors in behavior with dynamic psychologic and psychoanalytic concepts but should take account of historical, social, and philosophic influences in psychiatric diagnosis and therapy.

You are, of course, welcome to make any inquiries about me from any source whatever, although I would appreciate it if, after seventeen years at Northwestern, such inquiries reflect no disappointments or disloyalties to that University, since my relationships there have been productive and happy. May I also suggest that you and any other members of your Search Committee you designate then meet with me at some mutually convenient time.

Respectfully

How to get disinvited to comment on a proposed publication by a popular author:

February 8, 1963

Mr. Gordon Christiansen
Peace Education Division
American Friends Service Committee

Dear Mr. Christiansen:

I am honored by your kind invitation to join a select company of commentators on Erich Fromm's proposed manuscript on "The Psychological Causes of War," subheaded "Man: Sheep or Wolf?" which you apparently intend to publish. However, I must regretfully decline, because:

(a) I am repelled by supposedly titillating titles such as Mind *vs* Matter, Love *against* Hate, and Man—Sheep *or* Wolf?

(b) I am impatient with the naïveté of attempting to classify protean human transactions by giving them names such as "necrophilia" or "biophilia," animating these false reifications into "instincts" and then further classifying them as "traits of behavior," or worse, "types of personality." I had begun to hope that the shades of Gall, McDougall, and Lombroso had long since been decently exorcised from serious social or psychiatric discourse.

(c) When Fromm appeals to nature myths about animals (for example, directly contrary to Fromm's assertions, sheep can be quite "vicious" even to their young, and wolves quite kind to their kind), I can't help wishing he would become better acquainted with modern ethologic and comparative evolutionary thought (see my attached reprint on "Ethology, Biodynamics and Psychoanalytic Research").

(d) Finally, I am disconcerted that, while the world teeters, the American Friends Service Committee, with so much good work at hand, can seriously consider adding yet another pamphlet of pseudopsychoanalytic parlor patois, however nicely composed in eight-sentence cadences, to library shelves already replete with deservedly unread irrationalities. In effect, for the life of me—and it may amount to that—I can see no practical relevance or applicability to any of our pressing problems of Dr. Fromm's newest tax on taxonomic credibility.

An acknowledgement and a tribute:

July 29, 1963

Francis J. Gerty, M.D.
Director, Dept. Public Welfare
Chicago, Illinois

Dear Dr. Gerty:

Your retirement as director of the Department of Mental Health constitutes a culmination of only one aspect of your distinguished career and recalls several milestones which, through your efforts, were prominent in mine. To cite but five in the last quarter century:

Your personal welcome and encouragement when I came to the University of Chicago in 1935.

Your help in keeping me active in clinical teaching, administration, and research when I moved to Northwestern by appointing me to organize the Residency Training Program at Downey, eventuating in a long and friendly collaboration with Ben Boshes and my current co-chairmanship of the Department of Neurology and Psychiatry.

Your modest protests over my initiation of a campaign that rapidly snowballed into your election to the presidency of the American Psychiatric Association in 1959.

Your sense of professional probity when, as president of the board of psychiatry and neurology, you consulted me and the Academy of Psychoanalysis with regard to a sub-specialty board of psychoanalysis, and thus helped achieve equitable action on this important issue.

Your further affirmation of confidence in me when, as chairman of the Research and Training Authority, you confirmed my *pro tem* appointment as director of education at the Illinois State Psychiatric Institute, and your invaluable counsel and guidance during the crucial months that followed.

I could recount many more such markers, but these indicate my personal respect and gratitude.

Most sincerely,
Jules

To an editor of a psychologic journal who requested my comments on another unpublished manuscript critical of my work:

March 17, 1964

Mark Keller, Editor
Quarterly J. of Studies on Alcohol
Smithers Hall, University Heights Campus
New Brunswick, New Jersey

Dear Dr. Keller:

To put it as objectively as I can, Dr. S's long introductory polemics about the 1946 paper by Dr. Yum and myself on alcohol preferences in neurotic cats is somewhat misleading in that:

1. He himself cites only two references to our work, does so quite inaccurately, and has obviously not read either my book *Behavior and Neurosis* or the twenty or so technical papers in which we describe our methods in wearyingly precise detail.

2. Neither has he—possibly to be unique among workers in the field—troubled to view the easily available motion picture films in which our actual experiments and results are recorded for anyone to see and interpret.

3. He does not mention the confirmatory reports of Jacobsen, Seitz, and many others, or the fact that Professors Hoff and Schenker recently duplicated our entire studies at the University of Vienna and prepared a teaching motion picture film on them.

4. And most amusing of all, he comes out of it all with results essentially similar to ours (i.e., the effects of "conflict," alcohol, etc.), yet rejects the most parsimonious explanation of them: Namely, that alcohol disorganizes complex learned behavior, whether "normal" or "neurotic," into simpler previous patterns of integration and response. However, since every worker is entitled to his own premises (the usual euphemism for prejudices) this would not deter me from recommending the manuscript if the rest of it did not also consist in large part of a meandering, repetitious, and often self-contradictory dialectics, with occasional high points of semantic confusion such as attributing "neurosis" to "an organic [brain] lesion" (and incidentally misrepresenting Hebb's position on this point) or juxtaposing completely incompatible commentators in disparate fields such as Eysenck and Fenichel. Ordinarily, I would recommend rejection, but to be as encouraging to young authors as possible, you might return the paper with the suggestions that (1) it be cut to about a third of its size, (2) the experimental data be presented in better sequence and organization (3) the rationale, methodology, and conclusions be formulated more concisely, clearly and consistently, and (4) the discussion be less biased, acerbic, or clouded over with hyperbolic Pavlovian-Skinnerian jargon, and more guarded as to clinical parallels. Parenthetically, since when does the "same dose of alcohol produce the same effects in every human"?

If Dr. S doesn't accept these suggestions, we shall at least have done our Christian duty.

A peculiar interlude involving Hugh Hefner, High Priest of the Playboy Enterprises:

August 20, 1964

Mr. Hugh Hefner
Playboy Clubs International

Dear Mr. Hefner:

At the instance of our mutual friend Dan Schuffman, I

herewith invite you to be one of the principal speakers at the next annual meeting of the American Psychiatric Association, to be held at the Americana Hotel in New York May 3-7, 1965. The circumstances are these:

For the past several years I have arranged as a special feature of the annual program a plenary session on the arts and humanities, at which authors, musicians, artists, or movie and stage directors have addressed the association, using any illustrative material they chose on the relevance of their artistic insights and behavior. Since your own philosophy and enterprise seem to be in accord with the current swing toward an easement of social inhibitions and a zestful enjoyment of life, the association would be highly interested to hear your interpretation of this phenomenon. Is it an era of dissipation and decline under excessive stress, as in late Roman times, or is it a new sophistication and eagerness for life, as in the Greece of cynical Democritus and the frank and lusty Aristophanes? A whimsical title for your talk might then be: "Apollo *vs.* Dionysus—the Key Club to the Solution." But of course title content and illustrative material would be left to your judgement.

Please let me know, and I shall be glad to discuss further details.

To my consternation, the text of this personal letter was published in the next issue of *Playboy Magazine.* Since that involved the legal issue of abuse of privacy, I called Mr. Hefner, who invited me to his Chicago palace where I would presumably acquire broader, more tolerant views as to hedonistic as well as transactional amenities. I found him to be a concerned, intelligent and reasonable gentleman, quite willing to make amends, as instanced by the following public retraction:

October 27, 1964

American Psychiatric Association
Washington, D. C.

To All Concerned:

On August 20, 1964, Dr. Jules H. Masserman wrote me to inquire whether, because of the extensive writing I had been doing on the American sexual revolution, I would be interested in addressing the American Psychiatric Association on some aspect of our changing mores, especially as related to the communications and entertainment fields, of which I am a part. Dr. Masserman closed his letter with the suggestion that we meet in person, shortly thereafter, to discuss the details of such an appearance.

Whereas I thought this to be an official and public invitation to appear as one of the principal speakers at the next annual meeting of the association in New York in May, I now understand that it was intended only as a preliminary expression of interest in me, as a possible speaker on that occasion, and it could not be official unless and until all arrangements had been confirmed by the entire program committee, of which Dr. Masserman is the chairman.

Having misunderstood the true nature of Dr. Masserman's letter, I released it for publication, and it appeared in somewhat edited form in the October 1964 issue of *Playboy Magazine.* This action was taken in good faith as a positive expression of my own reaction to the invitation, but the letter appeared without Dr. Masserman's prior knowledge or permission.

Because I misunderstood the original intent of Dr. Masserman's letter to me, I am now fearful that its publication may be the cause of misunderstanding in some quarter, and be a possible cause of embarrassment for either Dr. Masserman or the association.

I would be extremely sorry if this proved to be the case, for the misunderstanding was clearly my own, and the subsequent impropriety in publishing the original letter from Dr. Masserman is totally my doing, also.

I am writing this letter, therefore, to express my deep

regret over this matter and to correct any misunderstandings that may have arisen over this episode.

Sincerely,
Hugh M. Hefner
Editor-Publisher
Playboy Magazine

October 29, 1964

Dear Mr. Hefner:

Since your letter constitutes the sincere and honest explanation of a gentleman, please be assured that I consider it completely acceptable and join you in regretting the misunderstanding. As an instance of this, I hope that we can get together at some mutually favorable opportunity (and in a less distracting milieu) to discuss the matter of your addressing the American Psychiatric Association at some future time.

Permit me to add my personal wishes for your health and welfare.

That future time has not yet arrived.

In reply to a *N. Y. Times* inquiry directed to me by the APA central office:

July 13, 1967

Robert L. Robinson
Public Information Officer
American Psychiatric Association

Dear Robbie:

It was apparently at your instance that *The Times* called from New York to ask about "the validity of a British statistician's conclusion that people whose names begin with letters from S to Z are four times as likely to develop neuroses as all others"; therefore, it would be only fair to apprise you of my unresearched, spontaneous but conclusive reply on the subject, to wit:

"That British statistician's inferences are just possibly valid, since surnames beginning with letters from S to Z are more likely to belong to Slavs, and according to upper-class British opinion, most Slavs are neurotic or borderline psychotic anyway. However, others could contend that certain qualifications could modify this generalization until disproved: namely, that it applied only to those born under the Sign of Aries when Jupiter is in conjunction with Mercury on the third Wednesday after Whitsuntide."

You may like to know that this serious and learned commentary was apparently taken down in long-distance shorthand, and you may therefore expect an official letter of thanks from the august *New York Times.*

July 17, 1967

Dear Jules:

I know you would come up with a scintillating response to Jan Brody's problem, and I think your bon mot may settle the question of alphabetical neuroses for all time. What would we do without you?

Robbie

Next, an encomium recommending one of my favorite science writers for the APA Writer's Award at their annual celebration:

March 25, 1968

Dear Co-conspirator Robbie:

As to Art Synder [science writer of the *Chicago Daily News*] herewith my Celebration:

His Contributions: Cogent, clear, calm, concise, contemporaneous, rarely censorious or condemnatory, and consequently calculated to carry conviction.

His Character: Cooperative, charitable, congenial, rarely

capricious or controversial, and convivial as well as charismatic.

If you concur, I'll compose a ceremonial concerto—appropriately in the Key of C—and play it on the cello while you cite these commendations at the ceremony.

Complacently

Mr. Snyder was given the award.

To a colleague who asked me to join him in a highly questionable plan for founding and developing a colony for retired scholars near Teneriffe:

August 22, 1967

Dr. Joshua Bierer
London, England

Dear Joshua:

I found your letter on my return from Spain and, as I promised, immediately consulted my trusted legal and financial counsellors as to your proposition. Unfortunately, their advice was completely adverse to my joining you in this venture, for a variety of reasons, among them these:

1. Possible profits: At my age (nearly 62) and financial position, the wise course is to conserve my funds for contingencies and for retirement (and for Christine after my demise) rather than to increase an estate already adequate for these purposes—all the more so since we have no heirs.

2. Milieu: Teneriffe, however salubrious its climate, would suit Mrs. Masserman and me only for annual or even less frequent social and professional visits with you and our mutual friends, but is far from our ideal as a locale of retirement when compared to our base in Chicago in summer and in tropical waters at other times.

3. Finally—and this may be adventitious and uncalled-for advice, but I offer it out of concern and friendship—it was also their sincere opinion that you should realize whatever profit you can on your option now rather than undertake to develop

the land yourself or with only a few partners of limited means, since (a) the necessary additional investment will be far greater than you anticipate; (b) the Spanish government is unreliable and may turn confiscatory tomorrow; (c) A very great deal of specialized administrative skill and effort will be required of those involved—and your next few years may be far more troubled with business concerns than you would wish.

I am therefore writing this immediately so that, if you still think it wise, you can offer others the opportunity you kindly offered me. In the hope that our other personal relationships can continue as pleasant and productive as previously.

With personal concern

I was asked to write a commentary on a research report by Stephen Milgram which purported to show that college students directed to administer electric shocks "to motivate subjects in a learning experiment" (the "subjects" were really laboratory assistants and the shocks actually remained minimal) would, despite "mounting, subjective tension," increase these shocks to near-lethal levels even though the "learners" seemed to suffer agonies and pleaded with them to desist. I declined to write a formal critique, and instead sent the following letter:

June 21, 1967

Mr. Seymour Weingarten
Associate Editor
International Journal of Psychiatry

Dear Mr. Weingarten:

I, too, was initially fascinated by Milgram's article. On further reflection, however, as has often been my reaction to much of Freud's writing, I recognized that I had been intrigued more by Milgrams' gracefully persuasive style than the heuristic value of his studies or the significance of his conclusions. My reservations arose from the consideration that, despite Milgram's tendencies to reifying his experimental "situation," he was manifestly dealing with a series of *triadic interpersonal relationships* in which:

(a) He may have seriously underestimated the influence of his own obviously charismatic (i.e., research-bent, grant-securing, subject-involving) personality and that of his similarly motivated and inspired associates.

(b) He may have overlooked the subtle non-verbal communication in which the "learner" informs the "teacher" that despite the former's histrionic moans, groans and protests, he is not really suffering—a message certainly reinforced by the necessarily false mimetics of the "sufferer situation."

(c) In the absence of measured psychosomatic correlates, Milgram may have also overestimated the socially-oriented reports of "anxiety" and "tension" in the "teacher."

These and other perhaps unavoidable nebulosities in Milgram's methods in no sense detract from his ingenious attempts to find measurable vectors in a highly complex interpersonal transactional matrix: However, they tend to promote escalations of "punitive" voltage not necessarily correlated with the infliction of actual pain. In analogous experiments, it has been shown that most "hypnotized" Trilbys will viciously stab a victim at their Svengalis' command, but only if, despite their professed denials, they really know the dagger is rubber, that little or no retribution will therefore follow, and that the demonstration will thereby end happily for all concerned.

In essence, I am heartily in favor of bold and original research in interpersonal transactions, and particularly enthusiastic about Milgram's esthetically clear and literate reporting. But even in humans, labile experiments must be viewed in the context of labored (as distinguished from laboratory) experiences. In this connection, some humans, like other gregarious animals may look for self-service through authoritative guidance even to the extreme of implementing directions to assault or destroy their fellow-man; however, Milgram's experiments do not necessarily demonstrate that even this pattern springs from innate motivations—i.e., sadism, viciousness, or cruelty—*sui generis.*

June 27, 1967

Dear Dr. Masserman:

Thank you very much for your letter to me regarding Milgram's paper. As it is a very specific letter, I wonder whether I might use it in the *Journal* either as a letter or in the form of a brief discussion with the title "Dubious Conclusions."

Sincerely,
Seymour Weingarten
International Journal of Psychiatry

In reply to an inquiry about a colleague being considered for a Chairmanship of Psychiatry:

Clifford Grobstein, Ph.D.
Vice Chancellor for Medicine and the Biological Sciences

Dear Dr. Grobstein:

I have known Dr. Arnold J. Mandell professionally and socially for over a decade as a broadly informed, original yet integrative thinker, as an ingenious and productive research worker, as a literate and highly respected contributor to the scientific literature, and as a teacher who invariably proved stimulating and inspiring whenever I have invited him to lecture at Northwestern University. These evaluations will, I trust, be apropos to most of your well-directed inquiries, with the possible exception of those concerned with his administrative abilities. As to these, of course, I have no direct data other than that I know him to be personally friendly, sincere, likeable, loyal and trustworthy and have only similarly favorable reports from his staff, students and academic colleagues.

Dr. Mandell was appointed to the chairmanship. Another, briefer recommendation for a full professorship:

January 26, 1969

Dr. Worden
The Center for the Health Sciences
University of California

Dear Dr. Worden:

My opinions of Dr. Judd Marmor, based on fairly intimate contacts with him over a period of twenty years, can be expressed in brief superlatives: an erudite scholar, an inspiring teacher, an academic gentleman, and a valued friend. UCLA could do no better.

Dr. Marmor was appointed full professor. And another:

January 27, 1969

Dr. John Field
Associate Dean
The Center for the Health Sciences
University of California

Dear Dr. Field:

Pursuant to your inquiry of January 20 and our telephone conversation on this date, herewith a brief evaluation of Dr. L. Jolyon West, presumably now under consideration for the Chairmanship of Psychiatry:

Intelligence: Quick, perceptive, encompassing and integrative; more importantly, also inquisitive, self-critical, unfettered by fading orthodoxies, and generative of original and pregnant concepts.

Personality: Warm, friendly, loyal and eminently likeable; tinctured with a restless urge for new contacts and esoteric explorations.

Social orientations: Courageously liberal, particularly as to the current problems of youth—even though his outspoken attitudes have occasioned some conflicts with the conservative powers that be as the price of maintaining his interests in and long-range influence on the what he has designated the "red" (political), "green" (drug) and "black" revolutions.

Professional: So well liked by his psychiatric colleagues in the American Psychiatric Association, especially those of his own and younger generations, as to have been elected by popular vote to the august board of trustees of that body. Also, sufficiently admired by his seniors so that, on my recommendation and undoubtedly those of others, he was granted a Fellowship at this Center [for Advanced Behavioral Studies] a year ago.

Pedagogic: An intriguing, dramatic and effective teacher on every occasion when I have invited him as Visiting Professor at my University, or observed him elsewhere.

Research: Has done commendable collaborative work in sleep, dreams, psychedelics and other fields that relate "normal" behavior to the borderland of the "deviant" and "irrational"; in these studies he readily acknowledges the need for more accurate controls and newer methodologies and attempts to supply them.

Administrative: As noted, excellent in departmental recruitment and rapport, although inclined to delegate to others what he might consider as onerous routines that inhibit his freedom and creativity.

Academic: Has, to my knowledge, been offered chairmanships of psychiatry in at least two other universities.

Herewith, then, an appraisal best summed up in a trenchant coda: I would personally recommend him to succeed me at Northwestern when I retire.

None of the above recommendations was really needed; all candidates were successful. Testimonial letter to another friend was sent on the occasion of his terminating his services as director of the Illinois Department of Mental Health:

Harold M. Visotsky, M.D.

Dear Hal:

Some time ago, in response to a request that I nominate the

most qualified candidates I know for the coveted Strecker Award for Distinguished Service in Psychiatry, I wrote to the award committee, without your knowledge, as follows:

> Herewith a copy of Harold Visotsky's *curriculum vitae,* reflecting his thorough training, excellent qualifications, manifest dedication to humanitarian science, and uniquely distinguished accomplishments for a colleague only half through his forty-fourth year. I am certain you and your committee are completely aware of the recognition, the confidence and responsibilities both the APA and our national government have accorded him, so that I need not add that he can be regarded not only as one of the pioneer planners of the social and community psychiatry of our immediate future, but also as a most talented and effective administrator who will bring those plans to reality. I reflect the sentiments of many that he be accorded the Edward A. Strecker Award for Distinguished Psychiatric Service.

I could not put in that letter what I shall add here: my deep appreciation of your warm friendship, my regret that I cannot be with you on this one occasion to join your many other friends in expressing my reciprocal feelings personally, and my hope that our academic and social relationships will continue into a future bringing you and your charming family all happiness.

When absence possibly made the heart grow fonder: Acceptance *in absentia* of the 1967 Wayne University Alumni Award for Distinguished Service to Science:

Dr. Preston Walker and Fellow Alumni:

It is with the deepest sense of disappointment that I must miss being physically present at one of the greatest honors ever accorded me: a Centennial Award for Distinguished Service from my Alma Mater Medici. And yet it was precisely here at

Wayne where I learned that duties must come above honors, and that therefore my concurrent obligation to preside at an International Psychiatric Conference in Boston as arranged many months ago must take precedence. Nevertheless, in spirit I am here with you to express my humble thanks and appreciation.

To a colleague and friend who wished to nominate me for presidency of the American Psychiatric Association:

January 21, 1969

Milton H. Miller, M.D.
Professor and Chairman
Department of Psychiatry
University of Wisconsin

Dear Milton:

There are some joys that become ever more fulfilling throughout life: literature, music, *natürfühlung* (including sailing and flying), and a few others—but the greatest are enduring friendships. Your letter really touched me, and I deeply appreciate it. I cannot pretend that I would refuse the honor you suggest, especially since I could then do more than was possible during my term in Council to inspire the inbred APA hierarchy by appointing more vital and creative people like yourself to key chairmanships such as those in organization, program or foreign liaison. However, reality remains; not altogether regrettably, Bob Garber, Milton Greenblatt, George Tarjan, and several others are senior to me, and are also fine and highly competent gentlemen. The most I should expect in the next few years then, would be one of the vice-presidencies, with the other office, as was the case with Brosin and Waggoner, far in the future if ever.

I would indeed also like to come to Madison again to converse with you and your staff, residents, and students, and if some Friday and Saturday would be suitable, I'll arrange it. The reasons for choosing a weekend are two-fold: I come to

Chicago about six days a month to keep the department running until we can get a full-time chairman, now being negotiated, and I have concurrent regrets about not taking fuller advantage of the remainder of my fellowship in the Advanced Behavior Studies at Stanford for yet more illuminating (and humbling) converse with geneticists, sociologists, mathematicians, historians, philosophers, et al. In fact, I have a counterproposal; both of you come stay in the extra bedroom in our luscious high-rise in Palo Alto, meet some of the other fellows, join in the Center activities, and so pave the way for your own year there when you would like it most.

At the farewell banquet for departing Fellows at the Center for Advanced Behavioral Studies:

There is, perhaps, one aspect of this unhappy celebration that we might thoughtfully reconsider; namely too much Dionysian revelry and not enough Apollonian esthetics. I therefore propose a toast to the most appropriate patron deity of our Center—Apollo, God of Literature and Science, a gentleman who, being not only wise, good, and dedicated, is also superbly virile and handsome, and therefore the very image of every Fellow assembled here this evening. Parenthetically, Apollo was also the father of Asklepios who at Apollo's direction was taught the art of medicine by the centaur Chaeron and transmitted it to Apollo's granddaughters, Hygeia and Panacea. However, I always wondered what so mixed up a creature as a centaur had to do with our medical genealogy until, at the end of my usual sixteen-hour workday in Chicago, I realize that many a physician has to be, like Chaeron, half man and half horse—though, as I tell my residents, they should always remember which end should be the man.

But Apollo has yet one more claim to our fealty, although this generation of Fellows, with only a trio of exceptions, was regrettably atheistic in that regard. Apollo was also the God of Music, and thereby of Pythagorean fitness, rhythm and harmony in this universe. And in that role I am privileged by my fellow Fellows to dedicate our gift to the Center—a modern version of the classical Aeolian harp, now called a piano. I will hasten to make the gift more acceptable by promising that Drs. Dodwell, Koopmans, and I, who constitute that trio, will not—I repeat, will *not*—impair this occasion by playing tonight. And now, the entire fellowship takes great pleasure in presenting to Met Wilson for the Center these plaques signifying our gift, one for the piano and one for the wall behind it. The piano plaque reads simply: "From the Fellows, 1968-69, With Grateful Memories."

May Apollo, God of Literature, of Science, and also of Music, continue to bless this Center—and like a good fellow, bring Venus, Minerva, or Aphrodite with him. Ladies and Gentlemen—to *all* good Fellows and their beauteous goddesses.

My departing report to the trustees of the Center for Advanced Study in the Behavioral Sciences, June 1969, "A Study of Advanced Behavior."

A quarter of a century ago, as part of an investigation of the psychologic effects of various drugs later classed as "psychedelic," I dosed myself with fifty micrograms of mescaline, and soon experienced what has since been tragically misnamed a period of "mind-expansion," to wit: Steam radiators breathed like accordions and sang cacophonies; people became literally and horribly transparent; and time accelerated, reversed, or stood terrifyingly still. The delirium passed, and I knew once again that the "mind" can be "expanded" only by reading, observation, travel—and best of all—by dignified dialogues in depth with dedicated colleagues in fields other than one's own. In the latter sense, the Center for Advanced Study in the Behavioral Sciences could be whimsically subtitled the Center of Scientific Psychedelia.

True, the uncluttered time, generous facilities and creative atmosphere throughout my fellowship at the Center also made possible the writing of a 400-page *Psychiatric Odyssey* (yclept, in smaller print, "Memoirs of a Maverick Psychiatrist"), the editing and proofreading of three other volumes (*Transcultural Problems of Youth,* Volume VIII of *Current Psychiatric Therapies,* and Volume XV of *Science and Psychoanal-*

ysis), and half a dozen papers, reports, and reviews that could not otherwise have received the careful research, thoughtful preparation and critical revisions good psychiatric literature requires. The Center also afforded the first sabbatical I had ever taken during four decades of pressing academic, research, administrative, and clinical duties—although, regrettably, continued commitments in these spheres still necessitated occasional absences. But, trite as the statement may seem, far transcending even these advantages were the stimulating contacts and conversations I was privileged to have with other Center fellows. To name only a few:

In psychology and related disciplines: Ray Birdwhistell, Peter Dodwell, John Crook, Robert and Pauline Sears.

In sociology and political science: James Barber, Lewis Coser, Kai Erikson, Ulf Himmelstrand, David Riesman, Charles Tilly, Robert Ward.

In jurisprudence, linguistics, and miscellaneous: Richard Falk, Leon Lipson, Norman Malcolm, Kenneth Pike, Ledyard Stebbins.

I also was privileged to invite several of these Fellows to participate in a conference on culture, law, and psychiatry under the auspices of my university. Other Fellows were similarly interesting and stimulating, though less intimately so. But these acknowledgements would not be complete without recording my indebtedness to the courtly, intelligent, inspiring guidance of the Center by Mcrcdith Wilson and his ever-accommodating staff.

Regrets? Only that I did not clear my docket of previous commitments so as to make possible a practically continuous stay at the Center.

Recommendations: That each Fellow be given one other precious privilege: after he had come to appreciate the Center more clearly, an invitation to return for from three to six months at some future time (at his own expense, in part or whole if need be) to take more full advantage of its unique opportunities.

Gratefully submitted,
Jules H. Masserman, Fellow

19. PREVIEWS, VIEWS, AND REVIEWS

As noted, psychiatrists who have attained some academic stature are not infrequently presumed also to be capable of evaluating the work and writings of their colleagues. Whether or not this presumption was valid in my case may be judged by the following sampling of reviews of books, films, and submitted manuscripts.

A few equivocal appraisals:

Review of Reik's The Haunting Melody

The principal theme of Theodore Reik's *The Haunting Melody: Psychoanalytic Experiences in Life and Music* is stated on page 10: "Melodies . . . may give the analyst a clue to the secret life of the emotions."

That auditory as well as visual, olfactory, gustatory, postural, and other perceptual configurations can be reassociated with repressed and seemingly forgotten events can hardly be doubted, since this is a matter of common experience. Unfortunately, Reik promptly proceeds to obscure this insight by techniques peculiar to much of the psychoanalytic writing of a passing era: looseness and turgidity of expression and fantastic postulates presented as valid demonstrations of universal psychologic truths. As to stylistic efflorescence, a single quotation from Chapter I may suffice: "In fleeting tunes whose wings have fluttered away into the unknown as on a melody that has a hold on you and will not release you for hours, that life, concealed from yourself has sent messages to the mental surface."

More serious than such verbal excrescences, however, are the author's tendencies to uncritical thinking and aphoristic dogmatism under the guise of analytic reasoning. A great deal of the clinical material of the book is admittedly fragmentary, discontinuous, or personalized. For example, while analyzing an attractive woman who planned to fly to India, Reik kept thinking of the melody of Mendelssohn's *Auf Flugein des Gesanges,* and associated: "Hence, to the banks of the Ganges/My loved one, oh fly with me."

Even more revealing—although, unfortunately, again about Reik rather than about music—is the rest of the book, which the author devotes mostly to a discussion of his musical alter ego: the conductor-composer Gustav Mahler. Reik admits that his wishful identification sprang from two characteristics he shared with Mahler: an ethnic sensitivity and an overweening personal ambitiousness. Several chapters are then devoted to elaborate speculations as to how a stormy relationship with J. B. Forster may have led Mahler to write his Second Symphony as an immortal tribute to his deceased friend. Reik then tirelessly takes up the question as to why, between December 25, 1924, and New Year's Day, 1925, he himself was "haunted by the melody . . . of the *Resurrection Chorale*"—a topic Reik seems to consider of cosmic importance. Fortunately, self-analysis again solves this momentous problem: It appears that at the time he felt guilty about the recent death of Karl Abraham, a prominent Berlin psychoanalyst who had befriended Reik, but had thought (perhaps correctly) that since Reik was not medically trained, he had best confine his analytic speculations to his profession of popular writing rather than to treating patients. However, the music of the Chorale, much as it eased Reik's conscience, did not resurrect Abraham, whereupon Reik was able to accept Freud's invitation to read a tribute to Abraham before the Vienna Psychoanalytic

Society. This, Reik implies, was a happy ending for all concerned.

The Haunting Melody is not all bad; indeed, the author is to be commended for his frankness, his prolific earnestness, and perhaps even for his dogged loyalty to a set of naive approximations and formulations about human behavior that Freud himself began to discard in his later maturity of thought. However, though the book may amuse and in places titillate trained psychologists and musicologists, it may seriously mislead others less sophisticated and experienced in either field. It is therefore recommended for students only if these reservations are kept in mind.

Karpman's The Sexual Offender and His Offenses

In Section I of this book, Dr. Benjamin Karpman presents a survey of the literature on the nature, distribution, and psychiatric classification of the sex offender and his offenses, the medicolegal questions involved, and various current methods of prevention and treatment. The style here is frequently telegraphic or cryptic, and the conflicting opinions of various authors are often merely assembled rather than integrated and analyzed. However, since the general field is covered and topically summarized, this section constitutes a valuable reference index to many publications in the field.

Section II, in which Karpman presents his own theories as to the psychodynamics of sexual offenses, begins with the following sweeping elimination of all other contributions: "Conventional psychiatry offers but little by the way of explaining the meaning of sexual offenses, their pathology and their treatment; not even clues. Other disciplines interested in the problem, such as psychology, sociology and so on, do not offer any better understanding or hope. . . ."

To fill the void thus created, Karpman submits that "sexual offenses are a direct descendant of the clinical condition known as perversion, or paraphilia, which dynamic psychiatry views as being essentially in the nature of a neurosis." Unfortunately, this pronouncement is not further clarified in the next 289 pages of somewhat ataxic writing, despite 300 case studies (described on the dust jacket as "meticulously reported") and a plethora of discursive commentaries. Under the heading of Topical Synopsis, Karpman scrutinizes certain psychiatric and legal concepts of "sexual psychopathy," again without reaching any consistent conclusions. The volume ends with a list of (sic) 312 questions to be asked the suspected sexual offender in a "psychogenic interview." It begins with: "Q. 1. Describe each of your paternal grandparents. If they are dead and you have no memory of them or had no childhood association with them, tell whatever you had heard about them from others . . ." And closes with: "Q. 312. Do you believe in birth control, or are you firmly opposed to it? If you believe in it, discuss the circumstances under which you consider it justified."

Presumably, after this ordeal, the most hardened sexual offender would go and sin no more.

Since this volume has an extensive bibliography and is well indexed, it will prove convenient to bibliophilic attorneys, sociologists, psychiatrists, and others interested in forensic sexology. However, since many sections of the text must be read critically, it is recommended only to those specially trained in this difficult field.

Wertham's Seduction of the Innocent

This book is another in Dr. Fredric Wertham's widely publicized series of diatribes against so-called comic books, on the customary theme that they constitute a "moral disarmament of our youth." Apart from the intriguing implications that "morality" constitutes an "armor," nearly everyone will agree with Dr. Wertham's indictment of these publications on the ground that they depict crime and brutality, are overtly pornographic, covertly glorify aggression and cruelty, and even advertise air-rifles and switch-blade knives by the aid of which lurid illustrations of robbery, rape, and murder may be translated into criminal acts. Besides, adds Dr. Wertham, they are examples of bad spelling, worse drawing, and unethical merchandising of breast developers and acne lotions.

All this has been well stated before, and may have deserved restatement in an adequately documented and illustrated pamphlet. But this particular *Seduction of the Innocent* extends over nearly four hundred stereotyped pages, replete with pithy, penetrating, patented phillipics such as: "In my own Don Quixotic crusade (against the comic book industry) I was fighting not windmills but paper mills" (p. 15). Or concise clarifications: "In our clinical research on crime comic books we came to the conclusion that *crime comic books are comic books that depict crime"* (p. 20, Wertham's italics.) Or portentous pronouncements such as: "We should be thankful that the big S (on Superman's uniform) is not an S. S." (p. 34). Or unforgettable unctions: "A member (of a Committee to Study Comics) said to me 'Somewhere right now a little boy has a gun and reads crime comics. That boy will be president some day. What do you say to that?' 'All I can say,' I answered, 'is that that is precisely what I would like to prevent' " (p. 347).

Dr. Wertham, of course, professes to consider his subject comprehensively and objectively; however, after a piercing glance over the field, he apparently decides there is no tenable position but his own. In Chapter 9 he therefore disposes of "experts for the defense" in a currently familiar fashion by implying broadly that most of them, including various nationally respected authorities, have been financially bribed and prostituted by publishers of comic books to endorse their corruption of the young. Dr. Wertham's comments on this score include a flight into whimsey in which he fantasies himself finally admitted into heaven because St. Peter, after discounting all of Wertham's other services and sufferings for humanity, acknowledges his special martyrdom in having read the "opposing experts." Then, without further discussion of the content or validity of their writings, Wertham's Goldwaterish rebuttal culminates in this polemic gem: "Neutrality—especially when hidden under the cloak of scientific objectivity—that is the devil's ally" (p. 351).

As to how to toss an inkwell at the devil he envisages, Dr. Wertham has but two suggestions: (1) desensitize (de-seduce?) the individual child, and (2) prohibit comic books by law. Of the first he gives only one clinical example, but this is again worthy of quotation. Said Dr. Wertham to a preadolescent girl of threatened virtue: "Suppose you get used to eating sandwiches made with very strong seasoning, with onions and peppers and highly spiced mustard, you will lose your taste for simple bread and butter and for finer food . . . If later on you want to read a good novel it may describe how a young boy and girl sit together and watch the rain falling. They talk about themselves and the pages of the book describe what their innermost thoughts are. This is what is called literature. But you will never be able to appreciate that if in comic book fashion you expect any minute someone will appear and pitch both of them out of the window" (p. 64). To relieve our breathless concern, Dr. Wertham then assures us "The girl understood, and the advice worked."

Next, reviewing the specific legal problems involved in controlling the distribution and sale of comic books, Dr. Wertham cites the case of an ordinance drafted by the Los Angeles Board of Supervisors to the effect that: "Comic books in which crime and violence were prominently featured could not be sold to anyone under eighteen;" subsequently, this ordinance was nullified by the Appellate Department of the California Superior Court on the grounds of violation of press freedom and other considerations. Wertham scrutinizes similar efforts in other localities which also came to naught and states that for an awful moment "It really seemed that Superman had licked me" (p. 340). Fortunately, however, Dr. Wertham soon recovered his crusading zeal and continued to investigate other opportunities for legal action.

In summary, Dr. Wertham expresses his rejection of the usual apologetics in this field in an impassioned plea: "Suppose for a moment a girl of nine is physically violated by an adult. Democratic justice demands the most rigorous determination: Did this violation occur? Is it established beyond a reasonable doubt that it was an adult who did it? But do we give this man the right to address the parents of the victim, expounding his view that from his investigations he had found that the girl liked it; that it satisfied a real innermost need of her own, that struggling against him helped her get rid of her own "aggressions"; that in her "humdrum" home and school life this was a way of psychologic "escape" for her; and that, after all, in this modern world of ours girls may get raped and he was helping her to become acquainted with it and adjust to "reality"; and that she will laugh it off and grow out of it; that the basic character is formed in the first few years, anyhow, so that rape when she is a little older than that can have no real effect?

"The simile is not far-fetched. This is precisely what we permit the comic book industry to do when they violate children's minds" (p. 271).

Here, perhaps, the reader would be most moved by Dr. Wertham's unexpected eloquence, and most inclined to agree with his sentiments. But sentiment or no, the fact remains that objective studies undermine the basis for even this earnest analogic appeal. For example, Karl Bowman and his associates, after prolonged research, submitted in their formal 1951 Commission report to the California Legislature the following disconcerting conclusions about "induced sex delinquency" in preadolescent girls: (a) as often as not, it is the girl who does the seducing, (b) the man is often a middle-aged passive, fairly well-meaning and friendly neighbor, and (c) there is no evidence that the experience itself causes serious harm to anyone, provided the situation is not complicated by horrified parents and vigilante social action.

Does Dr. Wertham have more positive proof of the degrading effects of comic books? Again, regrettably, the answer is no. Numerous "case histories" are scattered throughout the book, but all are of the form: "Jimmy (or Alice) committed assault (or robbery, arson, rape, prostitution or suicide) . . . Psychiatric investigation revealed that he (she) had been reading comic books daily, which had obviously induced this behavior."

On such anecdotal evidence, only slightly expanded to other juvenile or adolescent preoccupations, it could equally well be demonstrated that toy soldiers, tanks, and "atomic guns" given to children at Christmas lead to a life of crime, or that hippie dress and rock music have demonstrably diabolical influences. Granted also that the twenty million children who read comic books may graduate to twenty million adults who read Mickey Spillane, even this does not necessarily mean that the population of voyeurs, sadists and killers will increase correspondingly. All in all, one may admire Dr. Wertham's monothetic zeal and dedication, yet have uneasy memories of the eventually devastating results of Peter the Hermit's self-inspired mission, or concomitant fears for the fate of an overardent latter-day Savonarola.

Roche Laboratories Film, You Are Not Alone

The story line: The company president informs Mr. Simpson, a junior executive, that he has been passed over for a promotion. Mr. Simpson suppresses his resentment, but later explodes at his secretary; that evening he quarrels with his wife, and rebuffs his small son's plea for help in fixing a bicycle. At night Mr. S. suffers severe abdominal cramps despite an increased intake of antacid tablets, and is sulky, depressed, and inefficient at work the next day. He consults his family physician, who examines Mr. S. and reassures him as to his physical health; the doctor then gives his patient a ride home during which he attributes the young executive's symptoms to anxiety, probably springing from marital, familial, financial, or occupational stresses. Mr. S. admits that his wife doesn't understand him, but after a reflective walk, he soliloquizes ruefully while gazing at photographs of his wife and father, resolves to reform and, to the accompaniment of a somewhat awkward gavotte on the sound track, goes out to fix his son's bike. That evening he apologizes to his wife for venting his business troubles on her, whereupon she confides that she, too, occasionally loses her temper but loves him just the same. And so, this time without antacids or sleeping pills, they repair happily and quite literally to bed. A film trailer features the president of an insurance company assuring the audience that the film was made by his firm in "enlightened self-interest," after which a psychiatrist invites each viewer to inform him of his "emotional reactions" to this cinematic experience.

The emotional reactions charted in two mixed lay and medical audiences to which the reviewer exhibited the film were also mixed. Their appraisal confirmed the impressions of this reviewer that the film had a number of annoying defects: a script that was too contrived and telescoped, acting that was often amateurishly exaggerated and self-conscious, a "musical" background in which unremitting crescendos of minor thirds in the oboe and flute, intended to herald an actor's agony, more often evoked it in the listener, and a number of extraneous and psychiatrically fuzzy comments such as the recovered hero's monologue that "for the first time, my father wasn't my father." On the other hand, there were many commendable features: the personal and poignant pain of suddenly shattered self-esteem, the unpretentious, direct and effective therapeutic manner of the smalltown practitioner, and the reversibility of familial disruptions when their source was traced and ameliorated.

The final consensus was that the film achieved its primary objective of demonstrating that severe somatic dysfunctions can be caused by a variety of sociofamilial stresses, and that these and their interrelated behavioral and somatic effects can be relieved by the resolution of occupational, marital and social disappointments and conflicts through medical reassurance and friendly semi-directive counselling. For these purposes, the film can be recommended without serious reservations to both lay and professional audiences.

Other writings and films deserved more detailed reporting and occasionally fulsome praise:

Frank's Persuasion and Healing

At regrettably rare intervals in American psychiatry there appears a book which in scope of scholarship, originality of appraisal and clarity of presentation deserves the sincere appreciation of the entire profession. Jerome Frank has written such a volume, *Persuasion and Healing: A Comparative Study of Psychotherapy* (The Johns Hopkins Press, 1961). While no brief review can do it full justice, the following may indicate some of its merits.

In his initial survey, Frank defines the essentials of psychotherapy as the employment by a "trained, socially sanctioned healer" of "circumscribed contacts . . . words, acts and rituals" to relieve a "sufferer" according to *either* (sic) a "religio-magical" or "scientific" rationale. In permissive, democratic coun-

Review appeared in the *American Journal of Psychiatry* 118: 659-661, 1962.

tries "psychotherapy" may be extended to cover not only "mental diseases" but also "normal reactions to stress... eccentricities, and moral weakness." Psychotherapy may therefore be highly variable in method and application, but "convincing objective demonstrations that one form of psychotherapy produces better results than another is lacking": moreover, "the duration of psychotherapy seems to depend largely on the therapist's notion of how much treatment is necessary rather than on the patient's condition." The premise is therefore justifiable that the "similarity of improvement rates reported from different forms of psychotherapy results from features common to all."

In Chapter II, Frank explores the anxieties and adaptive maneuvers evoked when any man's "assumptive world . . . which varies widely with each individual's culture and experience" is threatened by doubt or stress, and the modes whereby his conduct then follows a set of "normal, neurotic or psychotic ... self-fulfilling prophesies." On this groundwork, Chapter III traces the biopsychologic and social roots of religious healing, from ancient shamanistic magic to the consummately developed and effectively modern pageantry of Lourdes—a healing shrine to which, as Weathered remarked, "a trip is never in vain." The clinical relevance of this discussion is brought home by a documented survey of the "placebo effect" in medicine and surgery (Chapter IV), after which Frank again broadens the readers' perspectives by a fascinating scrutiny of "thought reform" as practiced by the Russians and Chinese. Frank demonstrates that this method can profoundly, though contingently, modify behavior through the use of covert humiliations and threats subtly countered by seemingly "permissive" and inviting promises of reward if the subject "spontaneously" acquires "insight" into his past misdeeds, renounces his previous convictions, and adopts instead the interrogator's conceptual and operational universe. Frank broadly implies that these methods are disconcertingly relevant to many forms of psychotherapy which employ (a) isolation, (b) progressive disintegration of former frames of reference, resulting in (c) uncertainties enhanced by (d) self-doubt and helplessness, followed by (e) control of new sources of motivationally related information, and (f) the power of implicit group influences, leading to emotionally abreactive "confessions" and the seeking of new allegiances and securities.* Here Frank comments: "Since the English language lacks a common word for invalid, penitent, and prisoner on the one hand and shaman, evangelist . . . interrogator [or psychiatrist] on the other, the first categories will be referred to as sufferers, and the second as persuaders."

In Chapter VII Frank marshalls operant-conditioning and other experimental studies which demonstrate the deeply persuasive effects of role-playing, "spontaneity," indirect rewards, and especially the approval of the therapist and the patient's peer groups—either expressed as advice or equally strongly implied in the misnamed "non-directive counselling." Frank then selects for special examination psychoanalysis as a theory and technique, with which until recently the self-styled intelligentsia among psychotherapists seemed most entranced. Frank believes that this was true because psychoanalysis not only (a) conferred status and security to its practitioners, but also (b) constituted a quasi-religious cult which could neither be confirmed nor refuted by facts and (c) exacted from its students a high investment of time, money, and public dedication which most votaries could not easily abandon in favor of more inclusive views and practices. But whether or not a good psychotherapist is analytically trained, he must have "self-confidence, energy, and controlled emotional warmth: These qualities enable him to offer his patients a pattern of active personal participation which arouses their expectations of help and facilitates attitude changes."

Included in the methods of individual therapy (Chapter VII) are the use of physical and pharmacologic media which produce a "central excitatory state so intense as to be disorganizing, thereby paving the way for a new reorganization of attitudes." These effects are enhanced by the impetus of the perenially renewed enthusiasms of the physician and the experiences of "novelty" and hope for the patient; ergo, "all forms of treatment work best just after they are introduced." But even Redlich's "organic-directive" type of therapist adds sage advice or unabashed exhortations as to the changes his

*See Chapter 21 for an elaboration of these concepts.

patient should make in attitude and conduct. So also the "evocative therapies," though less openly and blatantly, likewise direct the patient into prescribed paths by means of inevitably biased inquiries, "interpretations," "reflections," and "summaries"—all of which derive their effectiveness less from rational understanding than from reeducation by, and reidentification with, the therapist and the social order he represents.

In Chapter IX Frank subjects the various "directive" (e.g., Alcoholic Anonymous) and "evocative" (e.g., socio-analytic) group therapies to a scrutiny which is again both incisive and integrative, and once more traces their strengths to the restoration of the patient's self-esteem, his renewed feelings of belongingness, and the sense of mastery he derives from help to others, including the therapist. Chapter X extends this survey to the operations of mental hospitals, which Frank somewhat arbitrarily divides into (a) "asylums," which employ alienation from home, personal isolation, humiliation, and systems of rewards or punishment leading to desired conformity in the manner of Thought Reform, and (b) "therapeutic communities," which aim to restore the patient to a fuller life through techniques of reeducation, esthetic, and intellectual growth, and social rehabilitation through democratic participation.

As may have been inferred, the text abounds with pithy purviews as well as astringent aphorisms, among which the following are other examples: "As a relationship in which one person tries to induce changes in another, psychotherapy has much in common with child-rearing, education and various forms of leadership. . . . Too many of the ablest, most experienced psychiatrists spend most of their time with patients who need them least . . . Psychotherapy is the only form of treatment which . . . appears to create the illness it treats . . . The psychotherapist assists much as a midwife might at the birth of a baby. What he does may make a lot of difference in how smoothly or rapidly the process occurs, but the extent to which he causes it [remains] uncertain."

As in all near-masterpieces, there are also minor defects in the book. To broaden the readership appeal of his volume, Frank has sometimes oversimplified his points and included details—for example, as to the institutionalized ritualism of psychoanalytic training—familiar to most physicians. As another concession to lay concepts, Frank occasionally speaks of "thoughts," "feelings," "emotions," "attitudes," etc., as though they were Kantian categories rather than dubious abstractions of highly protean behavioral processes—a short-circuit which has blacked out many an illumination. Further to avoid any appearance of pedantry, all references and footnotes are clustered in twenty-four pages at the back of the book—an arrangement that forced this reviewer, a confirmed pedant, to keep thumbing through text, footnotes, and bibliography at frequent intervals to check Frank's sources, references and comments. Nor does Frank always maintain the courage of his stated convictions: for example, after analyzing the mythical-magical nature of Freudian theory and linking the dynamics of prolonged analysis with those of brain-washing and faith-healing, he still feels impelled to pay somewhat indiscriminate tribute to psychoanalysis as "objective" and "scientific." Nor can the volume be said to be complete even within its self-imposed limits: on the one hand, Frank omits the highly significant contributions that ethology and animal experimentation have made to the theories of learning, adaptational and social conflicts and their "therapeutic" resolutions; on the other, Frank takes only passing notice of the burgeoning pretensions of current medico-metaphysical departures such as phenomenology, existentialism, autogenic training, logotherapy, etc. Finally, the index—a tail that occasionally wags the dog in every good reference work—does not do the contents justice and thereby diminishes the book's ready usefulness.

But again on the positive side, Frank's eye is sweeping and critical but never jaundiced, his quotations from Lewis Carroll are gems of the slyly apropos, his style nearly always a literary delight, and his chapters and summaries models of memorable condensation. Therefore, my personal appraisal: I shall recommend to all of my best students in the foreseeable future that they read *Persuasion and Healing,* think deeply about it, read it again, and continue to develop the profoundly important issues it raises for the rest of their lives. Those of my students who are less than the best I shall, regretfully, consign to inevitably more constricted and doctrinaire spheres of thought and therapy.

Stein's Contemporary Psychotherapies

Dr. Morris Stein merits congratulations for fulfilling well two of his principal functions as editor: selecting authoritative and articulate contributors to present their several fields and then ably editing their material to achieve a balanced volume, although exception might be taken to a chapter arrangement which still seems to imply that all techniques lead to the *Ultima Thule* of psychoanalysis. Nevertheless, the resulting book, though massive, is so trenchant a commentary on current pretentions, practices, and polemics among therapists who work wonders with words that each contribution deserved at least a thematic review.

The editor's brief historical introduction necessarily neglects the rich heritage of self-knowledge and self-healing that man seems to have acquired throughout the ages outside of any physician's direct supervision. Stein implies his own current bias toward existentialism, but quotes approvingly Meyer Maskin's observations that each psychiatric theoretician tends to overgeneralize from his special clinical interests: e.g., Freud modelled all behavior on Viennese hysterics, Adler on rebellious youth, Jung on other-worldly academes, Rank on nonconforming artists, Fromm on white-collar futility, Sullivan on jejune schizophrenics, and—adds Stein—Rogers on impressionable college students. But in all cases the goals of psychotherapy are, in Whitehorn's simple words, "To work well, to feel well, and to expect well."

Jerome Frank, with his characteristic clarity and urbanity, presents what is essentially a condensation of his book *Persuasion and Healing,* commended at length by this reviewer elsewhere.

In the two succeeding chapters, Rudolph Driekurs presents Alfred Adler's "individual psychotherapy," which he characterizes as "socially orientated . . . holistic and teleological." Its objectives are realistic: first, to establish "contact with the patient," next to re-examine his "life style" for the purpose

Review appeared in the *Archives of General Psychiatry* 7: 461, 1962.

of correcting his "basic mistakes" in his "conscious continuum," then to set mutually satisfactory alternative "life goals," and finally to elicit changes not merely in deceptive verbal professions of "insight," but in concrete behavior. Unfortunately, Driekurs' generally sensible discussions are repeatedly marred by his strident, contentious tone, by recurrent inaccuracies in drawing physical, philosophic, and ethologic analogies, and by his tendencies to startling self-contradictions. As but one example of the latter, he states (p. 75) that: "In general, awareness of motivation is very rare"—then adds a paragraph later "It is a great mistake to assume that the unconscious is to blame for most detrimental and antisocial actions." Despite these defects, Driekurs' contribution is an effective reminder of Adler's earthy and pragmatic but neglected contributions.

In the next section, Carl Rogers reiterates that his "client-centered therapy" is intended to achieve "more appreciation of, more expression of, more functional use of the latent inner resources of the individual." He then cites various studies by Baldwin, Whitehorn and Betz, Heine, Fiedler, and others in support of his thesis that only a "democratic," permissive, "non-intervening" relationship can achieve these ends. Ergo, the therapist must be (1) sincere; (2) "helpful to himself"; (3) feel "love" rather than "professionalism," but (4) be "separate"; (5) "let the patient be," yet (6) enter his world (7) unconditionally, (8) sensitively, and (9) nonjudgmentally so that finally (10) he can accept the patient's "becoming." After, in his own theologic tradition, enunciating these ten commandments to the former worshippers of Baal, Rogers proposes another sextet of criteria to measure therapeutic progress. These consist of (1) gauging how much the client's "feelings have been thawed . . . by the counsellor's warmth," so that (2) the client's experience becomes more "rich" and "vivid," despite (3) inevitable "inconsistencies" or (4) a contradictory "self" which may (5) "still have internal problems," but (6) has achieved better external relationships. Rogers claims that two of his associates, Walker and Roblen, could accurately rate a client's "progress" by these criteria merely by examining two pages of a transcript of any "non-directive" interview. Once again the reader is intrigued by Rogers' evident sincerity, puzzled by his naïve claims of objectivity, and a bit irritated by his hortatory unctiousness.

Otto Will takes as his text Harry Stack Sullivan's views that anxiety represents mainly "an actual or anticipated decrease in self-esteem" and that "mental disorder is a . . . cumbersome, expensive way of inter-personal relationships." Will's therapy is therefore based on these premises: (1) that all men "are more human than otherwise," (2) that they respond to interpersonal influences, (3) that "reality" (undefined) can be proved preferable to "fantasy," (4) that destructiveness "doesn't fit" in human relations, so that (5) cooperation eventually increases. Will then seems to follow Melanie Klein in his exposition of the prototaxic (prelogical) omnipotence of the infant, in the child's later concepts of the "good and bad nipple," the delay of "we feelings" until adolescence, and schizoid "parataxis" (conceptual deviations) and withdrawal under excessive frustration. Will then doubles Rogers' decalogue of therapy in listing his own technique as follows: (1) "identify" the anxiety; (2) establish the patient's anamnestic "identity"; (3) "clarify distortions"; (4) conserve a "residual of cruelty and pain"; (5) "interact emotionally," but recognize (6) the patient's defenses; (7) correct his inadequacies; (8) have a consistent frame of reference however many defects in it; (9) communicate corrective concepts but (10) accept dissociated material; (11) "expose yourself"; (12) convince the patient that self-revelation is not tantamount to subservience and that (13) life is real, not ideal; (14) that he must accept his family, yet remain independent; (15) that both the patient and therapist "give and receive" and thereby (16) play interchangeable roles and (17) use each other as models which are (18) both like and unlike so that (19) the cure is never "clear" ("in human relatedness lies both man's bedevilment and salvation"—p. 89) and finally, (20) that "every man . . . has values from which . . . he cannot be freed." Will's exposition, despite his tendencies to prolixity and redundancy, is based on searching and empathic clinical experience.

Roy R. Grinker, Sr. proposes a more inclusive "transactional" approach in which "the relationships among field theory, role theory and communication theory may be epitomized as transactional . . . involving non-dimensional space bounded by people enacting a variety of roles and traversed by verbal, nonverbal and paralingual communications." But the therapy [of deviant roles] "does not require focusing on and interpreting vast uncharted areas of the Unconscious; more important is effective transactional communication between patient and therapist as to mutually significant realities." Grinker closes his first chapter with the following therapeutic precepts: (1) Accept the patient; (2) alleviate his self-image of "badness . . . what the religionists call original sin"; (3) "permissiveness" should include the therapist's privilege of expressing disapproval; (4) the concept of "health" must depend on familial and social as well as individual requirements; (5) remain active: select the field and mode of discourse as indicated; (6) never let dream or symbol analysis interfere with more relevant communications; (7) "we do not invite, and we certainly avoid, the development of a transference neurosis"; (8) reorient the patient as to his optimal implicit and explicit social roles.

As to the patient involvement techniques of Whitaker and Malone, Grinker comments: "It is quite apparent that this . . . irrational therapy is quite dangerous, and probably requires the therapist to be as ill or as nearly psychotic as the patient."

Nathan Ackerman begins his contribution by enunciating his credo that "The family is the unit of living, the unit of experience . . . the family group can make or break mental health"—a dictum that some may think does not necessarily apply to those sectors of many cultures, including our own, in which familial influences are being progressively weakened. Ackerman then summarizes his methods of treating "all who live under one roof as a family unit" (1) by conjoint interviews; (2) "forthright intervention" in family affairs; (3) taking sides when necessary; (4) "choosing his own emotions"; and (5) extending this therapy to all patients except those temporarily alienated from their families by psychosis. Ackerman's views, though at times tending to the doctrinaire, offer corrective vistas to those who take pride in examining individual patients so closely that all peripheral and contextual vision is occluded.

Don D. Jackson's chapter on Interactional Psychotherapy, written in his customary open, engaging style, is perhaps the most entertaining part of the volume. Jackson first takes classical analysis to task not only for being internally oppressive on its practitioners but also for subjecting the patient to a variety of insoluble "double binds." As but one example, it is implicitly demanded that the analyzand follow many stringent rules, whereupon his cooperation is interpreted either as counter-aggression or masochism. However, some of the more "active" techniques that Jackson employs would make even a nonanalyst gasp, e.g.: He lent a "woman patient with masculine strivings . . . and plantar warts" his own pipe and tobacco and directed her to smoke it every evening after dinner with her husband; she refused to do so, but her warts cleared up. When another woman complained of a tic of the tongue, he transferred it by hypnotic suggestion to her toe "where it didn't annoy her husband as much"; predictably, it then disappeared. He advised an overconscientious old lady, guilty and depressed over the death of her alcoholic husband, to begin drinking a bit of bourbon herself; she did so under great protest, but "felt better."

Commendably, Jackson subtends a coda to the effect that "when the therapist does not know what is going on, [such] interventions should *not* be used" (italics mine). Jackson also advocates a more passively observant and mediating role than that described by Ackerman in the family treatment of schizophrenics.

In his exposition of Existentialism, Rollo May calls for a return to Liebnitzean phenomenology in preference to a Lockean preoccupation with causes and effects, and cites with approval Binswanger's critique that "Freud dealt with the *Umwelt* (environment) of man rather than with his *Mitwelt* (human empathies) or *Eigenwelt*" (inner self). In accordance with Tillich's dictum, each of us must have the "courage to be," yet we must "go out from self-centeredness... or perish." Since consciousness (knowledge of self) is deeper than mere awareness (wariness of threats), it includes all that has been repressed—ergo, "the Ego... cannot be fractionated" and is the main concern of therapy, in which "we help the patient to confront his anxiety and guilt constructively ... by being open, humble and by loving ..." True, "the patient after therapy may well bear more anxiety than he had before, but it will be conscious anxiety and he will be able to use it constructively." May closes with the admission: "I have proposed here a number of ideas which I realize are left hanging in the air"—Many readers would describe that atmosphere as the nonexistent interplanetary ether existentialists seem to breathe.

Aaron Karush's presentation next deals with the Adaptational Psychodynamics school of Rado, Kardiner, David Levy, et al. In their view "reparative psychotherapy," not always easily separable from analytic reconstructive techniques, consists of:

A *situation* in which (1) the patient knows he should change, (2) desires it, (3) has confidence in the therapist, and (4) is not too greatly disturbed by feelings of fear, rage, or sexual arousal.

A *process* which involves (1) sympathetic support, (2) the release of affect, (3) persuasion and suggestion, (4) direct intervention when necessary, and (5) the attainment of insight in action.

In the final two chapters, Arthur Miller presents a somewhat diffuse survey of the peregrinations and vicissitudes of so-called "classical analytic" therapy in accordance with Rangell's definition of this as a "a method whereby conditions are brought about favorable for the development of a transference neurosis in which the past is restored in the present in order that, through a systematic interpretative attack on the resistances which oppose it there appears a resolution of that neurosis, transference or infantile, to the end of bringing about structural changes in the mental apparatus of the patient to make the latter capable of optimum adaptations to life." Unfortunately, Miller does not point out, as this reviewer has documented elsewhere, that Freud himself had a much more transactional concept of the key terms "transference neuroses" than is currently being debated, nor are the semantic vagaries and vacuities of Rangell's definition subjected to further scrutiny. Instead, Miller proceeds to a conscientious review of other writings on psychoanalytic therapy with the net effect of revealing once again how crumbly and insubstantial the seeming monolith of psychoanalysis proves to be even when lightly tapped.

In summary, Stein's book has the virtues, faults, incongruencies, and promises of integration that characterize current psychotherapy, and is therefore precisely as intriguing, rewarding, and frustrating as is the field itself.

Miller's Systems Theory in Psychiatry

Dr. James G. Miller, because of his synoptic-integrative systematizations requires us as psychiatrists to have at our command an almost incredible grasp of nearly every level of organization from subatomic to socially sublimated. Let us glance at but a few of the stages between chromosome and cosmos comprised in his sweeping Systems Theory.

Cellular: Even if we skip the impenetrable mysteries of the molecule and proceed to micro-histology, we are faced with the Promethean task of decoding the double helices of adenine, guanine, cystosine and thymine in the DNA that mediates our heredity, including enigmas as to why 21-trisomy should lead to Mongolism, an extra sex chromosome to Klinefelter's syndrome, or the loss of one to Turner's. Nor can we ever rest secure in temporary tenets: *vide* Hsia's latest report that the diagnostic and dietary controls of congenital phenylketonuria are after all largely illusory.

Organic: At this next ordinal we must proceed from genetic defects to the behavioral consequences of infectious, traumatic and neoplastic diseases of the nervous, endocrine and other somatic systems. How many books and journals on physiology, pathology, neurology and medicine can one read between patients in preparation for yet another lecture on comprehensive psychiatry?

Organismic: Here we must comprehend and, when necessary, correct the failures of internal integration and maladaptive transactions of the total organism in its highly complex and constantly varying milieu.

Dyadic and Group Transactions: If we now compound the near-infinite number of reactive valences and vectors in any

Review presented before the American Psychiatric Association, May, 1967.

one organism with those that characterize one or more others, the problem of interactional possibilities would rapidly seem to transcend predictability, let alone control.

Socio-cultural: Finally, we must expand our matrix even further to comprise the ever more subtle and intricate influences of ethnic, historic, economic, and wishful-mythologic parameters, their teleologic and eschatologic implications, and, as open systems, their multidirectional interpenetrations. Let us take but one condensed clinical illustration:

> Mr. X, a middle-aged male patient, neglects a hormic-metabolic-somatic disorder—say, diabetes—which so affects his neurogenital "system" as to cause impotence. Seeking to restore his sociomarital functions, our patient, after some verbal and monetary transactions with a venal druggist, doses himself with a supposed aphrodisiac containing yohimbine, which unfortunately induces a superadded nephrosis. Young and unsympathetic Mrs. X engages in an extramarital affair, thus pyramiding covert and overt triadic conflicts in a social "system" involving a jealous husband and an understandably fearful lover. Depending on ambient legal, moral and religious contingencies, their further interactions may then lead to various eventualities ranging from a relatively resigned *ménage a trois* through a bitter court battle to homicide or suicide—all with expanding cultural reverberations. And yet the psychiatrist, called in at any stage of this developing drama in his various roles as physiologist, neurologist, internist, psychotherapist, marital counsellor, court alienist—or, even more lamentably, as autopsy consultant—is required to process all of these intersystemic penetrations and permutations and emerge with oracular dicta that imply a barely asymptotic approach to omniscience! I submit that, in view of such expectations, Freud's characterization of psychiatry (he spelled it psychoanalysis) as an impossible profession takes on a more poignant meaning in that, to use a medieval paraphrase, we often try to assemble an infinity of high-flown but intangible concepts on the point of a pen.

Survival Kit: How then, do we as putatively universal specialists retain a semblance of serenity despite this inundation of information, all of which must be processed at a rate ranging from a biochemical maximum of about 10,000 bits per second to a still-too-rapid rate of 4/sec. in human interactions? I submit we do so by utilizing one or more of the adaptive devices that Dr. Miller himself has described in previous publications. For another immediate illustration, we may bring these maneuvers down to the here and now of patterns of communication among psychiatrists as follows:

1. *Selection of Data:* Many of us take comfort in the soothingly familiar speeches at the classical psychoanalytic, ontoanalytic, biopsychiatric or other specialized meetings held during the weekend preceding more diverse scientific sessions of the APA—and then hastily depart for home rather than face the more variegated influx of information to follow. As Nobelist Medawar recently noted, a scientist's "interest and understanding and also in a curious way, his loyalties, tend to spread horizontally, along strata, rather than up and down."

2. *Deletion of Input:* As the avalanche of information grows, we not only attend fewer meetings, hear fewer reports and read fewer journals, but also more readily divest ourselves of unwelcome penetrations of data. As a temporarily immobilized listener once remarked to me: "Since your elaborate exposition seems contrary to what I had thought, I propose to sleep on it tonight and forget it in the morning."

3. *Queing:* During remaining overloads, input data that seem less urgent are deferred in the order of decreasing priority—as for example, postponing ancillary reading and writing to thereby vitiated summer "vacations." After some years of rationalized evasions I recall ballasting my yawl Naiad with piles of files and reams of notes, writing continuously in remote harbors for three summer months and losing 26 pounds while producing a handwritten manuscript of my *Practice of Dynamic Psychiatry* that, when registered for mailing weighed precisely twenty-six pounds.

4. *Approximation of Response:* However, when input and output cannot be so effectively balanced, the product of an information-processing system may become diffuse and impre-

cise—perhaps as illustrated by the peregrinating nature of most discussions of systems theory.

5. *Decentralization:* A corollary method of evasion is to defuse and diffuse (i.e., neutralize and scatter) new input; for example, the APA Council voted against a concentrated Task Force on Systems Theory and instead recommended:

6. *Multiple Channelization,* so as to distribute the threat and thrust of this overriding organon among tangential APA subcommittees which would not too readily subsume their special interests under this newer holism.

7. *Tolerating and Perpetuating Errors:* We may as well admit that in psychiatry as elsewhere, we persist in defending cherished orthodoxies or else modify them as slowly and with as many "compromising" formulae: so also did Ptolemaic astronomers cling to a geocentric cosmology of "epicycles" added to "epicycles" ("wheel within wheels") long after Copernicus, Brahe and Galileo proved the solar system to be heliocentric.

8. *Escape:* Or else, as suggested by K.M. Colby et al., we delegate not only our theory but our therapy to compliant computers while we contemplate taking off for Tahiti.

The Compleat Duodecalogue: However, if Dr. Miller will permit to add to the eight devices designed to dodge dementia he described, I shall, though necessarily very briefly, suggest four more:

9. *Overgeneralization:* Despite the poetic and often illuminating parallels between cell and society drawn by encyclopedic writers from Herbert Spencer through Peter Lillienfeld, J. T. Bonner and Ralph Gerard to Arnold Rapaport, the nutritive, restorative, integrative, communicative, affective, reproductive and other functions of a cell can be said to be analogous to those of a society only by virtue of the semantic overlays of the common terms employed, whereas it is equally tenable that there may be qualitative or quantum jumps rather than infinite gradations among organic, organismic, group and societal systems not easily bridged by the convenient prefixes *sub, para* or *supra* that Dr. Miller has employed. And yet so great is our human yearning for concepts of continuity and uniformity—and thereby predictability—that we insist on im-

posing superordinal systems upon disconcerting diversity.

10. *Reification:* An extension of this seeking for universals invites another wishful error to which Platonic philosophies have been perennially prone, but which Whitehead, Russell, Wittgenstein, and others deplore: namely erecting a verbal abstraction into a quasi-independent, quasi-willful *entity* which then somehow assumes an independent existence and function. In this context, systems theory can further be misconceived as lending some sort of "purpose" to the cosmos much as an Aristotelian or Drieschian "entelechy" was formerly supposed to "direct" animate behavior, or as an "autonomous Ego" is said to "control" a disruptive "Id" under the watchful concern of a pejorative "Superego," and so on into similarly homuncularized mythologies.

11. *Deification:* From this reification, it is but a small devotional step further to canonize vaguely panchrestic nouns until Systems Theory, now deistically capitalized, may tend to assume the cultist aspects of still another esoteric vocabulary, a prescribed ritual of thought and discussion, and a transcendency that orders all other knowledge. Thus did Comte, Eddington and Freud, as each over-extended his field, respectively erect sociology, mathematics and psychoanalysis into quasi-theologic systems.

12. *Delusion Formation:* Finally, faced with so many intertwining intangibles, we may resort to man's ultimate or *Ur*-faiths: irrational beliefs that he can trichotomize his milieu into physical, social and metapsychological systems and then master each through his sciences and technologies, his laws and mores and his philosophies and religions. But what would life be without such self-reassuring *hubris?*

To summarize: Systems Theory requires a panoramic breadth of vision and perceptive-integrative capacities of such high calibre that we, as mere mortals, may seek to escape by at least a dozen devices, diversions and deceptions. However, precisely for these reasons, we owe profound thanks to Dr. Miller and other logical positivists and systematizers for their Herculean attempts to clean out the Augean stables and get Antean behavior theory off the ground.

Why write reviews?

January 16, 1963

Dear Jules:

The exquisitely cut jewel necklace which reviews Stein's *Contemporary Psychotherapies* in *Archives of General Psychiatry* prompts me to write you in appreciation. This is another example of your rare combination of a comprehensive grasp of your subject, felicity of expression, and sound evaluative judgment. I wish there were more like you, and I also wish I knew you better.

Sincerely yours,
Alan Challman, M.D.

However, nineteen thousand other American psychiatrists did *not* write, and may have thoroughly disagreed.

20. INTERNATIONAL PSYCHIATRIC CONGRESSES, WITH FURTHER NOTES ON THE ARTS AND HUMANITIES

In 1966, the Fourth World Psychiatric Congress was scheduled to be held in Madrid. I had been invited to several international psychiatric conferences, had helped plan and conduct a world tour for the American Psychiatric Association, and thus had unusual opportunities to meet colleagues of diverse interests in many lands. As a member of the APA Council, I was therefore delegated to collaborate with Dr. Juan Lopez-Ibor, president of the World Psychiatric Association, in arranging the scientific program of the Congress, particularly with regard to American participation.

Two problems were immediately apparent:

1. How to choose, from among the hundreds of APA members who wished to attend the Congress, a score or so of speakers who would be representative of the best in American psychiatry.
2. In view of the probability that the National Institute of Mental Health would grant the travel funds requested by the APA, how to select fairly the 40 or so most deserving from the hundreds sure to apply.

To make the choice as equable and as inclusive as possible, the chairmen of the departments of psychiatry in each medical school and the directors of principal psychiatric training institutes and research centers in the country were invited to nominate for attendance to the Congress the three candidates whom each considered (a) most qualified to present either original work in, or comprehensive surveys of, special fields in psychiatry, and/or (b) most likely to acquire information and inspiration at the Congress that would benefit future psychiatric research, teaching, and therapy in the United States.

Progress was reported to the Council of the APA on December 9, 1965, as follows:

Committee Activity: Since my last report to the Council on October 29th, your chairman has:

1. Sent follow-up letters to all training centers which did not respond to our initial questionnaire as to speakers, topics, and travel funds locally available.

2. Received enough additional offers of participation to bring the total of institutions to about 75 and of volunteer speakers, on a wide variety of topics, to about 150. Contributions to travel remained at about 50%, with those who claim to be least solvent generally being most anxious to go.

3. Received bids to organize the following Joint Meetings, seminars, or workshops: Reparative Processes: Academy of Psychoanalysis; Psychiatric Liaison of East and West: Paris Psychiatric Society; Higher Nervous Activity: Johns Hopkins and the Research Studies in Psychic Trauma: Wayne University.

4. Kept Dr. Lopez-Ibor and his committee fully informed through a score of communiations as to all volunteer speakers, suggested topics, seminars and other data as soon as they became available. However, since reciprocal communication remained incomplete, my last letter to him read as follows:

> Since your last circular to our APA Mail Pouch, I am somewhat uncertain as to whether you wish volunteers to the Madrid Program to apply directly to you, or to be processed through our APA Ad Hoc Committee, which must also assign travel grants when available ... It would seem highly desirable for us to work out a much more complete understanding

> as to cooperative procedures, either by full correspondence, or perhaps by a joint meeting of the delegates from the Spanish and the APA Committees within the near future. What would be your pleasure in this matter?"

I have received no reply to date, which poses at least two serious problems: (1) A hundred and fifty American applicants will not know whether or not they are selected for places on the program (and therefore eligible for university allowances and tax deductions) until a bare six months before the Madrid meeting, and may therefore have considerable difficulty in securing university leave, planning travel arrangements, etc. (2) The Ad Hoc Committee's task of working out reasonably equitable travel support for the most qualified and deserving applicants—a project which would require a vast amount of calculation, correspondence and accounting, will be rendered all the more hurried and difficult.

Recommendations: I therefore recommend for Council consideration the following:

1. *Program:* That a cable be sent to Dr. Lopez-Ibor urgently requesting either an early conference to agree on American speakers, their topics, dates, etc., or a list of his own selectees as soon as possible.

2. *Conference Support:* That, although the NIMH grant was placed in my name, the support monies be placed entirely in the hands of Dr. Walter Barton and his Central Office Staff for full and accurate control and subsequent accounting to the NIMH.

3. *Travel Support:* That the following principles be adopted to govern the granting of travel subsidies: (a) Whereas the established luminaries of American Psychiatry should of course be represented, preferential financial aid be given to younger men who can contribute original research and stimulating ideas to the conference and return with information and inspiration for teaching and research. (b) To ensure fairness of academic and geographic distribution, the committee be empowered to call on impartial consultants who are best acquainted with volunteer speakers and their work in

universities and institutions in all regions of the country. (c) That secretarial and other facilities be provided in the central office for the very considerable clerical work involved. (d) That some way be found to compensate the members of the Ad Hoc Committee including myself for the hundreds of travel-disappointed friends they are sure to lose as a result of their foolhardy participation in this enterprise.

The Council regarded the last recommendation as impractical, but granted the others. I thereupon sent all the travel applications received to nine impartial authorities geographically distributed, with the request that they grade each candidate on the criteria listed on their forms as in Par. (1) above. On the basis of their consensus, fifty of the most highly recommended applicants were granted up to $400 each for travel to Spain.

The success of the Congress is recorded in its four weighty multilingual tomes of Proceedings. My final report to the APA Council and the NIMH:

Fourth World Congress of Psychiatry, Madrid, 1966

Selection of NIMH Grantees for Travel to the Congress was accomplished as follows:

1. The chairman or director of each of the leading psychiatric training or research centers in the United States was requested to recommend three of his staff who were most likely to contribute to, and benefit from, the scientific proceedings of the Congress, and bring back from it valuable data as to advances in training and research.

2. Formal applications from each candidate so recommended were graded on an equitable scale by the Ad Hoc Committee and by nine expert consultants distributed over the country who furnished information as to each candidate's background training, personality, current teaching and research abilities, and likelihood to return from the Congress with valuable knowledge and new directions for research, teaching and service.

3. On the basis of a careful review of all available data by the Ad Hoc Committee and its impartial consultants, ten senior

and forty junior psychiatric teachers and investigators, fairly distributed by universities and institutes over the country, were awarded $400 each toward their expenses to the Madrid Congress, with the provision that they (*a*) pay all other expenses involved; (*b*) attend a minimum of two-thirds of the Congress Sessions; and (*c*) submit an account of their experiences to the APA for evaluation and assembly into a final report to the NIMH.

The Congress: Since the scientific meetings were diverse and kaleidoscopic, I shall here review only the sessions in which I was particularly active as organizer and participant.

Human Values in Psychotherapy: Under the crisp, courteous chairmanship of Dr. Howard Rome and following his philosophically integrative introduction, several contrasting approaches were brought into sharp relief: evolutionary, secular, religious, socio-cultural, and psychiatric. Dr. H. W. Janz dealt with somewhat abstract Teutonic concepts of "deviated freedom . . . pathologic hope . . . phenomenologic anxiety . . . and the dialogue of emancipation." I followed with a cultural reexamination of the formerly postulated conflicts between the "materialistic technologies" versus the "humanities," and outlined the historical, comparative, and scientific bases for man's universal trilogy of ultimate (*Ur-*) values: (1) his concerns for his personal health, skills, and longevity; (2) his seekings for human alliances; and (3) his wishful convictions that his life has some transcendent meaning and significance.* Carlos Seguin of Lima next conceded the futility of certain classical modes of retrospective analysis and then launched on a panegyric to the asexual but unfaltering "love" that each therapist must feel toward his patient whatever the latter's trials and vagaries—a thesis that evoked wild enthusiasm and a clamor for copies of his speech from the female contingent in his audience. Less dramatically but more soberly, J. J. Prick of the Netherlands returned to a consideration of *Daseinanalyse* as an intimate experience in I-Thou relationships, somehow in turn based on chemico-physical "corporality"; separation in these spheres purportedly creates "existential crises" in human values. In formal discussion, Leo Bartemeier urged further thought and

*See Chapter 22.

research, B. Callieri of Italy equated values with platonic absolutes, and R. H. Vispo reviewed but only partially reintegrated the diverse approaches of the participants.

Concepts of psychiatry, East and West.

Dr. Leon Chertok of Paris and I, as co-chairmen of this session, had been rather unexpectedly successful in securing the participation of high-ranking psychiatrists from Russia (A. V. Snezhnievsky, whom we welcomed as third co-chairman, R. Lebedev, L. Saarma, N. Sapir, and four others), Czechoslovakia (F. Knobloch), East Germany (H. Rennert, D. Muller-Hegemann), Poland (A. Jus), and Yugoslavia (J. Schipkovensky), as well as from France (H. Ey, V. Gochkel), Canada (E. Wittkower), and the United States (H. W. Brosin, H. P. Rome, H. J. Tompkins, F. C. Redlich, and Z. Lebensohn). Dr. Rennert read a formal paper on "Eastern Concepts of the Etiology of Behavior Disorders" for the first period of the seminar and, substituting for Dr. I. Ziferstein, I later essayed a comparison of "Psychiatric Therapy, East and West." A typical case history also focused the discussion at both sessions which, together with preliminary statements by each speaker and audience participation, lasted over three and one-half hours. By my arrangement with the Congress secretariat, the entire proceedings were recorded on colored film and audio tape for subsequent editing and distribution.* The prolonged and variegated discussion cannot be readily summarized, but perhaps three convergences are worth recording:

Eastern psychiatrists generally rejected Freudian concepts of libidinal determinism, but were far from rigidly monothetic on any other parameter of etiology: biologic, Pavlovian, experiential or socio-economic. In fact, there were greater differences among psychiatrists from Leningrad (Pavlovian) and Moscow (more eclectic)—let alone Prague and Belgrade—than among those from New Haven and New York.

When an occasional Eastern psychiatrist (*e.g.,* Saarma) presented a particularly narrow approach, advocating, for example, that all psychoses be treated exclusively by diet, vitamins, or hormones, the most vigorous disclaimers or rebuttals

*See the film, *Psychiatry, East and West,* issued by the Fairview Hospital Foundation, as listed in the bibliography.

generally came from his own countrymen.

Co-chairman Chertok's well-meaning attempts to provoke "open controversies and differences of opinion between East and West" similarly met with what is currently becoming known as an attitude of "cool" on the part of nearly everyone concerned.

By arrangement with Dr. Shervert Frazier, an invitation was extended to all participants to continue their rapprochement at an evening panel planned at the 1967 APA meeting in Detroit. Official invitation would be issued, if needed, to help those who wished to come from abroad obtain travel grants from their respective governments or other sources.

Psychiatry in Morocco: Wherever available in my post-Madrid tour of that country, nurses, social workers, psychiatrists, and physicians in other specialties were interviewed, and the hospitals in Fez, Barraschid, and Salé were visited. In briefest summary:

1. Berber and Islamic cultural patterns were so foreign to Western understanding (e.g., the complete subservience of women, passive submission to "fate," an aversion to all but minimal physical activity, religious fanaticism, etc.) that the only private psychiatrist in all Morocco must confine "psychotherapy" to Western patients.

The central government and the local police considered psychiatric hospitals to be custodial institutions to be kept in marginal and generally deplorable condition. Psychiatrists lower in rank than hospital directors were paid a bare living wage, and have between 400 to 1000 patients assigned to them. Nurses, the rare social workers, and ward aides served under far greater actual personal hardships; for example, Mr. H. Rasspp—a most capable, intelligent and dedicated person who is chief nurse at Salé—received the American equivalent of $95 per month, some of which he spent on food and medication for his patients. And yet, as I had found in other African countries (e.g., Kenya and Ethiopia), many hospital personnel at all levels offered their services under almost incredible difficulties to the forgotten sick and poor placed in their charge.

Since Berber and Arabic patients keep their personal problems to themselves (even in the case of adolescent rebellions against the old order, often expressed by *grand hystérie* in girls and pseudocatatonic retreats in boys) and generally refuse any forms of occupational, recreational, or group approaches, hospital therapy—in the rare cases when any was available—consisted of drug allowances of two cents per day per patient, or of electroshock therapy. Insulin had long ago been abandoned as "too expensive."

Despite its proscription by the Prophet, alcoholism was a major problem among the Muslim population at all economic levels.

But perhaps of greater import to American psychiatry was the finding that the use of hashish—which is freely sold in any market place and smoked by a third of the poorer populace—within five to ten years produces an organic dementia in most consumers which, according to Dr. M. Dehrmann of the 3000-bed hospital at Barraschid, is characterized by progressive aphasia, amnesia, ataxia, and habit deterioration. If confirmed, this places some of our pot-smoking American youth in yet another cavalierly ignored peril.

The success of the Madrid meetings prompted me as a continued member of the APA Council to propose to that body that a Third International Conference on Psychiatry be scheduled in conjunction with the annual meeting of the APA in Detroit on May 10, 1967, after which the foreign invitees would proceed to Chicago for a Fourth Transcultural Conference on Family Therapy. The Council approved, and as also described in *Psychiatry, East and West,* the Detroit conference on Transcultural Approaches to the Problems of the Family was the best-attended session at the annual meeting; the follow-up meetings at the Forest Foundation near Chicago were equally successful.

An interim letter of appreciation from APA President Brosin encouraged subsequent plans and correspondence:

May 17, 1967

Dear Jules:

I have received yours of May 12 and the three enclosures and want to congratulate you upon your speedy activity in pursuing the interests of the APA for future meetings.

I want to congratulate you also upon the success of your various enterprises (the Transcultural Conference and the session on the theatre of the absurd) at the Detroit meetings. I hear nothing but praise for them. As I mentioned at the East-West symposium, I think that there was more basic understanding attained than in previous meetings. You may be very proud of the part you have played.

Cordially,
Henry W. Brosin, M.D.
President, A.P.A.

A subsequent Transcultural Conference on Problems of Youth was therefore planned for the 1968 APA meeting in Boston, again with continuation at the Forest Foundation in Des Plaines. Once more, the APA requested and secured an NIMH grant-in-aid in my name, again raising the issue of the equitable distribution of invitations, travel allowances, and honoraria for our foreign invitees.

September 6, 1967

Shervert H. Frazier, M.D.
Chairman, Committee on Program

Dear Sherv:

From still vivid past experience, I can well appreciate the position of a program chairman whose committee is neatly hung up on exactly opposite poles of every question, leaving him to make the final wise decisions. Herewith developments that may help in yours:

International Seminars: Walter Barton (medical director

of the APA) has again applied for an $8,500 foreign travel grant with the proviso that this year's topic be World Problems of Youth, and that only experts in the field be invited. Gene Brody is to select three invitees from Latin America, and I am going to Washington this Saturday, September 9, to check with Walter as to other invitees from Britain and Holland and some Asian countries to present a review of similar problems in widely differing cultures. Walter is leaving for Russia the following week and must have the names in to the NIMH as soon as possible.

Arts and Humanities: Since it would be disastrous to put any kind of session—symphony, ballet or whatever—on the bare 12 x 32 foot x 5 foot high stage of the Sheraton ballroom, I shall presume we must use the Memorial Auditorium; if the extra thousand dollars required can't be gotten anywhere else, I'll ask Fairview to come through or go into bankruptcy myself.

In accordance with your last directive—and with a tangential confirmation from Hank Brosin—I am counting on the Boston Ballet Co. for Tuesday evening, May 14th, with much good music, illustrative modern dance, and minimal verbal commentary. However, I would recommend to your committee that they have concurrent evening panels—an arrangement which leaves everyone free to choose what he prefers.

After full consultation with Dr. Frazier, APA President-elect Larry Kolb, APA Medical Director Walter Barton, the APA Committee on Transcultural Psychiatry, and the Forest Hospital Foundation, I proceeded with the necessary invitation to the foreign and domestic experts we had agreed upon, supplementing each form letter with a personal one suitable to the country and person involved. For example, as specially required by Soviet protocol, my formal letter to the titular head of Russian psychiatry who, since he spoke no English, had informed me through an interpreter in Madrid that he himself could not come to the United States:

November 20, 1967

Dr. Andrei Snezhnievsky
Academy of Higher Nervous Functions
Moscow, USSR

Dear Dr. Snezhnievsky:

You will recall our most productive and enjoyable East-West Seminar in Madrid, and will be glad to learn that a motion picture film of it has been released and that the conference proceedings are being published. I would now like to seek your invaluable aid to process the following request through the proper governmental channels.

The American Psychiatric Association will hold a Transcultural Seminar on Problems of Youth at its annual meeting in Boston, Massachusetts, on May 16, 1968, to be followed by a second seminar under the auspices of the Forest Hospital Foundation in Chicago, Illinois, on May 18-19. Dr. Walter Barton, medical director of the American Psychiatric Association, Dr. Stanley Yolles, Director of our National Institute of Mental Health, and other recent visitors to your country have suggested that, among others, any one of the following authorities on Soviet youth, all of whom also speak English, would make excellent contributions to these seminars: Prof. V. V. Kovalev, Dr. Maya G. Schirina, Dr. Marate Vartanian.

We would greatly appreciate it if you would arrange and expedite the attendance of any one of these respected colleagues, or any other suitable authority on Soviet youth, including yourself, and so inform me at the earliest possible time so that his or her name can be included on the program and proper arrangements made for travel and maintenance.

Most respectfully

The APA Council again gave me a free hand, but cross-cultural misunderstandings temporarily arose:

December 6, 1967

Tulane University
School of Medicine
Dept. Psychiatry and Neurology

Dear Jules:

I have just returned from participating in a meeting in Moscow, where I was advised that a bit of a problem has evolved as a consequence of invitations sent to a couple of members of the Institute of Psychiatry of the Academy of Medical Sciences to attend the APA meeting next May. Apparently invitations were extended to Maya G. Schirina, M.D., and Professor Marat Vartanian, but not to Professor A. Snezhnievsky who, as you know, is the head man. Snezhnievsky now very much wants to attend the APA and, as a matter of fact, it is doubtful if anyone could come from the Institute if he is not invited too. Someone at the Institute said that Snezhnievsky was invited to attend a previous meeting of the APA, but was unable to make the trip and this may be the reason that he was not reinvited for next May.

Anyway, I think the problem can be resolved if an invitation is extended to Professor Snezhnievsky—reinforced with some Masserman tact.

I should appreciate hearing if the invitation is sent since I am in frequent communication with the group in Moscow.

Kindest regards and best wishes for the holiday season.

Sincerely,
Robert G. Heath, M.D.
Chairman, Dept. of Psychiatry
and Neurology

December 11, 1967

Dear Professor Snezhnievsky:

As you are doubltess aware, I have been writing to Drs. V. V. Kovalev, Schirina and Vartanian requestiong them to clear with you as to their possible attendance at several International Seminars on Problems of Youth to be held in our country as described in the attached form. These invitations were extended to conform with the following conditions prescribed by the American Psychiatric Association and the agencies granting the travel funds: (1) That only one speaker from each country be provided with funds for travel. (2) That he be selected from a limited list of specialists in problems of youth that was furnished to me. (3) That each speaker be fluent in English, so that, without a translator being available, he could join freely in the various discussions planned in Boston and Chicago.

In view of these conditions imposed upon me, and despite my deep professional and personal respect for you, I could not at first directly invite you alone until I could guarantee your travel expenses and arrange for a translator. Most unfortunately, I am even not yet certain of additional funds available, although I shall continue to do my best to secure them for you. However, if this is not a necessary condition, then the person you select could act as your interpreter, and we could have the honor and pleasure of your attendance at the seminars.

The enclosures will furnish further details of the meetings and those in attendance, to whom I would be happy to add your illustrious name. Please advise by return mail or, better, by cable, and I shall proceed accordingly.

Most respectfully

At this juncture, the medical director of the APA thought he should assert his superior knowledge and interpersonal skills:

December 20, 1967

Dear Jules:

It may take several exchange missions negotiated between the United States and the Soviet Union to undo your letter of December 11, 1967, and ones that preceded it. If you will read the letter to Professor Snezhnievsky carefully, it says—you're an afterthought on invitation; we really don't want you because you don't speak English fluently and if worse came to worse you could share a travel grant.

It is not a gracious invitation observing protocol and sent through channels. In my opinion, when communicating with Iron Curtain country personnages, one first informs the State Department of intent. Next, the president of the association should write the Minister of Health extending a gracious invitation and suggesting the kind of competence required in the persons to be invited. The American Embassy in the USSR also must be informed of the extended invitation.

Quibbling over travel funds is in bad taste. Russia is a great and powerful nation, not likely to be beholden to the United States for travel funds. Should the Russian government reply to you in any form, will you please let me know? I may then take care of the courtesies with the State Department and the American Embassy. I shall be very surprised if you get any answer.

If you'd like to know why one writes to the Minister of Health, even though Dr. Heath is correct in his December 6th letter, I'd be glad to explain it.

Sincerely yours,
Walter E. Barton, M.D.
Medical Director

December 27, 1967

Walter E. Barton, M.D.
Medical Director
American Psychiatric Association

Dear Walter:

The tone of your letter is hardly that of a Christmas card, and a bit surprising in view of our long and friendly cooperation. To set the record straight:

1. I have had quite cordial relations and much personal correspondence with Prof. Snezhnievsky ever since our first international invitational seminar participation in Czechoslovakia in 1959, and my return bid directly to him to Madrid last year. Indeed, he awarded me the Order of Pavlov in recogni-

tion of my research, and has repeatedly invited me to visit his Academy and to tour the USSR. Knowing him, I doubt that he would interpret my respectful letter to him as anything but a warm, friendly reciprocal invitation to a highly honored guest. In fact, I enclose a copy of a note from Bob Heath, who saw him last, much to that effect.

2. Far from making an arbitrary personal selection among those I knew in Russia, and in pursuance of our desire to have someone represent Russian thought in our Transcultural Conferences on Youth, I requested the APA delegation that visited the USSR with you to make their own recommendations. On your return, I was advised to write V.V. Kovalev (preferred), Maya G. Schirina, or Marate Vartanian, and did so. Snezhnievsky was not mentioned on your list; however, knowing Soviet custom I wrote to each (see my letter to Kovalev) merely requesting information as to their interest and how best to proceed according to protocol, and in addition sent the attached earlier cover letter to Snezhnievsky fully recognizing his status and authority in the matter.

3. As to finances: it is true, as you say, that Russia is a "great and powerful nation" but it is also true that the Russian economy is so short and chary of American exchange that invitees here have to be given our own travel grants in American money or nearly starve. With full approval of the council, last year I arranged to obtain these from the Forest Hospital Foundation for our "Iron Curtain" (a phrase they detest) guests, all of whom came without any State Department difficulties at either end, and all of whom regarded their travel funds as essential. Even in Madrid, the Russian delegation including Lebedev, Saarma, and Snezhnievsky himself were so strapped for pesos, that they were frankly eager for complimentary meals—some of which Chertok and I provided. I again brought the matter of travel funds up at council three weeks ago and, since the NIMH grant was still not available, was directed to secure additional funds for only one of your Russian invitees from the Forest Foundation—and again did so.

4. More to the point is that ever since both the 1967 and 1968 international seminars were authorized by the council, I kept you as medical director (as well as Henry Brosin as president, Dr. Howard Rome as chairman of the Council on Interna-

tional Relations and State Department consultant, and Sherv Frazier as chairman of the program committee) fully informed in advance of all plans, and sent you complete copies of all correspondence. Hank Brosin and Howard Rome, personally and in letters, signified concurrent approval of my procedure, but this is the first time I heard from you that we should have gone through the State Department, the Soviet Ministry of Health, our American Embassy, *et al.* You know that I always carefully coordinate each step with you and the Council and would have been glad to have gone through any and all channels at any time you indicated.

Finally, although I of course regret any failures of communication, I do not believe that our Russian relations are at all strained or the situation as complicated as your letter implies. But I shall continue to keep you fully informed, and, as always, be glad to follow all further suggestions.

Best of Seasons' Geeetings anyway.

The follow-up note from Dr. Heath:

December 13, 1967

Dear Jules:

As usual, your note to Snezhnievsky was masterful. Best wishes.

Bob

Only two days later I received a cable from Prof. Snezhnievsky saying that he would be most happy to come to the Conferences in Boston and Chicago, and adding, with typical Russian warmth, that he especially looked forward to personal visits with me as "a most learned and famous American psychiatrist." I felt it a delightful duty to send a translation of the cable (omitting some of the overcomplimentary passages) to Dr. Barton, and to his credit got this reply:

February 19, 1968

Dear Jules:

Your charm overcomes international diplomacy. Congratulations on getting an agreement from the Soviets to be represented at the Transcultural Seminar on Problems of Youth!

Walter E. Barton, M.D.
Medical Director

February 23, 1968

Dear Professor Snezhnievsky:

Let me again express my great pleasure that you will honor us with your presence, and will be accompanied by Drs. Marate Vartanijan and Maya Schirina. I attach an amended schedule and form letter in the hope that it will help in your planning. As to the manuscripts requested, we would welcome all contributions from all of you; however, only one set will be sufficient if you so prefer.

Permit me also to repeat my invitation for you to be our house guests in Chicago, and my hope that you can accept.

As you requested, I am sending a copy of this letter and the attached material to the Foreign Relations Department of the Ministry of Health.

Most respectfully

Another form of invitation:

June 20, 1968

Ari Kiev, M.D.
The New York Hospital
New York, New York

Dear Ari:

My admiration for your clear, objective, and literate reports on Soviet psychiatry leads me to ask another favor. As you know, I recently organized the Transcultural Seminars on Problems of Youth, and invited several Russian psychiatrists. They accepted the invitation and seemed delighted by our extensive arrangements for their travel and comfort—and then, early in May, probably because of changed directives from on high to our own recently reviewed anti-Soviet policies abruptly notified us that they couldn't come. The other twelve speakers not only attended, but submitted manuscripts which, with some editing, well described the status, problems and future of youth in their respective countries; however, our projected volume on *Transcultural Problems of Youth* would be obviously incomplete without a chapter on the Communist countries. Would you, in your own admirable style, supply such a chapter by November or so, and include topics of world-wide interest such as youth protest phenomena, hippieism if any, whatever has happened to the Makarenko movement, and whatever else you choose from the rich data you already have at hand? The book will be widely read, and your own chapter much appreciated.

The conferences were held as scheduled both in Boston and Chicago, and their proceedings were published by Grune & Stratton in a book, *Transcultural Problems of Youth,* which I edited and for which I wrote the following preface:

Preface to Transcultural Problems of Youth

In a preceding volume entitled *Psychiatry: East and West,* I summarized four antecedent International Conferences in which widely distributed European and North American experts presented the causes, nature and modes of therapy of adult behavior disorders in their respective countries. Basic concepts and practices, *homo sapiens* being but a single species with a common Aryan-Hellenic heritage in the West, proved to be predictably similar, although superficial differences had developed between capitalist and socialist socioeconomic systems along the following lines:

1. Psychiatrists from communist countries generally rejected Freudian libidinal-individualist determinism, but were far from rigidly monothetic on biologic, Pavlovian, socio-

economic, or other parameters of etiology.

2. There were greater differences as to psychiatric nosology and therapy among psychiatrists from Eastern European countries including the U.S.S.R., than among those from the United States; indeed, when any psychiatrist advocated a particularly doctrinaire approach, the most vigorous disclaimers and rebuttals generally came from his own countrymen.

3. Soviet psychiatrists were inclined to temper their relationships to their patients with expressions of warm personal interest, reconstructive suggestions, and the direct utilization of educational, occupational, recreational and other rehabilitative resources not directly available to physicians in non-communist countries.

4. Nevertheless, no matter what theoretic or political orientation was propounded in whatever language, competently trained and experienced psychiatrists throughout Europe and the Americas generally treated their patients in very nearly the same biologically based, empathically insightful, dynamically individualized, socially-culturally oriented, and essentially humane manner—and with about the same results.

5. Every conferee agreed, moreover, that "we must look to the future" and—since in a future as near as 1970 half the world's population will be under twenty-five years of age—that the future lay with our youth.

Accordingly, the American Psychiatric Association and the Forest Hospital Foundation, in collaboration with Northwestern University, sponsored a Fifth International Conference on Transcultural Problems of Youth, to which we invited authorities not only from the West, but from countries and cultures as remote as Indonesia, Guam, Ceylon, Japan, and Thailand. Each participant was requested to prepare a manuscript which would furnish data and commentaries along the following lines: (a) The historical, socio-cultural, religious, economic, and other influences on the youth of the country. (b) The range of what is considered "normal" with regard to familial, educational, occupational, sexual, marital, and parental behavior. (c) The use and abuse of alcohol and drugs. (d) The dynamics of personal and group protest, including vandalism, juvenile crime, gang formations, and mass movements. (e) The modes of dyadic, familial, and social prevention. (f) The availability of private, social agency, and governmental programs of treatment, including the special training and availability of competent therapeutic and supervisory personnel. Or, to put it more whimsically, each expert was invited to answer these questions: (a) Is youth a pandemic disease with similar causes and symptoms everywhere or are its problems endemic and specific to particular cultures? (b) In either case what, if anything, need or can be done about its current vagaries and deviations?

Every contributor to this book has attempted to answer these questions seriatim in his own way, minimally modified by editorial stringencies; accordingly the reader will find the diversity on the one hand, and the scope and comprehensiveness on the other, equally fascinating. And he will emerge from these hegiras into transcultural understanding with this among many insights: Youth is everywhere changing our world, and we had best comprehend and collaborate while yet we may.

The following more personalized report on the fifth conference was published by the Argentinian delegate Dr. Mauricio Knobel in *Psiquiatría y Psicología de America Latina* (1968). The translation by Nelson Borelli is here reproduced unaltered except for the deleting of excessively kind compliments to me—unlikely as that editing may seem to be.

Two North American Conferences on the Transcultural Problems of Youth

"The annual Congress of the American Psychiatric Association, attended by several thousand specialists from the United States and foreign guests, brought up to date a most diversified selection of subjects. Pure investigation, animal and pharmacologic experimentation, community psychiatry, psychotherapy, psychoanalysis, hospital organization, problems of violence and delinquency, applied psychiatry as a speciality in different ages (infant, adolescent, geriatric), administrative aspects, military psychiatry, and even political conflicts were among the many subjects, all of which reached a high level of scientific discussion in the Congress.

"Masserman was there, vivacious, inquisitive and articulate. His experimental work with animals enabled him to demonstrate the effects of distorting and disadapting external influences on all behavior, in that uncertainty with regard to events important to the organism induces various degrees of neurotic maladjustment in both laboratory animals and human beings. As a training analyst, his observation about the clinical basis of psychoanalytic theory and therapy allowed him to emphasize the value of psychoanalytic contributions to contemporary psychiatry, without sacrificing pragmatic objectivity: he confirmed the value of experimentation, but did not believe that human problems could be solved through technology alone. He advocated the integration of psychoanalytic and social knowledge for a greater reach into the community. He was able to understand the student revolts as a revitalizing protest and he placed them in the frame of reference of social psychiatry. He did likewise with the claims of the black people and the "black power" problem, a psycho-social-economic movement which requires objective study and response. . . .

"Later, in Des Plaines, Illinois the International Seminar on Adolescence found in Masserman a dynamic leader, profoundly acquainted with the problem on a transcultural level. He was always appropriate and respectful of his foreign colleagues whom he stimulated and supported so that they could freely express themselves without embarrassment. His goal was clear: to integrate psychiatry. The classic psychodynamisms were not unknown to him; he collaborated with those of us with psychoanalytical orientation. On the other hand, other subjects such as social, religious and ethical questions of the society in crisis were brought to discussion, constantly to the point and with knowledge of sociology, economics and politics. With respect to treatment he also showed mastery through comprehensiveness of his approach. It was intriguing to listen to a psychoanalyst and an investigator such as Masserman discuss with ease subjects related to group psychotherapy, family therapy, psychopharmacotherapy and hospitalization. He uses precise psychiatric language and refined sociologic terminology.

"We said goodbye to Masserman at a party given for the foreign represenatives by him and his fine wife in their own home in Chicago. There we knew another Masserman. A frank, generous, congenial host, he let us view a colored television program as long as we wished, and his comments were those of a common man, whom all human manifestations touch. He then dazzled us with his musical knowledge and aptitudes, creating an artistic climate in which Dr. Knobloch of Czechoslovakia was induced to play the piano. Masserman then captivated us with several musical performances on his viola and violin, solo and in duets with Dr. Knobloch. The owner of two valuable antique musical instruments, he played them with the hands and feelings of a maestro. But it was not only the classics that came out of those instruments; from them appeared Masserman the composer, suave, tender, profoundly human.

"I will remember his music, his graceful wife, his row of 30 books which he wrote or edited, his library of the classical texts of the literature, his good liquor and excellent food and his view of Lake Michigan facing his apartment and showing his anchored yawl, which was waiting for the next morning when the sportsman would leave all this behind. Jules Masserman is a paradigm as a scientist, professor, and therapist, who gives much to those that can come close to him."

My three-year term on the APA Council expired in 1968, but at the May meeting that year the program committee once more requested that I arrange the Arts and Humanities Session and the Transcultural Conferences for the 1969 meeting in Miami. In follow-up:

June 11, 1968

Shervert H. Frazier, M.D.
Chairman, APA Committee on
Programs

Dear Sherv:

At a meeting of the Forest Hospital Foundation last evening I was authorized to offer its financial support for a fifth set of international conferences to be held during the APA meeting in Miami and the following weekend at the Forest Hospital. These plans were tentatively recommended:

Topic: Transcultural Aspects of Socio-Forensic Psychiatry.

Foreign Invitees: Limited to six representatives from contrasting socioeconomic cultures throughout the world: (e.g., Anglo-Saxon, Latin, Slavic, Muslim, Indonesian, Chinese, African) and not more than two from the United States or Canada.

Purpose: To examine (a) how various ethnic and economic factors are expressed in unwritten customs and written laws as to class privileges, sexual conduct, marriage, abortion, euthanasia and crime, (b) how social sanctions, modes of trial and guilt, institutionalization, punishment, and other social instruments exert control, (c) how these affect the growth and development of children, adolescents, and adults, and (d) how the implicit codes and explicit rules correlate the conceptual dynamics of individual behavior and affect the therapy of its social deviations.

Publications: As in the two preceding international conferences, prepared papers by the panelists and abstracts of the discussions will be published.

You will recall that at the last meeting of the program committee in Boston, President Brosin spoke for the council in recommending the continuation of these international conferences as well as the arts and humanities sessions. After further liaison with Drs. Alspach and Hibbs of the arrangements committee, I shall write you separately about the arts and humanities session, but I hope that the preliminary thinking about the international conferences meets with your approval.

Once again, my hearty congratulations for a superb Boston program.

An invitation to Olympus:

The Honorable Earl Warren
Chambers of the Chief Justice
Supreme Court of the United States
Washington, D.C. 20543

Dear Mr. Warren:

Nearly half a decade ago, as program chairman of the American Psychiatric Association, I had the honor (or *hubris?*) to invite you to give the academic address to the May 1965 annual meeting of that association, and in a most courteous letter you declined because of your paramount obligations to the President's Commission on the Assassination of President Kennedy. May I most respectfully call your attention to the enclosed projection of a Transcultural Conference on the Relationships of Psychiatry, Law and Culture, which is to be held under the auspices of Northwestern University and the Forest Hospital Foundation near Chicago on May 10 and 11, 1969? May I also inquire whether it would be at all possible for you to honor us by your presence?

You may wish to know that several highly authoritative sociologists, historians, political scientists, and psychiatrists have tentatively accepted the invitation to constitute a panel of about ten knowledgeable and communicative participants, and that all would be most appreciative of any contribution you may wish to make to the symposium. The audience will be by invitation to professionals only, and publicity, if any, will be confined to what is authorized by yourself.

Rest assured that if you can spare the weekend, every effort will be made to make your visit intellectually interesting and personally useful and enjoyable.

Most respectfully

With the graciousness of the great, Justice Warren replied:

Dr. Jules H. Masserman, Chairman
American Psychiatric Association

Dear Dr. Masserman:

I regret very much circumstances are such that I must decline your cordial invitation to deliver the Convocation Address at the annual meeting of your association next May.

For almost a year I found it necessary to share my time between the Court and the President's Commission on the Assassination of President Kennedy. As a result, I was forced to lay aside many of the things which constantly confront me as Chief Justice. In order to now catch up, I feel that at least during the present term I should devote all of my time and attention to the Court work. I know you will understand.

It was thoughtful of you to invite me to participate in your program, and I appreciate it. I trust that your annual meeting will be an enthusiastic and interesting one.

Sincerely,
Earl Warren

However, an illustrious Associate Justice accepted:

Justice William O. Douglas,
Supreme Court of the United States

Dear Justice Douglas:

It is, of course, redundant to inform you that the legal and psychiatric professions are delighted that, Supreme Court duties permitting, you will participate in the Northwestern University–Forest Foundation Seminars on Culture, Law and Psychiatry at Des Plaines, Illinois, next May 10th and 11th. The sole purport of this letter, therefore, is to assure you that every effort will be made to render your stay not only intellectually interesting but personally enjoyable as well, and to invite you to inform us as to any special arrangements as to hotel accommodations, transportation, free periods, special guests, etc. you may wish us to make.

With our personal respects and best of New Year's Wishes.

Respectfully

As did another famous jurist:

David L. Bazelon
Chief Judge
US Court of Appeals
Washington, D.C. 20001

Dear David:

Delighted that you will come if at all possible, but it's new to me that you take such assignments so seriously. No "formal papers" need to be read at the conference—only whatever you wish to say, with or without notes, on any aspect of the broadest of topics: culture, law and psychiatry. And as to the publication of the Proceedings in the inevitable Book, any relevant manuscript you have—even of one previously published—would do.

As to my Cartesian Center at Stanford: I think I think, therefore I am here.

At this juncture, again a bit unaccountably, the APA medical director elicited from Dr. Lawrence Kolb, then president of the APA, a letter with a copy to me to the effect that "all arrangements for all parts of the annual program of the APA," including the Arts and Humanities and the Transcultural Sessions, must be made "only" by the program committee and that all foreign guests should be invited "directly" and "only" through the "office of the president" or the "central office." I replied:

Dear Dr. Kolb:

Your letter to Dr. Barton, the copy of which I just received on my return from an absence of some weeks, was, to put it euphemistically, once more disconcerting. Let me review the following:

1. As chairman of the program committee from 1961 to 1964, I myself, after repeated recommendations entered in its minutes, helped convince the council to discontinue sections, perennial joint meetings, etc., and entrust the program entirely to my successors on the program committee.

2. Since leaving that committee on election to the council, I have conscientiously abided by that ruling. Specifically, no arts and humanities sessions and no international seminars were ever planned, arranged, or conducted without the prior and continuous approval of the program committee and Dr. Walter Barton, supplemented by running reports invariably accepted by council (see its past minutes), and liaison with the current arrangements committee. As to the last international seminars, I have such correspondence—including cordial exchanges with our Russian colleagues—to supplement copies previously sent to you at the time for your information and approval. I also trust you received a copy of *Psychiatry: East and West,* covering the previous seminars; if not, I shall be glad to send one to you.

3. At its last meeting on Friday morning, May 17, Dr. Henry Brosin—who, I presumed, was speaking for the council—urged the program committee, in accordance with his eloquent Presidential Address, to continue the international seminars indefinitely. It was at that meeting that I was again specifically commissioned by unanimous vote of the program committee, in Dr. Brosin's presence, to arrange both the 1969 Arts and Humanities Session and the International Program. Once more I agreed to do so only if I could continue to secure the advice and approval of the Committee for each step taken.

4. I have again carried out this policy, and only with the consent both of Sherv Frazier and Alan Lipton by telephone and letter did I: (a) Have the Fairview Hospital Foundation consider a contract (for about $6000) with the Columbia Artists

Management for a presentation on "The Evolution of Musical Synesthesia"—a performance of high intellectual and esthetic merit that has received very favorable reviews in *The New York Times* and elsewhere—at our Miami meeting, at a time and place designated by Drs. Frazier and Alspach. Again, this entails no financial obligation whatever by the APA other than council acceptance of a grant and the usual footnote of acknowledgment to Fairview. Just as you were co-chariman of the session in May, I hope Dr. Waggoner will so serve in 1969. (b) Secure other funds ($5000 to $10,000) for the next international seminars, the general plan of which I proposed in the attached letter to Dr. Frazier, which he also approved. Every subsequent step will again be in full consultation with him, Dr. Barton, Dr. Waggoner and, if you wish, yourself.

And now let me add that although these sessions in the past have demanded literally full weeks of my time and from a thousand to two thousand dollars of personal expenses for telegrams, long-distance calls, site travels, extra secretarial work (not counting missed income) every year, I continued to arrange them when requested because I had reason to hope, from many expressions of appreciation, that it was one of the ways I could continue to serve the APA. Indeed, for the academic year of 1968-69 I have accepted a fellowship at the Center for Advanced Behavioral Studies and a travelling professorship in Australia and New Zealand, and had looked forward to a sabbatical from many of my usual academic, research, and administrative duties. If then, the program committee, the central office, the Council or you would like someone else to take over these tasks, I shall be most happy to relinquish them.

Dr. Kolb wrote that he had apparently misunderstood the situation, whereupon:

August 19, 1968

Walter E. Barton, M.D.
Medical Director, APA

Dear Walter:

As a follow-up of my last letter to Larry Kolb, I called him as to how he now wished to proceed about next year's international seminar and arts and humanities session. He replied that there had apparently been some failure of communication between Sherv and yourself as to the program committee having once again assigned these to me, and my acceptance on condition of continued close collaboration with all concerned.

Since I thought the matter was cleared, I secured promises of grants for both sessions for Council acceptance as in previous years. However, it is now necessary to proceed with the selection of invitees, officers, time, content, and other program arrangements for the international seminar, so please check with Sherv directly as to these matters, and be assured that, although I have suggestions as to international participants, time, place, content, etc. (see copy of my previous letter to Sherv), I shall be happy to have Larry, Sherv, or yourself proceed in any way you think best.

However, since cooperation was again being so long delayed as to threaten essential preparations for the conference:

August 30, 1968

Lawrence C. Kolb, M.D.

Dear Larry:

I hope and trust that by this time you have fully recovered from the surgery you told me about in our last phone conversation. Since I must meet with the Forest Hospital Foundation on September 4th about the grant they have already offered the APA in support of travel to the 1969 Transcultural Seminars (as always, subject to program committee approval of personnel and scheduling, and with only a footnote of program acknowledgement), would you please let me know how you wish these to be arranged? Sherv Frazier has again confirmed their assignment to me, and Henry Brosin, who was present and recommended that course, may inform you likewise. However, in view of Walter Barton's letter I would appreciate specific instructions so that I may proceed or not as you wish.

A full month later, Dr. Kolb wrote to inquire as to "progress" and to suggest that the Transcultural Seminar consist of prospective "Dutch and World Health Organization visitors to the annual meeting." On rereading my reply, I can detect an overtone of more than mild impatience:

September 25, 1968

Lawrence C. Kolb, M.D.

Dear Larry:

1. As to the Arts and Humanities Session, there seem to be no problems. I shall preview the performance of the New York Company by making a special trip from here to the University of Wisconsin on October 8, and if all is satisfactory, secure the relevant program and brochure data for Drs. Frazier, Barton, and Alspach, and send it on to them.

2. The international sessions, however, now present two complications. (a) The topic proposed by the Forest Foundation: "Culture, Custom, Law and Psychiatry," as submitted to and approved by Sherv Frazier, may not be the main field of interest or competence of those likely to attend from the Dutch or other WHO societies. As per the prospective letter Sherv approved, a copy of which I sent you, we had thought of a much wider sociocultural sampling: Hindu, Muslim, African, etc., to make the comparative study truly significant. (b) If we wait until after the program committee meets next month, it may be impossible for highly desirable invitees to make all the complicated arrangements to come to Chicago and Miami next May; in fact it is already quite late.

The Forest Foundation may, therefore, decide that in view of the fact that it had already sponsored two highly successful international seminars, with published proceedings, and had, with preliminary authorization, publicly projected another for 1969, it might be best to proceed to invite its own foreign speakers independently of the APA for a sixth conference on the weekend preceding or following our May meeting, thus technically not interfering with us. I would regret this; and when I meet with the officers of the Foundation next week, I shall urge them: to wait still longer, until after the program committee meets; or failing that, to submit a preliminary list of possible invitees to Sherv for his and your selections; or in any case, to inform you as soon as possible who among the invitees are coming, so that you and Sherv can issue parallel invitations over your signatures to those you choose for an international seminar at the APA.

September 30, 1968

Dear Jules:

Just a brief note to acknowledge receipt of your letter of September 25 to Larry Kolb. It does seem to me that you covered the subject thoroughly and I have no suggestions for any change. I am sure that your letter will be considered at the fall committee meetings at the end of October.

I do hope that you and Chris have a delightful trip to Australia.

Raymond W. Waggoner, M.D.
APA President-elect

With official follow-up:

October 8, 1968

Shervert H. Frazier, M.D.
APA Program Chairman

Dear Sherv:

You will again recall that at its last meeting the program

committee, with Dr. Brosin present, directed me once more to seek subsidies for and make preliminary arrangements for the 1969 Transcultural Seminars. Since then, changing directives from APA officialdom, with all of which I have tried to comply, have so delayed even the initial steps that it now appears too late to correspond with expert advisers in far countries, select those most suitable from those recommended who can arrange to come, seek substitutes for those that cannot, and clear all the other innumerable details involved. At a meeting of the board of directors of the Forest Foundation, it was therefore decided:

1. To retain the general seminar topic of "Social Order, Law, and Psychiatry" for a Transcultural Seminar to be held at the Forest Hospital on the weekend of May 10 and 11, 1969.

2. To take advantage of their presence this year as Fellows at the Center for Advanced Study in the Behavioral Sciences at Stanford of the following experts in these related fields: Kai Erikson, Yale University, sociology; Richard Falk, Stanford, comparative law; Marc Franklin, Stanford, forensic science; Leon Lipson, Yale, Soviet order and law; Nadav Safran, Indonesian cultures; and S. J. Tambiah, Thai and related cultures. In addition, Dr. Falk who has a world-wide acquaintance with many other authorities, suggested Ali Mazrui, for Africa; Raman Suvastava, for India; and George Abi Saab, for Islam—with Julius Stone of Sydney, Australia (whom Richard Falk described as "probably one of the foremost thinkers in the world on the general significance of legal norms in human affairs"), and/or Gertrude Leighton of Bryn Mawr and Harold D. Lasswell as moderators. Finally, among knowledgeable, approachable, and probably available Russians we have Aleksandr Borisovich Sakharov, Boris Nikolaevich Nikiforov, and Aleksei Adol'fovich Gertzenson, with additional recommendations of Leo Festinger of the University of Minnesota Law School and Jerome Cohen of Harvard as additional moderators. Naturally we would add to this list of possibilities various APA corresponding fellows, such as T. Lambo of Nigeria.

The foundation is aware that the APA is extending special courtesies to the Dutch and Puerto Rican societies in 1969, and would welcome to its Chicago seminars one representative each as selected by the program committee, expenses fully paid.

To expedite the work of the program committee, I shall request the Center for Advanced study in the Behavioral Sciences, of which I am also a fellow this year, to send you the *curriculum vitae* of all the Fellows listed above, and shall also request Drs. Falk and Lipson to send you the addresses and other information about the experts they suggested.

From among this list the program committee can then choose six (the usual number at a symposium) as speakers and/or discussants for a Transcultural Seminar on Social Order, Law and Psychiatry as envisaged in our previous correspondence, with officers of the session also selected by the committee. All invitations to these selectees will then be sent by the program chairman, plus foreign invitations sent by Dr. Kolb.

All additional expenses of travel to Miami (before the Chicago seminars) for those selected by the program committee will also be paid by the Forest Hospital Foundation, with only the usual footnote acknowledgement.

I hope that this new arrangement is fully in accord with the revised procedures of the APA. I am now en route to a month of academic lectures in Australia and New Zealand, but Dr. Mortimer Gross and Mr. Morris B. Squire of the Forest Hospital remain available, and I assure you of further full cooperation on my return.

The sixth international conference was held despite intercurrent APA politics, proved as illuminating as its predecessors, and is being published as a volume entitled, predictably, *Culture, Law, and Psychiatry.*

21. BIODYNAMIC PSYCHIATRY AND THE UNCERTAINTY PRINCIPLE

In this penultimate chapter, I can do no less than try to restate, as clearly and succinctly as possible, those residues of reified reflections in library, clinic, and laboratory with which I have filled threescore years of a full and perhaps only partly futile life. I cannot pretend that the theoretical product of these triune experiences is any parallel to Einstein's tri-termed $E = mc^2$, except that my formulation as to the interrelationships of the causes, phenomena, and control of behavior again consists of but three reciprocal sets of concepts, each again triply divisible, to wit:

First, that man's ultimate (*Ur-*)sources of concern are: (1) his physical health and longevity, (2) his social securities, and (3) his existential significance.

Second, that whenever these primary cares escalate to *Ur-anxieties* and become manifest in excessive and disabling somatic and behavioral aberrãtions, man seeks a corresponding triad of therapies designed (1) to restore his physical well-being, (2) to recultivate his social alliances, and (3) to reconstitute his faith in life's meaning and values.

Third, that these statements can be explored heuristically by recourse to the three epistemologic sources of all sciences:

(1) the historical, (2) the comparative, and (3) the experimental. Let us review each briefly.

I. Historical Approaches to the Essentials of Therapy

Physical: Since paleolithic times, man has tried to mitigate his fears of his inimical universe through his sciences and technologies. In two of the most important of these he has sought to find means to cure his ills and restore his skills by empiric medicaments ranging from herbs and minerals to the first specific use of quinine for malaria in 1820, and by various surgical procedures ranging from the ancient binding of fractures to the modern embedding of plastic hearts. Psychiatry, too, as a branch of medicine, has always explored pharmacologic, surgical, and other modes of relieving man's material fears and their somatic reflections and, fortunately, is once again intensely developing this important rubric of therapy.

Social: Scientific and technical advances, however, have historically proved inadequate for man's eternal quests for security, inasmuch as: (1) Expanding knowledge revealed mysteries and challenges ever beyond man's puny powers, however much he learned and applied. (2) Each man realized that the tools his neighbors developed could be as or more lethal than his own.

Ergo, man began to seek ever more inclusive human alliances, ranging from parental and familial ties through allegiances to the clan, tribe, city and state to their present limits in highly uncertain international pacts. Within all of these aggregations, specially selected men were given specific trusts and tasks toward enhancing group welfare: kings* and constables for internal government, soldiers for territorial safety (which is still thought to require external conquest), and medicine men, who as proto-physicians treated illness and as proto-psychiatrists prevented or corrected excessive deviations from locally accepted norms of conduct—a reintegration of medical and community function that is also being revived in modern psychiatry.

Mystical: But these irregular and sometimes inchoate

*Our term "king" (German *Koenig*), head of state, is derived from Anglo-Saxon *cyning*, head of kin (Perry).

strivings, even when combined with man's pyramiding technical knowledge and skills, have never yet been enough to allay a third and even broader concern, since no group of human scientists, however large or learned, has ever been able to control the heavens, guarantee the future, explain the nature or meaning of life, or mitigate the certainty of physical death. Man has therefore always postulated transcendent cosmic systems presumably operated by super-natural beings whom he could conveniently control either directly or through special mediators here on earth. Designated as such were magicians and priests who were thus wishfully charged with this third task: not only to minister to the physical and social needs of men, but also to influence in their favor the occult goals and gods of the universe.

Classical Roots:

It would obviously require too long a series of ponderous tomes to deal in detail with these triple trepidations of man throughout history, but perhaps a brief recall of how, with both conscious and intuitive skill, each aspect of a corresponding therapeutic trinity was intuitively invoked during one enlightened period—for example, in the Asklepiad sanatoria of Greece and Rome—may serve to illustrate the general thesis. In brief, the methods employed in these classically effective mental health centers mitigated man's *Ur*-anxieties as follows:

By restoring physical well-being: After the patient had left his contentious home and travelled to one of the sanatoria in the salubrious environs of Cos, Memphis, or Knidos, he was welcomed not by a clerk or social worker but by no less a parent-surrogate than the Head Priest or Priestess, who then further cheered and reassured him by conducting him past piles of discarded crutches and bronze plaques bearing testimonials from grateful ex-patients. Immediate attention was then concentrated on restoring the patient's physical well-being through rest in pleasant surroundings, nourishing and appetizing diets, relaxing baths and massages, and the carefully measured administration of nepenthics—drugs that resembled modern ataractics in that they served to tranquillize both the patient and the physician. Indeed, the Greek word *therapeien* itself meant service, just as later the Latin *curare,* to care for, gave rise to our term "cure."

By recultivating human relationships: In accordance with this objective, equal effort was expended in counteracting the patient's second *Ur*-anxiety as to social alienation as follows:

1. *Confidence in the physician:* Then as now, the patient was encouraged to relate to his therapist: (a) As a kindly and protective parental figure who provided a source of security and comfort. (b) As a learned and experienced teacher, whose counsels for more restrained and balanced and, therefore, healthier and happier modes of life could be followed on rational and practical grounds (*e.g.,* as in the various Stoic schools). (c) As a more personal mentor uniquely interested in the supplicant's complaints ("present illness") and willing to explore their relationship to the patient's past experiences (psychiatric history), their meanings and values (symbolisms), and acquired patterns of goal-directed action (operational analysis), in order that the intellectual understandings (verbal "insight") so derived would lead to more satisfying, lasting, and useful (emotional, or better, operational) adaptations. Socrates required his students to work through their own perplexities under his mentorship, and Plato interpreted the significance of dreams and symbols. In other anticipations of "modern" psychoanalysis, Aristophanes, in his delightful comedy *The Clouds,* had Socrates, while symbolically suspended in the air in a basket, instruct the distraught merchant Strepsiades to "speak all thoughts freely . . . omitting none." Through free associations twenty-three centuries before Freud, Strepsiades thus revealed his fantasies about controlling the phases of the moon so that the lunar month would never end, his bills would never fall due, and his problems would then be solved. As to less passive forms of therapy, Soranus records the cure of a case of "hysteria" in a virginal bride by a form of enforced erotic disinhibition (i.e., "lighting the torch of Hymen") that would shock many a modern marital counsellor. (d) Finally, the needful dependence of the patient on the physician (transference) that was thus cultivated also led to an avid acceptance by the patient of the efficacy of the physician's quasi-scientific, quasi-mystical remedies, some of which

were covertly punitive for, and thereby comfortingly expiative of, social and religious transgressions implicit in the patient's illness (a term related to Anglo-Saxon *yfel,* evil). Among these were not only a vast variety of unpleasant purgings, bleedings, coolings, roastings, and broilings, but even more direct physical and surgical interferences with cerebral function, such as the Egyptian practice of trephining the skull and incising the cortex, thus anticipating Moniz by three millennia, or, as described by Pliny the Elder, anticipating Cerletti by subjecting the patient to convulsive therapy by discharging electric eels through the head. Hippocrates condemned the ignorance and superstition inherent in many of these "false remedies" but this alone indicates how widely practiced, then as now, they must have been.

2. *Group therapies:* But the patient's social rehabilitation was not confined to dyadic transactions with his physician; concurrently, his essential group relationships and skills were also recultivated through the following modalities: *music,* which provided esthetic expression and encouraged conjoint rhythm and harmony; *calisthenics and dancing,* which afforded similar possibilities of interaction and communion; *competitive athletics,* not only for the joy of healthy exercise but for public recognition through nondestructive competition and public reward; and *legendary dramatics.*

Here the poetic psychiatrist (and there can be no other) may well ask: What writings better explore or epitomize basic human relationship than the classic Greek myths or the plays of Sophocles, Euripides, Aeschylus, or Aristophanes? For example, was Narcissus "in love with himself," as Freud would have it, or did he become so enamored of his vaguely reflected *image* that his friend Almeinas and his mistress Echo forsook him? Again, whether or not, as T. S. Eliot asserted, mourning became Electra, it certainly became fatal to her mother Clystemnestra, her mother's lover Aegisthos, nearly so to her brother Orestes, and to practically everyone else involved. But perhaps the most inclusive and poignant of man's perennial vicissitudes are dramatized in Sophocles' trilogy on Oedipus—a succession of legends which, far beyond epitomizing merely a middle-class Viennese son's supposed desire for coitus with his mother countered by Freudian fear of his father's terrible swift sword, deal much more deeply with nearly all human travail and triumph from childhood survival to the ultimate denial of death. Let us recount the story:

> Laius, King of Thebes, is warned by an oracle that his son will slay him—as indeed all children inevitably displace their elders. Torn by doubt and fear, Laius avoids the onus of direct infanticide and, as many parents do, hobbles his offspring by pinning together the ankles of the newborn Oedipus (Greek, *swollen feet*) and leaving him in a basket—there being no Mosaic bulrushes about—on Mount Cathaeron. However, Oedipus is found by a kindly shepherd and adopted by Polybus, King of Corinth—as indeed our own rejected children are partially rescued by babysitters, nursery teachers, pedagogues, and other surrogates. But Oedipus is never certain that he is "really" the true Prince of Corinth, cannot get satisfactory assurances from King Polybus or Queen Merope (for that matter, who *can* be absolutely certain of his paternity?), and is further perplexed when he learns at Delphi that he is destined to kill his father and marry his mother. Trying to escape his fate (as who does not?) he vows never to see his putative parents Polybus or Merope again, and leaves Corinth to wander in search of what Erik Erikson would call his "true identity." At a crossroads outside Thebes an old man blocks his right-of-way and is killed in the ensuing battle—as all oldsters who dare too long to challenge imperious youth will be disposed of in their turn. To display his intellectual as well as physical vitality, Oedipus then also conquers a Sphinx whose "riddle" (the old nursery puzzle about the quadri-, bi-, and tripedal locomotion of aging man) he easily solves, and thereby emancipates the Thebans from years of sphincteric terror. For reward he is given the vacant throne of Thebes and marries the widowed Queen Iocaste.
>
> But nagging doubts remain (who is free of them?) and Oedipus, after more years of restless searching,

> learns from the shepherd who rescued him the awful truth that he had indeed killed his father and cohabited incestuously with his mother—an "awful truth" only because he fears that others regard it so. With due public histrionics, he blinds (not castrates) himself in expiation (and thereby secures the advantage of being a pathetic rather than a reprehensible figure), curses his unwanted sons Eteocles and Polynices, and then preempts the lives of his daughters, Antigone and Ismene, in further wanderings throughout Hellas—as many an aging parent since Agamemnon sacrificed Iphigenia still tries to do. Finally, at the Grave of Colonus outside Athens he defies the Fates, and himself becomes a demi-god—thus acquiring the archangelic status we all believe we deserve.

There are, of course, many variations of these legends, not only in Greek, but in Hungarian, Romanian, Finnish, and even Lapland folklore. In one classic version, Homer has Iocaste commit suicide, after which a more sensible Oedipus completes his reign in relative peace. But the stories are never naively monothetic; instead, they portray almost every nuance of the imperative, ceaseless seekings that imbue the human condition—and the temporary triumphs, tantalizing traumata, and terminal tragedies that would be unbearable unless men can fancy that they exist in a covertly rational cosmos or else can believe themselves to be superhuman.

The Greeks cherished these tragedies and comedies for their deep human empathy and ageless significance, endlessly varied their themes, and were personally involved as actors, chorus, or affectively moved audience.

3. *Metaphysical.* Finally, the Greeks also recognized the third Human *Ur*-necessity of a belief in some metaphysical but Transcendent Order—and accordingly, demanded that Socrates pay the ultimate penalty for threatening man's trust in the existence of Celestial Beings. To capitalize on this ultimate faith, the Asklepiad sanatoria, like many hospitals today, were built and operated by one or another religious cult which added the following powerful factors to therapy:

A "divinely revealed" doctrine in which all believers could feel an exclusively self-elevating bond of fellowship.

A reassuring ritual which, through millennia of empiric refinement, included such exquisitely gratifying procedures as:

The symbolic eating and drinking of the parent-god's body in the forms of mystically potentiating food and wine (as exemplified in the ancient worship of Melitta and Mithra).

The temple hymns, sung and played in the simple, repetitive hypnotic cadences of a mother's lullaby—and often resulting in "temple sleep." Such escapist trances were then varied with food, drink and Dionysian sexual indulgences to be triply enjoyed, since they also honored one's permissive and accommodating gods.

The "anointing" or "laying on of hands" to cure an injured bodily part—a direct reminiscence of the soothing parental caressing of an injured child, as ever since exemplified in the healing powers of the King's Touch, exploited in the seventeenth century by Greatrakes the Stroaker, and still sought by the emotionally immature and physically deprived avid of massage and chiropractic.

The ethereal, elevating emphasis on the spiritual—a concept as fundamental to life as is the neonate's first breath (L., *spiritus.*) Every human indeed *as*pires, is variously *in*spired, acquires an *esprit de corps,* may become *ex*asperated or *dis*pirited, and finally *ex*pires so that his immutable *spirit* can begin life anew. And here, too, the physician-priest functions in knowing the Spiritual World, purveying professed contrition and remorse to the Spirits of our Fathers, and requiring only a gratifying small tithe and penance with which to avoid the horrors of eternal punishment. Meanwhile, the temple then as now furnished a divinely protected sanctuary from earthly stresses and problems, much as Mecca and Lourdes are havens of comfort and healing today.

Finally, the priest also mediated the supreme promise of all religions—or, for that matter, of all "scientific" systems: the conquest, through life eternal, of man's most grim and implacable enemy—death itself.

These, then, were the ancient—and the eternal—practices that embody what physicians have intuitively known for centuries: that although no man can ever be certain of his health, friends, or philosophy, the illusions of security in each of these spheres are essential to his welfare; and that all methods of medical-psychiatric therapy are effective only insofar as they restore physical well-being, foster more amicable interpersonal relationships, and help the patient amend his beliefs so as to render them more generally acceptable and useful.

II. The Comparative Approach to the Essentials of Therapy

To supplement this historical survey, it would require still another five-foot shelf to review the current and equally illuminating anthropologic, ethnic, and trans-cultural studies of Gillin, Margolin, Lambo, Kiev, and Leighton, *et al.,* to cite Ziferstein's and my own comparisons of Soviet and American techniques,* or to acknowledge the contributions of other socio-psychiatrists who have sufficient breadth of interest and objectivity to investigate therapeutic practices on a global scale; moreover, it would take an integrative genius to demonstrate that all of these fall into the familiar rubrics of physical, social, and metaphysical readaptation. However, even if we do not go so far afield, perhaps a more parochial reexamination of the various modes of thought and therapy in our own culture, from colonic lavage to Christian Science, may demonstrate a similar triune efficacy. This, of course, requires an unusual willingness to concede that concepts, conjectures, cults, and conceits other than our own might be operationally equivalent or even superior to the ones we personally cherish—a challenge that few of us are willing to accept. Nevertheless, playing the role of a pre-henbane Socrates in a peripatetic dialogue with my psychiatric residents and analytic trainees, I have sometimes proposed some outrageous postulate such as: Resolved, that electroshock therapy and psychoanalysis are essentially more alike than different in their basic therapeutic actions and effects.

In the past, though not so much recently, this usually evoked a storm of protest that the two methods were manifestly incomparably different: EST was "physical," "enforced," "impersonal," "stereotyped," "rigidly conducted,"

*See *Psychiatry, East and West* (listed in the bibliography).

"suppressive," "antimnemonic." "intellectually impairing" . . . *whereas,* in diametric contrast, psychoanalysis was "psychologic," "voluntary," "exquisitely interpersonal," "flexible," "evocative," "restorative of memory," and "designed to explore the Unconscious so as to develop to the full the patient's cognitive and adaptive capacities" through "insight."

At this juncture, I occasionally pointed out that the last catechism directly begged the question inasmuch as, in the historical and comparative contexts in which I had posed the question, "insight" itself could be defined only as that transiently ecstatic state in which patient and therapist temporarily shared the same illusions as to the cause and cure of each other's difficulties. With this additional goad, some of my residents began to explore subtler dimensions of therapeutically operative similarities between electroshock and analysis, and came up with the following disconcerting symmetries:

Physical parameters: Both methods offer an escape from the mundane stresses of external reality onto a sensorially isolated bed or couch (Gk., *klinikos*) provided by society and protected by a parental surrogate for about the same total number of recumbent hours in hospital or office. Both methods also serve to disorganize current patterns of deviant behavior: EST by direct cerebral diachises followed by synaptic reorganization, analysis by semantic and symbolic alterations of concept and reaction.

Interpersonal influences: In both methods, the patient, whether "voluntarily" or by equivalent "external" pressure *selects the method of therapy and the therapist* he regards as most suitable for his needs. Reciprocally, the therapist sympathetically accepts the patient as more or less helpless and "ill," is convinced of the special validity of his own therapeutic theories and the efficacy of his techniques—and thus rounds out an operationally effective *folie à deux.*

Social parameters: In both methods, there are covert but inevitable physical, economic, legal, and other punishments for the persistence of abnormal conduct: in EST, longer incarceration, exclusion of visitors, more quasi-lethal experiences with post-shock headaches, and other ostensibly beneficent punishments; in analysis, more time, more expense, more patronizingly disillusioning "interpretations" without the privilege of effective repartee, the induction of a discomfiting "transference neurosis" (which Freud himself deplored as "an artifact of poor technique") plus the ever-present Kafka-esque threat of having an "unanalysable character disorder" *i.e.,* being labelled by the therapist as incurably obnoxious. Conversely, there are highly desirable rewards for changes in behavior more in accord with the therapist's standards as eventually sensed by the patient (the "patient compliance" of Ehrenwald): *e.g.*, after "successful" EST, expanding hospital privileges, escape from eventually resented institutionalization, and restored familial and social status; or, after analysis—at least until recently—an assumption of cryptic wisdom privy only to the initiate, acceptance in the sophisticated elite of the "thoroughly analyzed" in the suburban cocktail circuit, and for Institute trainees, official admission to and referrals from the local psychoanalytic society which, until recently, supposedly guaranteed economic plenty, high social status, and serene metapsychologic transcendence.

Mystical: In the latter sense patient and therapist in both methods join in an essentially worshipful belief either that Bini and Cerletti on the one hand or Freud on the other brought providentially inspired salvation to ailing mortals, attainable through somewhat differently prescribed rituals of suffering, expiation, enlightenment and reacquisition of metaphysical grace. Any agnostic who, at national meetings, has attended the section on electro-convulsive therapy or—usually at another hotel at a discreetly non-communicative distance—a seminar of psychoanalytic theory and therapy, will have experienced the unmistakable aura of sacerdotal devotion as well as the purportedly scientific import of both proceedings.

Similar operational parallels can, of course, be constructed, say, between vitamin therapy and "non-directive" counseling or between *Dauerschlaff* and psychodrama. Such comparisons should, of course, never obscure the specific attributes and special clinical applicabilities of each modality, but outside the bounds of reductionist sophistry, incisive comparisons may help clarify the universal factors of therapy we have been considering, to help the patient realize that his formerly cherished modes of conduct in the three spheres of physical, social, and philosophic adaptation are no longer either necessary or profitable, and to teach him by exploration and personal experience, what new ones will prove more personally pleasurable, socially advantageous, and existentially compatible.

III. Experimental Validations of the Essentials of Therapy

This brings us to our final heuristic resource: the experimental approach to the study of "normal" behavior and the treatment of its deviations. In the words of Adolf Meyer, every friend and patient can be studied as a ready-made "experiment of nature," but for more adequate controls and precise analysis, animal research becomes necessary. Since the latter aspect of biodynamics has been my especial concern for a third of a century, we may here consider, first, the relevance of animal research to psychiatric theory and therapy, next, four testable propositions as to normal and abnormal behavior, and third, significant laboratory observations and their possible clinical analogues.

Animal Behavior and Psychiatry

As to the relevance of animal research, two issues are usually phrased somewhat as follows: "Are animal experiments *really* [sic] applicable to the subjective and social complexities of human behavior?" Or, in a more subtly patronizing vein, "Must we not be careful about *anthropomorphizing* animal data and be on guard against drawing false clinical inferences?" Such questions—Darwin, Pavlov, Simpson, Tinbergen, Harlow, and heaven be thanked—are now seriously raised far less frequently than formerly, but in briefest riposte may be respectively considered thus:

Neurophysiologically, just as the human central nervous system, although manifestly more highly developed in some respects, is nevertheless of the *same basic design* as that of other chordates, so also is human conduct more responsive to complex communicative and social influences—and thereby more contingent and versatile *but not different in basic adap-*

tational patterns—than the behavior of man's somewhat less pretentious, preemptive, pompous, and pugnacious fellow-creatures.

Epistemologically, no "datum" (L., given) whether labelled "material," "experiential," "experimental," "intuitive," "existential," or whatever, is ever really presented in pristine purity by a gracious cosmos; instead, since "data" can never be more than man's incomplete, exceedingly fallible and artificially categorized perceptions of his supposed universe, terms such as "real," "objective," "subjective," "anthropomorphic" become tautologic shibboleths, meaningless to the modern logical positivist rationale of science. Possibly out of misplaced pride in their own species, some psychiatrists may continue to insist on the precious uniqueness of human neuroses, but even they may find the following studies in animals disconcertingly reminiscent not only of the developmet of individual and social conduct in man, but significant to the therapy of his neurotic and psychotic deviations. Since "science" then, is but a testing and refinement of contingent premises, can such postulates be formulated for the most complicated field of all: animal behavior?

Biodynamic Theses

I have essayed to test in our own work the following four relatively simple and parsimonious hypotheses, respectively applicable to motivation, learning, adaptability, and neurotigenesis, and operative in both animal and human conduct:

1. *Motivation:* The actions of all organisms are directed toward satisfying physiologic needs, and therefore vary with their intensity, duration and balance.

2. *Perception and response:* In seeking these fulfillments, organisms conceive of and interact with their milieu not in terms of an absolute "external reality," but in accordance with their genetic capacities, rates of maturation, and unique experiences.

3. *Range of normal adaptation:* To maintain adequate levels of satisfaction, higher animals develop a broad range of adaptive techniques by employing versatile methods of coping

with difficulties or by modifying or changing goals as necessary.

4. *Neurotigenesis:* In its original formulation, this hypothesis held that when physical inadequacies, environmental stresses, or motivational conflicts exceed an organism's innate or acquired capacities for adaptation, internal tensions (anxiety) mount, neurophysiologic (psychosomatic) dysfunctions occur, and the organism develops over-generalized patterns of avoidance (phobias), stereotyped behavior (obsessions and compulsions), aberrant conspecific and extraspecific transactions (social deviations), and regressive, hyperactive, hostile or bizarrely "dereistic" (hallucinatory, delusional) responses analogous to those in human neuroses and psychoses. I would now add that the various forms of "conflict," whether postulated as an impasse among counterposed attractions and aversions, or between mutually exclusive attractions or equally balanced fears, may be subsumed under an even broader etiologic rubric: Namely, that in each instance the organism apprehends a failure to predict and control events important to its welfare—a parameter that, to paraphrase Heisenberg, may be called the Principle of Neurotigenic Uncertainty.

These "biodynamic principles," always subject to modification by further data, have emerged from the work conducted by my associates and myself during the past three decades, as briefly reviewed here:

Ontological studies

Phases of development: Our records and films of individual animals of various species from infancy to adulthood have confirmed the thesis that their young, as Piaget and others have shown for the human, normally evolve through an orderly succession of stages during which sensory modalities are distinguished and resynthesized, *individualized* concepts of the environment are developed, manipulative skills are refined, early dependencies on parental care are relinquished in favor of exploration and mastery, and peer, sexual, and hierarchic relationships are evolved. Infants given a stimulating early milieu, opportunities for continuously nutritive and protective contacts with parents or their surrogates, and later with peers, manifest progressive self-confidence, acquire motor and social skills, and develop "group acculturations" insofar as, by trial and error, their adaptations become experientially (L. *ex-perio,* that which pierces through), more competent and secure. Conversely, these expansions of the organism's concepts of physical and social "realities" also render its choices more perplexing and fallible and thereby potentially neurotigenic.

Learning and symbolism: During this development animal young show patterns of dependency, exploration, play, fetishism (e.g., continued attachment to objects such as rubber gloves used in early feedings), "tantrumy" rebelliousness, gradually more effective adaptations, and other characteristics significantly parallel to those in human children. In this process, the parents or surrogates involved, even when the latter are not of the animal's species, impart their own traits to the adopted young. As one instance, a rhesus raised from birth in the investigator's home learned to respond sensitively and adequately to many intonations of language and patterns of human action, but never acquired some of the aversions (e.g., a fear of snakes) supposedly "innate" in rhesus monkeys raised by their own mothers.

Early deprivations: In contrast, young animals prevented from developing adaptive capacities by prolonged periods of solitary confinement, even though otherwise physically well cared for, do not develop normal initiative, physical stamina, or adequate social relationships.

Character deviance: Unusual early experiences may engram peculiar characteristics which persist through adulthood. For example, if a young animal is taught to work a switch that sends increasingly intense electric shocks through its paws as a necessary preliminary to securing food, for the rest of its life that animal, apparently to avoid the uncertainty of other modalities, may continue to seek ways of experiencing such shocks to the point of tolerance even in the absence of any other immediate reward, and may thus appear to be inexplicably "masochistic" to an observer unacquainted with its unique experiences.

Neonatal brain injuries: A remarkable finding was that adequate care and training could in large part compensate for extensive brain damage in the newborn. Monkeys subjected to the removal of both temporal or parietal cortices at birth but given a protecting and non-conflictful home environment thereafter suffered minor kinesthetic and adaptive impairments which could be revealed only by elaborate tests (e.g., variable oddity selections) or during periods of sensory deprivation, but developed otherwise adequate individual and social adjustments. On the other hand, in the absence of such special care and training, bilateral lesions in the thalami, amygdalae, or in cerebral areas thirteen, twenty-three, and twenty-four impaired adaptive capacities more seriously in young than in adult animals, and did not ameliorate experimentally induced neurotic behavior as effectively as in the case of adults.

Early "psychological" traumata: These were even more devastating: If the young animal was subjected to unpredictable or severe conflicts among counterposed desires and aversions, or placed in situations that presented disturbing uncertainties as to whether or not expected and necessary rewards would be attainable, the animal developed deeply ingrained inhibitions, fears, rituals, somatic disorders, conspecific maladjustments, and other aberrations of behavior which became highly elaborate and more difficult to treat than those originating in adulthood as described below.

Social relationships

Animal societies in the laboratory as well as in the feral state organize themselves in hierarchies of relatively dominant and submissive members, with leadership and privileges generally preempted not by size or strength alone but in accordance with special aptitudes and "personality" skills. However, these relationships could be modified in the following significant ways:

Parasitism, industrial strife, and technological solutions: Cats or monkeys could be trained to operate a switch mechanism that dropped a reward of food into a distant food box. When two conspecific animals so trained were placed together, in most pairs each would for a time alternate in working the switch while the other fed; soon, however, one would begin remaining near the food box in an attempt to subsist solely on its partner's labors. This usually occasioned a sit-down strike on the part of the worker whose rewards had been preempted, but eventually a fairly stable "worker-parasite" industrial relationship would be established in which the "worker" operated the feeder energetically and sufficiently to provide enough pellets for both. Significantly, two such workers among fourteen pairs proved to be sufficiently "intelligent" (i.e., possessed of unusually high perceptive-manipulative capacities) to jam the switch so that the feeder mechanism operated continuously, thus solving a social problem by a form of technological automation.

"Altruism": Some monkeys continued to starve for several hours—though never more than half a day or so—rather than pull a lever to secure readily available food if they perceived that this also subjected another monkey to an electric shock. Such "succoring" behavior was apparently less dependent upon the relative age, size, or sex of the two animals than on (a) their individual "character," (i.e., relatively constant patterns of presumed conceptualization and observed response) and (b) whether or not they had been "well-adjusted" cage-mates, who had developed mutually predictable and favorable interactions.

Aggression: Conversely, actual fighting between members of the same species to establish various privileges was minimal; primacy and dexterity manifested by only occasional gestures of preemption were nearly always sufficient to establish dominance and priority. Indeed, physical combat appeared only under the following special circumstances: (a) When an animal that had attained a high position in its own group was transferred to one in which it came into direct conflict with new rivals themselves accustomed to dominance, and thereby had to adapt to unaccustomed challenges. (b) Similarly, when a dominant animal was subjected to an unexpected territorial rebellion by an alliance of subdominants. (c) When a female with increased social status derived from mating with a dominant male thereafter turned on members of her group that had previously oppressed her. (d) When a dominant animal, by being made experimentally neurotic, fell to a low position in its own group and thereafter expressed its frustrations by physical attacks both on animate and inanimate objects in its environment.

Experimental neuroses and psychoses

Methods of induction: As stated in the earlier versions of the fourth biodynamic principle, marked and persistent deviations of behavior could be induced by stressing the animal between mutually incompatible attractions and aversions: as, for instance, subjecting a cat to an *unpredictable* electric shock during conditioned feeding, or requiring a monkey to secure food from a box in which, on several occasions, he had *unexpectedly* been confronted with a toy snake—an object as representationally dangerous to the monkey as a live one, harmless or not, would be. Yet counter to early Freudian doctrines of neurotigenesis, neither actual nor anticipated fear of injury need to be involved at all, since, as noted, later experiments demonstrated that equally serious and lasting neurotigenic effects could be induced by facing the animal with difficult choices among mutually exclusive satisfactions—situations that parallel the disruptive effects of prolonged indecisions among equally attractive alternatives in human affairs. More recently, Dr. Marvin Woolf and I have found that variably delayed auditory or kinesthetic feedback of the animal's own vocalization or movements also render its physical milieu unpredictable and thereby also anxiety-provoking and neurotigenic.

Finally, we have used experimental techniques that even more specifically demonstrate the devastating effects of sequential or temporal uncertainty; for example, if a monkey is taught to operate a series of switches, plus a final lever in a given order to secure food or avoid shock, and is then faced with bewildering variations in the required sequence and timing of the switches and lever, it becomes highly disturbed, refuses to feed or escape, attacks the apparatus and develops other striking aberrations of behavior as described below; significantly, these adverse reactions are minimized if, during the experiment, the confused and thereby disorganized animal is permitted to profit by the guiding example of a monkey-like automaton in an adjoining compartment programmed to work the final lever in proper order and time and thus mitigate the observing monkey's trepidations as to operation and outcome.

Any of these stresses, when they exceeded the animal's adaptive capacities, induced physiologic and mimetic manifestations of anxiety, spreading inhibitions, generalizing phobias, stereotyped rituals, "psychosomatic" dysfunctions, impaired social interaction, addiction to alcohol and other drugs (v.i.), regressions to immature patterns of behavior, and other marked and persistent deviations of conduct.*

Constitutional influences: Animals closest to man showed symptoms most nearly resembling those in human neuroses and psychoses, but in each case the syndromes induced depended less on the nature of the conflict—which could be held constant—than on the constitutional predisposition of the animal. For example, under similar stresses spider monkeys reverted to infantile dependencies or catatonic immobility, cebus developed various "psychosomatic" disturbances including functional paralyses, whereas vervets became diffusely aggressive, persisted in bizarre sexual patterns, or preferred hallucinatory satisfactions such as chewing and swallowing purely imaginary pellets while avoiding real food to the point of self-starvation.

Factors that accentuated neurotic symptomatology: Experimentally, these were precisely those that also exacerbated the loss of control over, or prevented escape from, the stressful situation: namely, an increase in either hunger or fear or forced transgression of the phobic, compulsive, or regressive patterns described above. Under such circumstances anxiety mounted to panic, inhibitions became paralyzing, and psychosomatic disturbances grew serious enough to threaten the life of the animal.

Procedures that ameliorated neurotic aberrations: It would be inaccurate to state that the choice of methods selected for investigation was not influenced by my psychiatric and psy-

*The experimental techniques and results here described are recorded in a succession of motion picture films distributed by the Psychological Cinema Register, Pennsylvania State University, Audiovisual Services, University Park, Pa. The latest of these illustrates its title, "The Neurotigenic Effects of Manipulative Unpredictability."

See as listed in the bibliography. Cf. particularly those on social interactions, experimental neuroses, effects of brain lesion, induced alcoholism, and the influence of various drugs on normal and deviant behavior.

choanalytic training and clinical experience, since certain preferences, consciously or not, undoubtedly remained operative. Nevertheless, various techniques of "therapy" were investigated as objectively as possible, of which the following, with brief mention of their possible clinical parallels, were found most effective:

1. *Satiation of one of the conflictful needs.* If a neurotic animal with marked inhibitions of feeding and spreading symbolic aversions was tube-fed, its neurotic symptoms were temporarily relieved, only to recur when the necessity and the fear of spontaneous feeding returned simultaneously.

To cite a single clinical comparison: directly or implicitly enforced sexual relations may temporarily relieve repressed erotic desires but may exacerbate symbolic conflicts generalized to other spheres of behavior. It will be recalled that such clinical complications forced Freud to abandon his early attribution of the neuroses to quasi-physiologic "toxic accumulations of repressed libido."

2. *Prolonged rest away from the neurotigenic situation.* This blunted the other horn of the dilemma by removing the animal from the original environs of conflict. It is significant that this form of relief was minimal in monkeys in which, as in the case of man, neurotic reactions quickly became generalized; moreover, animals which were returned to the laboratory even after a year of relatively peaceful sojourn elsewhere soon redeveloped their neurotic patterns, even though the original traumata were not repeated.

Clinically, "rest cures" and vacations away from disturbing situations may alleviate acute symptoms, but do not necessarily dispel the underlying and potentially disruptive tensions. Soldiers with "combat neuroses" may feel relieved when removed from immediate danger, but unless the impasse between self-preservation versus military duty is effectively resolved, exposure to any situation reminiscent of this conflict almost inevitably spells the reappearance of neurotic reactions.

3. *Forced solution.* When hunger was maximal (from one to three days of starvation), food was made particularly attractive and openly available and no escape from the temptation was possible, some neurotic animals broke through their feed-

ing or other inhibitions, began eating spontaneously, and showed gradual relief from the various neurotic symptoms originally engendered by the hunger-fear conflict. On the other hand, animals with lesser readaptive capacities, when placed in similar situations calculated to break the motivational impasse, reacted instead with an exacerbation of phobias, somatic dysfunctions, destructive aggressivity, or a retreat into a quasi-cataleptic stupor.

Thus, also, actively directing patients paralyzed by confusion and anxiety into some decisive course of action is occasionally necessary and effective, but may likewise present the danger of further bewilderment, panic, or even psychotic reactions if the predictive and adaptive capacities in space, time, and modality are seriously exceeded.

4. *Spontaneous reexploration and solution.* Animals which had been trained merely to respond to an automatic food signal and which were then subjected to a counterpoised fear of feeding remained neurotic indefinitely since, without special guidance, they had no way of reexploring the traumatic situation. Markedly different, however, was the case of animals that had been taught to manipulate various devices that actuated the signals and feeder, since in this way they could exert at least partial control over their environment. This stood them in crucial stead even after they were made neurotic inasmuch as, though for a time they feared almost every aspect of the apparatus, when their hunger increased they gradually made hesitant but spontaneous attempts to reexplore the operation of the switches, signals and food boxes, and grew bolder and more successful as food began to reappear. If the fear-engendering situations were prematurely repeated, their effects were even more traumatizing, but if each animal's efforts were again rewarded with food as in its preneurotic experiences, it eventually became, to all appearances, as confident and effective in its behavior as ever.

This, perhaps, is a paradigm of how most conflicts and uncertainties—and "larval neuroses"—are resolved in most instances by spontaneous re-exploration of the problem situation, leading to the immensely reassuring discovery that something temporarily feared either does not recur, or may be mastered if it does. Pertinent also is the necessity all of us feel for acquiring a large variety of techniques to control our environment, not only for normal living but also as a means of trial reentry after retreat or flight. Explicitly, we invoke this principle in preparing our children for a wide range of contingencies; pragmatically, we employ "occupational therapy" or "job training" in our correctional institutions and hospitals to give our patients the skills, whether major or minor, which they can later utilize to meet social challenges in the world outside. Implicitly also, a comparable process is at work in psychoanalysis as the analysand, in a protective, permissive situation, re-explores his conflictual and deeply repressed interpersonal desires and fantasies both verbally and through his transference relationship (vide infra), finds himself not punished or rejected as he had, consciously or not, feared he might be and thus, gaining confidence and aplomb, retransfers and "works through" his relationships with things and people in the real world everywhere around him.

5. *"Transference" therapy.* This leads to the question: but what about animals that had been trained to respond only to external signals and had not been taught manipulative or social skills; or if so taught, were later rendered too inhibited to use them? In such cases, it was found possible to alleviate the neurotic behavior through the more direct influence of the experimenter, who could assume the role of a reorientative trainer or "therapist." Dynamically, this influence itself was derived from the circumstance that the animal had been raised in a provident, kindly manner either in the laboratory by the experimenter himself, or elsewhere by someone who also liked animals. Indeed, if the latter were not the case, when the animal came to the laboratory the first requirement was to dispel its mistrust of human beings and to cultivate its confidence; in effect, to convert an initial "negative transference" into a "positive" one. Whenever possible, all experimenters dissociated themselves (though such disassociation was rarely complete in the case of dependent dogs or the highly perceptive monkeys) from the animal's traumatizing experience by having the latter administered either by remote control or by an automatic electrical governor on the apparatus. Signifi-

cantly, some experimenters were not able to secure this favorable relationship in normal animals, and were correspondingly unsuccessful in helping neurotic ones. In my laboratory, this was particularly true of an assistant who had himself been raised in an oriental country where cats and dogs were kept as guards or as scavengers, sometimes eaten, but almost never liked, respected, and protected.

If, however, the animal's expectancy with regard to the experimenter, based on its experience with him *or his surrogates,* became predominantly favorable ("positive transference"), that expectancy could be utilized "therapeutically" for retraining and rehabilitation, however minimal the initial steps. For example, even the most "neurotic" animal, huddled in cataleptic rigidity in a dark corner, might be led by gentle petting and coaxing to take food from the experimenter's hand. Once this initial receptivity was established, the animal might be induced to eat from the floor if the apparatus of the experimenter remained near the cage; later, it sufficed that the "therapist" was merely in the room. At any stage of this retraining premature repetition even of a faint feeding signal could reprecipitate the conflict and disrupt the animal's recovery, perhaps irrevocably. However, if the experimenter exercised gentleness and patience and did not at any time exceed the gradually regained tolerance and capacities of the animal, he could eventually induce it in successive stages to open the food box, begin again to respond to signals and manipulate switches, and thus to reassert its former skills and patterns of self-sustenance. The retraining could then be continued to include acceptance of previously traumatic stimuli, so that eventually the animals would welcome even an airblast or electric shock (though not the toy snake) as itself a harbinger of food or other rewards. After such patterns were in their turn reestablished, the therapist could complete the process by gradually withdrawing from the situation as the animal reasserted its self-sufficiency, until finally his personal ministrations or presence was no longer necessary.

To claim sweeping identities between the mechanics of these experiments and the almost incomparably more complex dynamics of clinical psychotherapy would be an obvious over-

simplification; however, certain parallels need not be overlooked. The therapist, too, is preconceived as a parental or helpful surrogate, else his aid would not be sought at all. Wishfully endowed by the patient with anticipatory concern and competence (though often this is explicitly denied), the properly trained and experienced clinician gently but effectively approaches the patient in his neurotic retreat, fills his needs personally in so far as practicable, permits him to re-explore, retest, and reevaluate experiential symbols and their disruptive conflicts, first in the protected therapeutic situation, then gradually—and never more rapidly than the patient's anxiety permits—in the outside world, and finally fosters and redirects his personal relationships onto people and activities that can play a favorable and permanent role in the patient's future. This done, the therapist may relinquish his Vergilian role of guide and mentor as the patient relinquishes his dereistic fantasies and escapist or frustrating behavior in favor of more socially adaptive and creative conduct, and thus no longer needs the psychiatrist personally except, perhaps, as another friend among a new-found many.

Words, of course, are facile but sometimes deceptive instruments of communication, and abbreviations of statement should not imply abrogations of fact; nevertheless, in a field more plagued by over-obfuscation than by over-simplification, these comparisons and parallelisms are more than merely rhetorical.

6. *"Social" therapy.* In some animals, the effectiveness of a sixth method dubbed, debatably but conveniently, "social" therapy or "therapy by example" indicated that one factor in the process of so-called transference therapy was the relatively impersonal one of making the solution of a motivational or adaptational impasse seem easier or at least possible. In this procedure, the neurotic animal was simply placed with a well-trained normal one and permitted to watch the latter work the switches and signals and then feed unharmed. After from one to several days of such observation, about half the neurotic animals would begin to approach the food box, cower less at the signals, tentatively try the switches, and finally "emulate" the normal animal in resuming effective feeding patterns.

Once the conflict was thus resolved, its other neurotic expressions were also in large part—but never completely—mitigated, and the animal, aside from minor residuals such as slight furtiveness, restlessness, or tension, appeared to be recovered.*

Though the method was simple and certainly took the least effort on the part of the experimenter, it seems most difficult to formulate theoretically, especially since the convenient fiction of a postulated "interanimal relationship" or "identification" was dispelled when, in a control series of experiments, the neurotic animal could, as noted, also be induced to resume feeding when an appropriately furred, scented, and activated automaton mechanically "answered" the signals, opened the food box, revealed the presence of tempting pellets, and otherwise changed the neurotic animal's external and internal milieu.

Perhaps, as implied previously, this is the solipsistic nidus of all "interpersonal relationships." But whatever the dynamics, we utilize such influences empirically in our clinical work. To cite but one instance, we place a neurotic child in a foster home or a special school in the hope that our young patient may be favorably influenced by the "example" of normal children being duly rewarded for patterns of behavior we wish our patient, too, to acquire. Unfortunately, psychoanalysis has long neglected group theory and practice, though these are fundamental to the development of social and community psychiatry.

7. *Employing electroshock or other methods of producing cerebral anoxia and diaschisis* to disintegrate the neural basis of conflictful conceptualizations and their disruptive and regressive effects on behavior—*a method that may be utilized in human depressions, although never without some impairment, however subtle, of future capacities.*

8. *Performing various brain operations* to induce similar neuropsychologic disorganization; in monkeys, lesions corresponding to cortical areas twelve, twenty-three, and twenty-four were, as noted, most suitable for this purpose. However,

*Illustrated in the films on delayed closure and exemplification of behavior in monkeys; cf. Bibliography, F30. and F35.

our work in this field indicated that the after-effects of any brain operation depended less on its site and extent than on the preceding experiences and resultant characteristics of the operated subjects. For example, our early neurobehavioral studies demonstrated that the hypothalamus does *not* "originate motivation" or is "a center for the experience of affect." At higher diencephalic levels, bilateral lesions of the dorsomedial thalamic nucleus impaired the learning capacities of a normal animal but left it gentle and tractable, whereas the same operation rendered an animal, previously made experimentally neurotic, irritable and vicious.

9. Finally, *various drugs could also be used for the temporary disorganization of disturbing perceptions and conflictful reactions,* thus facilitating other methods of therapy. Additional pharmacologic observations were as follows: (a) Effectiveness: Most of the commercially promoted "tranquillizers" (meprobamates and phenothiazines) were less generally effective than drugs long tested in clinical therapy; e.g., alcohol, paraldehyde, and the barbiturates and bromides. (b) Preventive action: the latter drugs, if administered in mildly obtunding doses *before* subjecting an animal to stress or conflict, would also partially prevent the after-effect of an otherwise traumatic experience.

By analogy humans, too, are apt to take an alcoholic "bracer" or a trusted "tranquillizer" to narrow the conceptual field of threatening possibilities before asking for a raise, proposing marriage or contemplating some other potentially hazardous undertaking. (c) Addiction: However, a neurotic animal permitted to experience the partial relief from inhibition produced by alcohol would learn to prefer alcohol to nonalcoholic food and drink, and thus develop a "dipsomania" which would persist until its underlying neurosis was relieved by other means.*

In man, similar psychopharmacologic effects of addictive drugs are demonstrably operative but are, of course, com-

*The experiments recorded in my motion picture film, "Neurosis and Alcohol," distributed by the Psychological Cinema Register, State University, Pennsylvania, have recently been confirmed at the University of Vienna and re-recorded in color and sound in a clinical film on Alcoholism by the Pfizer Pharmaceutical Co., Newark, N.J.

plicated by highly individualized ethnic and culturally symbolic influences.

In and Out of the Laboratory

These observations added to those of Sechenov, Pavlov, Gantt, Delgado, Skinner, Mirsky, Brady, and many others cited in my previous reviews of the literature, may have helped to clarify basic issues relevant to both "normal" and "deviant" behavior; however, since man's perceptive, mnemonic, symbolic, and adaptive capacities are undeniably much (though not by necessity "infinitely" or "by quantum jumps") more complex than those of any other animal, it is obvious that ethologic or experimental studies alone cannot furnish data that completely "explain" human conduct. As already indicated, man seems to differ from all other animals in having developed three ultimate (*Ur-*) axioms, beliefs, assumptions, aspirations, categorical imperatives—no term quite expresses their ubiquitous dynamics—that are indeed uniquely immanent in human motivations and transactions. In briefest form we may review them once more as follows:

First, an urgent seeking for the knowledge and technology with which to control the material universe and, hopefully, conquer disease and death.

Second, a persistent need for human relationships that, despite debacles of distrust, have led from the primal mother-child dyad, through loyalties to the family, clan, tribe, state, and nation, to a growing imperative toward the brotherhood of man.

And finally, an existential faith that man's being has an enduring dignity and significance in some universal teleologic, theologic, or eschatologic system that extends beyond the here-and-now into eternity.*

*In this (*Ur-*) context, the animal analogs of our modes of psychiatric therapy may be correspondingly regrouped as follows: *Physical:* Gratification of somatic needs, relief of stress, pressure to adapt, reassertion of skills, and the use of drugs, electroshock or other cerebral alternatives (experimental methods 1,2,3,4,7,8 and 9). *Social:* Dyadic retraining or conspecific group rehabilitation (experimental methods 5 and 6). *Metaphysical-Existential:* Implicit in a primal joy in life, or a dog's faith in, and devotion to, its glorified human Master.

Applications to Clinical Therapy

Here enters a disconcerting thought that, despite Heraclitus' doctrine of external change to the effect that "No man can step into the same stream twice," perhaps all I have said has merely been a redevelopment of ancient wisdoms. We have always implicitly known that, although *no sentient human can ever be completely certain of his health, friends or philosophy,* adequate modicums of security in each of these spheres are essential to his welfare; consequently, all methods of medico-psychologic therapy have been effective only insofar as they restored physical well-being, fostered more amicable interpersonal relationships, and helped parochial man amend his beliefs so as to render them more locally acceptable and useful without stultifying his individuality, infringing on his essential freedoms, or stereotyping his intellect, imagery and creativity.

How, then, can these broader genetic-physiologic-ethnic-cultural (i.e., *biodynamic*) orientations serve to modify some of the more narrow and stultified therapeutic rituals of our recent past? Let us restate more specifically the fundamental uncertainties for which patients seek our succoring and reassuring services (*therapies*).

Ur-need I. Since physical well-being is primary, regardless of whether the patient's complaints are considered as "organic," "psychosomatic," or "neurotic," his bodily discomforts and dysfunctions should be ameliorated by every medical and surgical means available. Psychopharmacologically, conservatively prescribed and frequently changed sedatives and hypnotics can be used to dull painful memories, diminish apprehension and quiet agitation; for these purposes I continue to find, clinically as well as experimentally, that the barbiturates, bromides, aldehydes, and other well-tested drugs will in many cases be found preferable to some of the widely promoted but dubiously effective "ataractics" and "tranquillizers." Our first concern, then, should be to restore our patient's physical comfort, zest, and joy in living.

Ur-objective II. But since no man is "an Island intire of itselfe," the compleat therapist, whatever his "specialty," must also recognize that his patient may be deeply concerned about marital, sexual, career, and related interpersonal problems. As outlined in Chapter 15, this requires an exploration, always discerning and tactful rather than unnecessarily disruptive and prolonged, of the patient's characterologic assets and vulnerabilities, the attitudes, values, and incentives he has derived from his life experiences, the channelling effects of former successes or the disruptive remains of past and current tribulations, the residues they left in patterns of effective (normal), culturally ineffective (neurotic), or bizarrely disruptive (psychotic) conduct, the ways in which he presumes that these patterns relieve or exacerbate his present difficulties, and which of them are most accessible to various methods of inclusive biodynamic therapy. It is customary here for the psychiatrist or psychoanalyst to warn everyone else off his esoteric preserves; instead, let me confess that it has been my gratifying experience that in many instances other properly trained, sensitive and dedicated therapists can, with medical consultation when indicated, conduct the essential psychotherapy required. In brief, this will consist of using gentle reasoning, personal and group examples, and progressively reorientative experiences to help the patient reexamine and correct his prejudices and misconceptions, abandon infantile or child-like patterns of behavior that have long since lost their effectiveness, revise his values and objectives, restore his initiative, recultivate his occupational, socio-cultural and creative skills, acquire new ones, and in general adopt a more realistic, productive, and lastingly rewarding ("mature") style of life. In this skillfully guided reeducation, the enlightened cooperation of the patient's family, friends, employer or others may, with his consent, be secured and utilized to the full. By such means, his interpersonal readjustments will be strengthened by renewed communal solidarity and security—a *sine qua non* of comprehensive treatment.

Ur-need III. Lastly, to mitigate the third or cosmic *Ur*-anxiety, the patient's religious, philosophic or other convictions, instead of being deprecated and undermined, should be respected and strengthened insofar as they furnish him with what each of us requires: a belief in life's purpose, meaning, and value. In this sense, medicine, being a humanitarian science, can never be in conflict with philosophy or religion, since all three seem to be designed by a beneficent providence to preserve, cheer, and comfort man, and thereby constitute a trinity to be respected by any physician deeply concerned with man's health and sanity. Indeed, with respect to these latter concepts, it is of historic-philologic significance that the term *sanatos* implied to the ancients the indissolubility of physical and mental functions (*mens sana in corpore sano*) and that the very word "health" can be traced to the Anglo-Saxon root *hal* or *hol,* from which are derived not only physical *haleness* and *healing,* but the greeting, *"Hail, friend!"* and the concepts of *wholeness* and *holiness.* Ergo, once again Greek, Roman, and Gaul have bequeathed to us, in the rich heritage of our syncretic language in which wish and "reality" merge, their penetrating recognition of the indissoluble physical, social, and philosophic components of comprehensive therapy.

Implicit in this also is a subtle and profound insight, namely that we cannot and need not ever abolish man's ever-precious "delusions." Instead—and only when necessary for his own and society's welfare—we must help him gently to evolve culturally compatible convictions and more creative applications of them. In effect, as man's physicians, we must transcend the more simplistic concepts of various biologic, reflexologic behavior and early analytic theories in order to deal adequately with that most intricately constituted, sensitively reactive, and complexly vulnerable of living creatures—man in his physical, social, and philosophic milieu. The wise psychiatrist and psychoanalyst therefore soon learns—along with the devoted teacher and the good minister—that the essence of therapy is to help troubled men rebuild, largely on their own terms, their confidences in themselves, in their fellow men, and in their wishfully conceived "scientific" and religious systems. As mortal therapists, we can do no more.

22. THE SEARCH FOR CERTAINTY

But what about human esthetics, goals, inspirations?

It has sometimes been said that there are two types of human beings—one of which presumes to believe that there *are* two types of human beings. For example, C. P. Snow dichotomized men according to their contrasting values—and thereby their differing life interests—as *either* physico-mathematicians *or* humanists, and inferred that these "two cultures" may indeed meet, but rarely blend. In dialectic opposition, we have seen that *every* man, whether or not he has scientific or humanistic pretensions, cherishes the *same Ur*-values, here ultimately reviewed as his basic needs for health, skill, and longevity so that he may explore and control his material milieu; his deep desires for human friendships to ameliorate his tragic loneliness and cement his communal welfare, and his search for the significance of his existence in relation to some cosmic or religious system.

We may now develop contrapuntally these triple themes by showing:

1. That the "physical sciences" too, have evolved from primitive "materialism" toward an acceptance of these humanistic longings.

2. That, on the other hand, the "humanities," by a more

adroit use of Occam's razor, *entia non sunt multiplicanda praeter necessitatem,* can correlate their sometimes polyglot and protean concepts with these more simple and generalized formulae. Let us, therefore, first attempt a brief non-mathematical excursion into the psychological aspects of theoretical physics to indicate that, even in this esoteric field, we never relinquish the familiar sphere of human values, their therapeutic import, and their significance for the future of mankind.

The value of a wave-particle

Twenty-three centuries ago, Democritus, with classic confidence, wrote, "Sweet and bitter, cold and warm, as well as all the colors . . . exist but in opinion and not in reality; yet, reflecting man's eternal search for physical certainty." Democritus added, "What really exists are unchangeable particles, atoms, and their motions in empty space." Galileo, too, postulated a solid physical substrate for the subjectivity of color, taste, smell, sound, touch, and pain; so also, Locke, while admitting the evanescence of such "secondary sensations," once more insisted on an external reality in which "shape, motion, and solidity were primary qualities inherent in the object itself." The German mathematician Leibniz likewise maintained the eternity of his "monads" but began the modern return to subjectivism thus: "I am able to prove that not only light, color, heat and the like, but motion, shape, and extension, too, are merely apparent qualitics." Then despite the mysterious ubiquity of Planck's constant *h,* quantum physics glimpsed our ultimate uncertainties which, according to Barnett*

> ". . . demolished two pillars of the old science, causality and determinism. For by dealing in terms of statistics and probabilities, it abandons all idea that nature exhibits an inexorable sequence of cause and effect . . . and the hope that science . . . can forecast the history of the universe."

With this, other tangibles of sense and sequence likewise disappeared; again, to quote Barnett:

* *The Universe and Dr. Einstein,* ed. by L. Barnett. New York: Mentor, 1954.

> "A scientist can do no more than report his observations. And so if he performs two experiments with different instruments and one seems to reveal that light is made up of particles and the other that light is made up of waves, he must accept both results, regarding them not as contradictory but as complementary. By itself neither concept suffices to explain light, but together they do. Both are necessary to describe reality, and it is meaningless to ask which is really true. For in the abstract lexicon of quantum physics there is no such word as reality . . . It is futile, moreover, to hope that the invention of more delicate tools may enable man to penetrate much farther into the microcosm. There is an indeterminacy about all the events of the atomic universe which refinements of measurement and observation can never dispel."

And James Jeans admitted that theoretical physics led even further into affective solipsism by acknowledging that "It is probably as meaningless to discuss how much room an electron takes up as it is to discuss how much room a fear, an anxiety, or an uncertainty takes up."

Thus vanished "external reality." Yet precisely because man could not withstand the anxiety of a world in which objectivity and certainty were thus made ever asymptotic, nebulous, and unattainable, he continued to place a high value on the concept of formulated predictability. Einstein himself, in aspiring to a Unified Field Theory, wrote: "The ground aim of all science(s) is to cover the greatest number of empirical facts by logical deductions from the smallest possible number of hypotheses or axioms."

Einstein, however, was always explicit as to the inescapable anthropocentricity of both "fact" and "value": ". . . concepts are free creations of the human mind and are not, however it may seem, uniquely determined by the external world." Alfred North Whitehead put it more poetically: "Nature gets credit which in truth should be reserved for ourselves: the rose for its scent, the nightingale for his song, and the sun for its radiance. The poets are entirely mistaken . . . Nature is a dull affair, soundless, scentless, colorless; merely the hurrying of material, endlessly, meaninglessly." Freud, too, discerningly commented in an early discussion of the Vienna Psychoanalytic Society: "Our understanding reaches (only) as far as our anthropomorphism." So also Heisenberg, despite his exquisite demonstrations of the mathematical ineffability of "ultimate substance" (as extended recently to all epistemology by Godel) cherished the fact that the cerebral equations of quantum physics yield probabilities far more reliable (as witness gross thermo-nuclear reactions) than any arcane physical model such as a "wave-particle."

A curious by-product of these psychologic considerations was the revivification among physicists of the concept of free will. To quote Barnett once more: "A wave electron, a proton, a wave of probability, cannot be visualized; they are simply symbols useful in expressing the mathematical relationship of the microcosm. [But] if physical events are indeterminate and the future is unpredictable, then perhaps the unknown quantity called 'mind' may yet guide man's destiny among the infinite uncertainties of a capricious universe."

The Ur-faith in common endeavor

With materialistic certainty thus negated, man understandably sought a second *Ur*-defense against his primal anxieties: namely, alliance with his fellows for comfort and security —but unfortunately, again with only equivocal success. It has been said in diverse ways that we still live in an age when one must call his neighbor "friend", yet *act* as though he were a rival and perhaps an enemy; or, in cultural-evolutionary terms, the anthropologists in their search for the missing link between anthropoid apes and civilized man, have discovered it in *us*.

And yet man continues to long for human fellowship, both by historical loyalties to his predecessors and by improved communications and accords with his compatriots across space and culture. In the advance of knowledge, there is no better example of this than the communal endeavors of nearly all scientists themselves for the general enlightenment of mankind. Medieval scholars and "naturalists" increasingly acknowledged their common debts to the classical Greeks. In physics, Newton attributed his broadened perspectives to "standing on the shoulders of giants," and Einstein derived the inspiration for his General Theory of Relativity from the revolutionary experiments of Michelson and Morley and from the Lorentz Transformations. In ecology and economics, Malthus, Marx, Engels, Lenin, *et al.*, extrapolating Plato, Hobbes, and Machiavelli, proposed that by regulating man's power struggles, they could achieve earthly Utopias. Immanuel Kant preserved the values of individual will and freedom but included the categorical imperative of social commitment by insisting that each human must act in ways that could be "generalized as norms for all mankind." Bronowski (1956) added the semanticist's touch: "Sentences constructed with *is* usually have a verifiable meaning, but sentences constructed with *ought* never have . . . [but if man] accepts no evidence and no judgment except his own, he has no tools with which to frame an answer." Bentley Glass came even closer to the basic humanistic sources and values of all science: "By examining critically the nature, origins, and methods of science we logically arrive at a conclusion that science is ineluctably involved in questions of values, is inescapably committed to standards of right and wrong and unavoidably moves . . . toward social aims . . . Man's own values grew out of his evolutionary origins and his struggle against a hostile environment for survival. Our highest ethical values—the love of the mother for her child and the man for his mate, and the willingness to sacrifice one's own life for the safety of the family or tribe, and the impulse to care for the weak, the suffering, the helpless—all of these, too, had the same primitive beginnings . . . [The] primary function of science is not simply that of appeasing the individual scientist's curiosity about his environment—on the contrary, it is that of adjusting man to man . . . Somehow there has crept into our writings . . . that science is 'objective' while the humanistic studies are 'subjective.' What a profound mistake! . . . The scientist is a man, through his science doing good and evil to other men, and (deservedly) receiving from them blame and praise."

In our own field, we honor the medical *montagnards,* miracle-workers, and martyrs for whose cooperative and cumulative work humanity can be eternally grateful; indeed, physicians and psychiatrists, being both scientists and humanitarians, can thus especially well understand how inextricably fused are the respective values in both fields.

The Ur-faith of existential meaning

However, mundane knowledge and mortal alliances—the first two *Ur*-defenses—still could not adequately resolve the agonizing anxieties of individual existence and cosmic significance; ergo, men of all "cultures" have always resorted either to various forms of narcissistic self-sufficiency, or to their projections into transcendent systems variously labelled philosophies, cosmologies, or religions. As to the first or introspective mode of this third *Ur*-defense, nearly two dozen centuries before Husserl or Camus, Plato wrote: "The true lover of knowledge is always striving after *Being* . . . he will not rest at those multitudinous phenomena whose existence is appearance only."

Projecting homocentrism to the astronomic sphere, Kepler and Copernicus believed that the very stars were intimately concerned with mortal man, and that, therefore, his dealings with his fellows were astrologically written and predictable. But since the stars themselves were presumably but the puppets of God, Bishop Berkeley thus brought man into contact with Divinity:

"All the choir of heaven and furniture of earth, in a word, all those bodies which compose the mighty frame of the world, have not any substance without the Mind . . . so long as they are not actually perceived by me, or do not exist in my mind, or that of any other created spirit, they must either have no existence at all, or else subsist in the mind of some Eternal Spirit."

In an even more frankly anthropomorphic vein, we may recall that Eddington conceived of God as a "master mathematician" in the image of Eddington, whereas in a poignant extension of dyadic devotion, the encyclopedist Auguste Comte, who had founded the formal science of sociology, spent the last year of his life as the high priest of a religion which worshipped his dead wife Clothilde as the Queen of

Heaven. But perhaps it was Einstein, superb scientist, humble humanist, and profound philosopher, who put man's third Ur-faith most eloquently:

"I cannot believe that God plays dice with the world . . . The most beautiful and most profound emotion we can experience is the sensation of the mystical. It is the sower of all true science. He to whom this emotion is a stranger, who can no longer wonder and stand rapt in awe, is as good as dead. To know that what is impenetrable to us really exists, manifesting itself as the highest wisdom and the most radiant beauty which our dull faculties can comprehend only in their most primitive forms—this knowledge, this feeling is at the center of true religiousness."*

History teaches that history cannot teach us; and yet . . .

With so many consistencies between past and present, can we also extrapolate the values of the future? Let us again group tentative predictions about man's behavior around our now familiar *Ur*-trilogy.

Ur-preservation in the future: Despite the perennial legends of Pandora, Golem, Frankenstein, et al. in almost every mythology—and the knowledge that we now have at hand enough nuclear explosives to kill every human on earth ten times over, I doubt—I *must* doubt—that our race is really hell-bent on suicide. Rather, we shall discover dimensions and forces yet unconceived; we shall distill the ocean and dessicate its fish for tasteless food; we shall conquer cancer and induce new diseases; we shall explore the planets and find them cold corpses or incendiary infernos; in short, we shall continue to match our puny technologies against a universe ever beyond man's finite ken or control—and probably be only a very little less bewildered by the endless cosmos than ever.

Ur-society in the future: A world community is the only alternative to Armageddon, and since *Homo sapiens* is a single, universally fecund species, differences of "race" or "color" will eventually become about as distinguishable as Lombard, Hittite, or Etruscan strains now are in their Mediterranean de-

**Albert Einstein, Philosopher-Scientist,* ed. by Paul A. Schelpp. New York: Library of Living Philosophers, 1949.

scendants. Men will become more alike—and perhaps a little friendlier.

Ur-theology of the future: Finally, we shall develop a deeper sense of cosmic existence that will transcend the symbolic legends, rituals, and theocracies of our current religions further than they have progressed from the animistic worship of our savage ancestors. And when man achieves this breadth of vision and depth of understanding, he may also become humbler, kinder, wiser—and perhaps a bit happier. Amen.

EPILOGUE

This has been a curious year.

Here I sit again at my desk at the Center for Advanced Study in the Behavioral Sciences, once more gazing reflectively at distant San Francisco Bay as my hi-fi copes inadequately with Mahler's *Resurrection Symphony.* The surrounding mountains, sere with arid autumn when I began this odd odyssey, are now emblazoned with oestral emerald, and my desk, also cleared of the fallen quarto leaves of yesteryear, is bright with the sunshine of spring. What reflections on the winter's writings, now neatly entombed in a thousand double-spaced pages stacked neatly before me?

A few questions arise: Are my reminiscences elusive, overrationalized, ritualized? Have I done no more than hint shyly at the doubts, disappointments, and occasional depths of despair that have adumbrated my life? True, I alluded, however indirectly, to the social and sexual frustrations of an isolated and overtaxed adolescence, to the ever-present dread of renal invalidism and death that hung over my twenties, to the ineradicable remorse that followed Jeannette's passing, to my academic disillusionments at Wayne and Stanford, and to the harrowing misgivings I experienced when previously trusted friends or mentors seem to turn, however transiently, against me. But I have avoided almost all mention of a disastrous two-year marriage to a vixen social worker named Doris during my Alexanderian analysis; nor have I dealt even indirectly with the occasionally dramatic vicissitudes of twenty-seven conjugal years with the haughtily spirited, highly intelligent Christine McGuire who, as my constant companion almost everywhere, has been considered by many to be the perfect epitome of personal and professional helpmate—and who, on her own account, has achieved worldwide academic status for her research in medical education. For example when, in 1965, she was invited to teach at the University of Durban, it took her prospective hosts a fortnight to discover that I was her husband and to invite me also to present a series of lectures in South Africa. We are still remarkably happy, and perhaps here as elsewhere biographic ecdysis should stop before stripping away the ultimate coverings of privacy.

As to the rest, I have immodestly recorded that I attained various academic heights, that I was simultaneously elected president of three national scientific societies, and that the coveted Lasker Award for Scientific Research hangs inconspiciously in my study. I have written ten books, edited thirty, and crowded the literature (cf. Appendix) with about twenty-score more research reports, reviews and recondite reflections—averaging, heaven forgive, one publication about every seven weeks since I left kindergarten. And yet I must admit that, transcending all these transient triumphs, more memorable moments of exhilaration occurred at times such as these:

When my first composition, a romantic fantasia in simple harmony, was played at my graduation exercises by the high school orchestra with myself as concert master.

When I was conceded a draw by United States Chess Champion George Baker when he was playing twelve others concurrently in a college exhibition match.

When for the first time I navigated my own leaky little sloop through the Golden Gate, moored it to a Pacific entrance buoy (not knowing it was locally contrary to maritime regulations to do so) and then sailed it back on flood tide to the San Francisco Yacht Basin.

When, after making an obviously incredible hole-in-one at

a private golf club, I had sufficient presence of mind to remark casually to the gaping foursome who had let me play through, "Goodness, I almost missed that!"

When, after months of collaborating with marine designer and builder Elmer Olson and working personally as mechanic, carpenter, welder, electrician, and upholsterer on her hull, we launched our 32-foot steel yawl and christened her "Naiad, Nymph of the Lakes."

When Robert Kagan, the Chicago connoisseur of fine instruments, glowingly approved my selection of a silver-voiced 1709 Albani violin in preference to a more prestigious but less eloquent Stradivarius, and then secured for me a superb 1712 Albani viola so that I could be the proud—and undeserving—possessor of the only two perfectly matched Albanis in the world.

(Later, friend Kagan arranged for me to play the Albani viola in a string quartet with David Oistrakh, and Al Lipton included me in a similarly incredible ensemble with Eric Friedman, pupil of, and probable successor to, Jascha Heifetz.)

When, on my sixtieth birthday, a surprise party arranged by Christine and my eternal friend Lester Rudy was attended by over three hundred colleagues and former students, many of whom had travelled hundreds of miles to be on hand to present me with a magnificently bound volume of personal testimonials.

When, during a recent invitational lecture as Roche Visiting Professor to the universities of Australia and New Zealand, a prominent psychiatrist who was also a firm believer in native Maori lore showed me, in great confidence, an ancient jade sword sacred to the Supreme Deity Kane, the Earth-Mother Papa, and the Sea God Tangaros. My host explained, with complete sincerity, that this priceless object was so charged with *tapu* (mystic power for both good and evil) that ever since it had been brought to New Zealand by intrepid Maori seafarers in 1050 it could be possessed only by the greatest chiefs, whereas lesser men who had dared to preempt it had either died violent deaths or committed suicide; so also, an airplane in which a collector-purchaser had tried to export it had promptly crashed on take-off, killing its unqualified and therefore highly transient owner. At this point my new-found friend, again in all solemnity, showed me how to wield the sword in a secret ritual—a procedure he now considered safe because he had concluded from observing me that I possessed sufficient *mana* (thaumaturgic knowledge, prestige, and potency) to withstand its evil *tapu* and instead increase my own longevity and power. My host (and I repeat, he is internationally respected as a psychiatrist and ethnologist) also told me about a patient of his, a robust Maori girl who, having been told by her tribal seer that she would die two hours after delivering her first child, expired promptly on schedule despite the best of specialized hospital care throughout which all her clinical and laboratory findings had remained normal; moreover, autopsy had revealed no cause of death. I did not ask why he had not published this and other such clinical observations; I knew he thought me among the few sufficiently empathetic to believe him whether or not he had had expert witnesses (in this case, both an internist and an obstetrician were in continuous attendance) to confirm observations he did not dare report formally to a predictably unbelieving scientific audience.

And finally when, on my sixty-fourth birthday, I was permitted to fulfill another life-long ambition by soloing a light plane over the California mountains to qualify for a private pilot's license.

But how many more of such highlights can I anticipate as the road narrows, speed slackens, and sunset approaches? I still golf, fly, and sail, but tennis singles are about over. The Albanis are cherished possessions, but hardly any longer instruments of virtuosity. Convinced that younger men can better serve, I have retired from my departmental administrative duties at Northwestern, and from other executive responsibilities in various national, state and municipal bodies other than a four-year term as president of the International Association for Social Psychiatry. My role in the American Psychiatric Association is now confined to the chairmanship of the Committee on Transcultural Psychiatry and to perennial mentorship of the Arts and Humanities Sessions. I rarely attend a meeting of the American Psychoanalytic (and then only as an amused observer); and in the Academy of Psychoanalysis I remain active only as editor of its semi-annual *Science and Psychoanalysis* series. On my desk at this moment are bids to lecture again in the USSR, Bulgaria, Hungary, Greece, Israel, Argentina, Colombia, and Ireland—but what have I left to say? I could make more explicit my most sweeping inferences that all basic anxieties and their attendant deviations of behavior spring from what may be variously conceived as unpredictable and uncontrollable threats to one's physical, social, or philosophic securities—but should that not have been always obvious?

For thirty years I have tried to define "biodynamics" (never conceptually capitalized), as merely a term applicable to attempts to correlate and integrate the historical, comparative, investigative, and clinical data of behavior, whereas the term "school," in the sense of medieval scholasticism, should more appropriately be applied to the unidirectional dartings of aggregations of fish than to the individualized thought and behavior of scientists. Can I, then, really appreciate the whimsey that among the sections on Freud, Horney, Sullivan, et al., in most recent textbooks of psychiatry or psychology there now appears a separate chapter headed "The Masserman School of Biodynamics"? Freud is said to have remarked that he deplored being called a doctrinal Freudian; am I, at whatever lesser level, also to leave so misinterpreted a heritage?

But perhaps I can take comfort in another empathetic aphorism: Adolf Meyer's dictum that one's happiness does not depend on what one possesses, but rather on the ratio of what one has to what one wants. In that sense, during most of my life I have been given *almost* as much as I wanted, and have therefore been *relatively* content. And since my remaining wants seem moderate: for the pleasant sights, sounds, and sensations with which the world still serendipitously abounds, for the companionship of old and ever new friends, and for what remaining time there may be for wider learning and more leisurely creativity—perhaps I may have still a few more years of tranquil appreciation. Selah.

CURRICULUM VITAE

BIRTH:

March 10th, Chudnov, Poland.	1905
Emigrated	1910

EDUCATION:

Sandusky College of Pharmacy	1922
Pre-Medical: Wayne University, Detroit	1923–26
Wayne University School of Medicine, M.B., 1930, M.D.	1931
Internship: San Diego County General Hospital	1930–31
Residencies: Stanford University, in Neurology	1931–32
Baltimore Psychopathic Hospitals, and Clinical Assistant in Psychiatry, the Johns Hopkins University Hospitals	1932–35
University of Chicago Psychiatric Clinics	1935–46

PSYCHOANALYTIC TRAINING:

Rockefeller Fellow, Chicago Institute for Psychoanalysis	1936–1940
Certified in analysis and member of the Chicago, American and International Psychoanalytic Associations	1940
Founding Fellow of the American Academy of Psychoanalysis	1957

SOCIETIES:

American Medical Association, American Psychiatric Association (Program Chairman, 1962-65; Member of Council, 1965-68; Chairman, Committee on Transcultural Psychiatry, 1969), American Board of Psychiatry and Neurology (Diplomate 1939), Chicago Neurological Society, Society for Research in Psychosomatic Problems (Executive Councillor, 1943-46), Illinois Society for Personality Study (President, 1945-47), Illinois Psychiatric Society (President, 1952), Assn. for Research in Nervous and Mental Diseases, Society for Psychoanalytic Medicine (New York), Illinois Society for Mental Hygiene, American Society for Group Therapy (President, 1957), Society for Biological Psychiatry (President, 1958), American Academy of Psychoanalysis (President, 1959), International Association for Social Psychiatry (President, 1969-73)

WAR SERVICE:

Chairman, Morale Advisory Council; Chicago O.C.D., Special Psychiatric Advisor, Illinois Selective Service Sys-

tem, Psychiatric Instructor to Military Personnel, 6th Army District	1942–45

RELIGIOUS AFFILIATIONS:

Special Consultant to: Board of Foreign Missions, United Lutheran Church in America, Methodist Associated Medical Missions, Board of the United Christian Missionary Society

EDITORIAL:

Senior Editor, Grune and Stratton; *Progress in Psychotherapy*	1958–60
Associate Editor, *Psychosomatics*	1959–
Editor, *Biological Psychiatry*	1957–
Editor, *Science and Psychoanalysis*	Annually from 1957–
Editor, *Current Psychiatric Therapies*	Annually from 1961–
JAMA and other professional journals; book and motion picture reviews	
Editorial Advisory Board, International Mental Health Research *Newsletter*	1961
Consulting Editor, *British & International Journals of Social Psychiatry*	1964–
APA Psychiatric News	1965–
Music Therapy	1964–
Transcultural Psychiatry	1960–
Int. J. Group Tensions	1969–

ACADEMIC APPOINTMENTS:

University of Chicago: Full-time instructor to Assistant Professor and Research Associate at Otto Sprague Institute	1937–46

Northwestern University Medical: Assistant, then Associate Professor of Psychiatry & Neurology	1946
Professor and Co-Chairman of Psychiatry	1952–
Director of Education, then Senior Consultant, Illinois State Psychiatric Institute, Chicago	1959–65
Honorary Professor, National College of Education	1969

AWARDS AND HONORS:

Phi Lambda Kappa National Award in Pathology	1929
Sigma Xi	1931
Presidential Award for Selective Service	1946
Lasker Award for Research in Mental Hygiene, with Citation: "for outstanding contribution to advancement of mental health through experimental investigation on the field of behavior deviation."	1946
Various other awards including the G. Lyman Duff Honorary Lecturer, McGill University; Karen Horney Lecturer, New York; Camp Memorial Lecturer, Chicago; Canadian Medical and Canadian Psychiatric Associations; Honorary Lecturer, Roche Lecturer to Australia and New Zealand; Argentine Psychosomatic Society	1950–69
Fellow, Center for the Advanced Study of the Behavioral Sciences	1968–69
Wayne Distinguished Alumnus	1969

OTHER APPOINTMENTS:

Scientific Director, National Foundation for Psychiatric Research	1947–
Senior Consultant in Psychiatry, VA Hospital, Downey, Ill.; U. S. Naval Hospital, Great Lakes, Ill.	1947–
Consultant in Neuropsychiatry to Secretariat of the UN World Health Organization, Geneva, Switzerland	1951–
Member (appointed by Governor Kerner) of the Illinois State Research and Training Authority (1957); Vice-Chairman (1957-1965); Chairman (1965-69)	1957–
Councillor, Hunter College, New York	1950–
Executive Councillor, Youth for Tomorrow	1961–
Medical Advisory Councillor, Center for Psychotherapy, N.Y.	1963–
Annual Professorial Lecturer, NY Postgraduate School of Psychiatry, St. Luke's Hosp., St. Vincent's Hosp., NY	1955–
Program Chairman, American Psychiatric Association,	1962–65
Chairman, Advisory Council, National Assn. for Music. Therapy	1964–
Research Advisory Board, Institute for the Study of Drug Addiction	1963–
Chairman, Council of Stone-Brandel Mental Health Center	1966–
Chicago Council on Mental Health (chairman)	1965–68
National Advisory Council of State Depts. of Mental Health	1965–

LECTURES AND APPOINTMENTS ABROAD

West European Lectures and Seminars: Conducted under the auspices of the World Health Organization of the United Nations. Talks and seminars in England, France, Denmark, Finland, Sweden, Norway, Germany, Switzerland, and Italy; the universities of Oxford, Cambridge, London, Sorbonne, Helsinki, Copenhagen, Stockholm, Oslo, Bergen Zurich, Heidelberg, and Rome; the Royal Society of Medicine, the British, Swedish, French and Italian Psychoanalytic Societies; and lectures and seminars before the Swedish Medical Assembly, the Swedish Psychiatric Society and the West German Medical Society and Psychiatric Society. 1951

South American Lectures and Seminars: Invitational and Auspices of the State Department; lectures at universities and medical, psychiatric and psychoanalytic societies in Brazil, Uruguay, Argentina, Chile, Peru, Venezuela, Panama and Costa Rica. 1955–56

East European Lectures and Seminars: Invitational and auspices of the WMHO at the First Czechoslovak International Congress at Jesenik, and at universities and psychiatric and psychoanalytic societies in Austria, Yugoslavia, and Greece. 1958

International Congress on Peace and Democracy: Represented American Psychiatry at conference in Athens, November 11-18 1961

Official representative of the American

Psychiatric Assn., the Academy of Psychoanalysis and the U.S. State Department in invitational lecture tour to Japan, Hong Kong, Bangkok, New Delhi, Israel, Cypress, Lebanon, Turkey, Bulgaria, Romania, Hungary, and Poland.	1963
Invitational Lecturer and Official Representative of the APA and AP to South Africa, Kenya, Ethiopia and Egypt	1964
Program chairman, Joint Meeting of the APA and the Royal Medico-Psychologic Association, Edinburgh, Scotland and Program Chairman, Joint Meeting in Madrid, Spain	1965–66
Honorary President, Psychosomatic Congress, Buenos Aires	1970
President, Third Congresses of Social Psychiatry, Moscow, Leningrad, Budapest, Zagreb and Dubrovnik	1970

BIBLIOGRAPHY

Books

The Thyroid: Its Role in Development and Disease. Doctoral Thesis. Wayne University College of Medicine. The Lambda Kappa National Undergraduate Award, 1929.

Behavior and Neuroses: An Experimental Psychoanalytic Approach to Psychobiologic Principles. Chicago, University of Chicago Press, 1943.

Principles of Dynamic Psychiatry: Including an Integrative Approach to Abnormal and Clinical Psychology; with a Glossary of Psychiatric Terms. Philadelphia, W. B. Saunders, 1946.

Practice of Dynamic Psychiatry. Philadelphia, W. B. Saunders, 1955.

With Moreno, J.L. (Eds.): *Progress in Psychotherapy.* Vol. II, *Anxiety and Therapy.* New York, Grune & Stratton, 1957.

Tommy the Tipsy Tabby (illustrated by Eloise Smith). Alcoholism Res. Foundation, 9 Bedford Rd., Toronto 6, Canada, 1957.

(Ed.): *Science and Psychoanalysis.* Vol. I, *Integrative Studies.* New York, Grune & Stratton, 1958.

With Moreno, J.L. (Eds.): *Progress in Psychotherapy.* Vol. III, *Techniques of Psychotherapy.* New York, Grune & Stratton, 1958.

(Ed.): *Biological Psychiatry,* Vol. I. New York, Grune & Stratton, 1959.

With Moreno, J.L. (Eds.): *Progress in Psychotherapy.* Vol. IV, *Social Psychotherapy.* New York, Grune & Stratton, 1959.

(Ed.): *Science and Psychoanalysis.* Vol. II, *Individual and Familial Dynamics.* New York, Grune & Stratton, 1959.

With Moreno, J.L. (Eds.): *Progress in Psychotherapy.* Vol. V, *Review and Integration.* New York, Grune & Stratton, 1960.

(Ed.): *Science and Psychoanalysis.* Vol. III, *Psychoanalysis and Human Values.* New York, Grune & Stratton, 1960.

Residency Training Brochure, Illinois State Psychiatric Institute. Springfield, Ill., Ill. Dept. Public Welfare, 1959.

Residency Training Brochure, Northwestern U-Vet. Adm. Downey, Ill., Veterans Administration Press, 1959.

Principles of Dynamic Psychiatry, 2nd Ed. Philadelphia, W. B. Saunders Co., 1961.

(Ed.): *Science and Psychoanalysis.* Vol. IV, *Psychoanalysis and Social Process.* New York, Grune & Stratton, 1961.

(Ed.): *Current Psychiatric Therapies,* Vol. I. New York, Grune & Stratton, 1961.

Modern Concepts in Psychoanalysis (with Leon Salzman). New York, Philosophical Library, 1962. Also paperback by Citadel Press and republished in London by Peter Owen, Ltd., 1962.

(Ed.): *Current Psychiatric Therapies,* Volume II. New York, Grune & Stratton, 1962.

(Ed.): *Science and Psychoanalysis.* Vol V, *Psychoanalytic Education.* New York, Grune & Stratton, 1962.

Northwestern University—V.A. Residency Training Program, Downey Illinois, VA Press, 1963.

(Ed.): *Science and Psychoanalysis.* Vol. VI, *Violence and War, with Clinical Studies.* New York, Grune & Stratton, 1963.

(Ed.): *Current Psychiatric Therapies,* Vol. III. New York, Grune & Stratton, 1963.

(Ed.): *Current Psychiatric Therapies,* Vol. IV. New York, Grune & Stratton, 1964.

(Ed.): *Science & Psychoanalysis.* Vol. VII, *Development and Research.* New York, Grune & Stratton, 1964.

Behavior and Neurosis, 2nd Ed. (Classics in Psychiatry) New York, Hafner Publishing Co., 1964.

(Ed.): *Current Psychiatric Therapies,* Vol. V. New York, Grune & Stratton, 1965.

(Ed.): *Science and Psychoanalysis.* Vol. VIII, *Communication and Community.* New York, Grune & Stratton, 1965.

Residency Training in Psychiatry. Northwestern University Graduate Center. Evanston, Illinois, Northwestern U. Press, 1965.

Modern Therapy of Personality Disorders. Iowa City, Wm. C. Brown, 1966.

(Ed.): *Science and Psychoanalysis.* Vol. IX, *Adolescence and Psychiatric-Psychoanalytic Training.* New York, Grune & Stratton, 1966.

Code of Procedures and Grants Manual of the Illinois Psychiatric Training and Research Authority. Springfield, State of Illinois Press, 1966.

Therapy of behavior disorders. In Vernon, J.: *Self-Selection Textbook of Psychology.* Des Moines, Iowa, Wm. C. Brown, 1966.

(Ed.): *Current Psychiatric Therapies,* Vol. VI. New York, Grune & Stratton, 1966.

(Ed.): *Current Psychiatric Therapies,* Vol. VII. New York, Grune & Stratton, 1967.

(Ed.): *Science and Psychoanalysis.* Vol. X, *The Sexuality of Women.* New York, Grune & Stratton, 1967.

(Ed.): *Science and Psychoanalysis.* Vol. XI, *The Ego.* New York, Grune & Stratton, 1967.

The Biodynamic Roots of Human Behavior. Springfield, Ill., Charles C. Thomas, 1968.

(Ed.): *Science and Psychoanalysis.* Vol. XII, *Animal and Human.* New York, Grune & Stratton, 1968.

(Ed.): *Psychiatry: East and West.* New York, Grune & Stratton, 1968.

(Ed.): *Science and Psychoanalysis.* Vol. XIII, *The Dynamics of Dissent.* New York, Grune & Stratton, 1968.

(Ed.): *Current Psychiatric Therapies,* Vol. VIII. New York, Grune & Stratton, 1968.

(Ed.): *Youth : A Transcultural Approach.* New York, Grune & Stratton, 1969.

(Ed.): *Science and Psychoanalysis.* Vol. XIV, *Childhood and Adolescence.* New York, Grune & Stratton, 1969.

(Ed.): *Science and Psychoanalysis.* Vol. XV, *Dynamics of Deviant Sexuality.* New York, Grune & Stratton, 1969.

(Ed.): *Current Psychiatric Therapies,* Vol. IX. New York, Grune & Stratton, 1969.

(Ed.): *Science and Psychoanalysis,* Vols. XVI and XVII, and *Current Psychiatric Therapies,* Vol. X. New York, Grune & Stratton, 1971.

Articles

Pathologic changes in the thyroid gland during various diseases. *J. Detroit College Med. & Surg.* 1:59, 1929.

Report on the principles and uses of two new instruments of physical diagnosis. *J. Detroit Coll. Med. & Surg.* 2:18, 1931.

Two new instruments of physical diagnosis: stethoscope and electric resonator. *Cal. and Western Med.* 35:44, 1931.

Simplified encephalography technique. *Cal. and Western Med.* 37:249, 1932.

Intracranial hydrodynamics. I. Experiments on human cadavers (with Walter F. Schaller). *Arch. Neurol. & Psychiat.* 29: 1222, 1933.

Intracranial hydrodynamics. II. Influence of rapid decompression of the ventriculo-subarachnoid space on the occurence of edema of the brain (with Walter Schaller). *Arch. Neurol. & Psychiat.* 30:107, 1933.

Dinitrophenol: its therapeutic and toxic actions in certain types of psychobiologic underactivity (with H. Goldsmith). *JAMA* 102:523, 1934.

Psychogenic factors in some epilepsies. *J. Nerv. & Ment. Dis.* 79:377, 1934.

Effects of intravenous administration of hypertonic solution of dextrose: with special reference to the cerebro-spinal fluid pressure. *JAMA* 102:2084, 1934.

Intracranial hydrodynamics. III. Central nervous system shock and edema following rapid fluid decompression of the ventriculo-subarachnoid spaces. *J. Nerv. & Ment. Dis.* 80:138, 1934.

The relationship of the bromide content of the lumbar fluid to that of the cisternal fluid after the Walter-Bromide Test. *Am. J. Physiol.* 109:193, 1934.

Cerebrospinal hydrodynamics. IV. Clinical experimental studies. *Arch. Neurol. & Psychiat.* 32:523, 1934.

Effects of the intravenous administration of hypertonic solutions of sucrose with special reference to the cerebrospinal fluid pressure. *Bull. John Hopkins Hosp.* 57:12, 1935.

The blood-cerebrospinal fluid barrier, with special references to the changes in general paralysis and in dementia praecox. *Psychiat. Quart.* 9:48, 1935.

Cerebrospinal hydrodynamics. V. Studies of the volume elasticity of the human ventriculo-subarachnoid system. *J. Comp. Neurol.* 61:543, 1935.

Cerebrospinal hydrodynamics. VI. Correlations of the pressure of the cerebrospinal fluid with age, blood pressure and the pressure index. *Arch. Neurol. & Psychiat.* 34:564, 1935.

Cerebrospinal hydrodynamics. VII. Effects of the intravenous injection of hypertonic solutions of dextrose. *Arch. Neurol. & Psychiat.* 35:296, 1936.

Effects of Sodium Amytal and other drugs on the reactivity of the hypothalamus of the cat. *Arch. Neurol. & Psychiat.* 37:617, 1937.

The influence of hypothalamic stimulation on intestinal activity (with E. W. Haertig). *J. Neurophysiol.* 1:350, 1938.

Destruction of the hypothalamus in cats. Effects on activity of the central nervous system and its reaction to Sodium Amytal. *Arch. Neurol. & Psychiat.* 39:1250-1271, 1938.

Diagnosis and prognosis in psychiatry, with a follow-up study of the results of short-term general hospital therapy of psychiatric cases (with H. T. Carmichael). *J. Ment. Sci.* 84:893, 1938.

The effect of strychnine sulphate on the emotional mimetic functions of the hypothalamus of the cat (with E. W. Haertig). *J. Pharmacol. & Exper. Therap.* 64:335, 1938.

The clinical application of phantasy studies (with Eva R. Balken). *J. Psychol.* 8:81, 1938.

Results of treatment in a psychiatric outpatient department—a followup study of 166 cases (with H. T. Carmichael). *JAMA* 113:2292, 1939.

The psychoanalytic and psychiatric significance of phantasy (with Eva R. Balken). *Psychoanalyt. Rev.* 26:343, 1929.

The psychoanalytic and psychiatric significance of phantasy. II. The psychiatric significance of the phantasy material (with Eva R. Balken). *Psychoanalyt. Rev.* 26:535, 1939.

Effects of morphine sulphate on the hypothalamus of the cat. *Proc. Soc. Exp. Biol. & Med.* 43:315, 1939.

An automatic apparatus for the central conditioning of small animals. *J. Comp. Psychol.* 28:201, 1939.

Action of Metrazol (pentamethylenetetrazol) on the hypothalamus of the cat. *Arch. Neurol. & Psychiat.* 41:504, 1939.

Effects of analeptic drugs on the hypothalamus of the cat. *Assoc. Res. Nerv. & Ment. Dis. Proc.* 20:624-634, 1939.

The language of phantasy. III. The language of the phantasies of patients with conversion hysteria, anxiety state and obsessive compulsive neurosis (with Eva R. Balken). *J. Psychol.* 10: 75-86, 1940.

Stimulant effects of ethyl alcohol in cortico-hypothalamic functions (with H. H. Beal and Rose Sanders). *J. Pharmacol. & Exper. Therap.* 70:450, 1940.

Hypothalamic lesions and pneumonia in cats. With notes on behavior changes (with E. W. Haertig). *J. Neurophysiol.* 3: 293-299, 1940.

Effects of ethyl alcohol on the cerebral cortex and the hypothalamus of the cat (with L. Jacobson). *Arch. Neurol. & Psychiat.* 43:344, 1940.

Use of phantasy tests in differential psychiatric diagnosis (with Eva R. Balken). *Arch. Neurol. & Psychiat.* 43:1249-1255, 1940.

Hypnotic treatment of acute hysterical depression: The dynamics of hypnosis and brief psychotherapy. *Arch. Neurol. & Psychiat.* 40:488, 1941.

Psychodynamisms in manic-depressive psychoses. *Psychoanalyt. Rev.* 28:466, 1941.

Psychodynamisms in anorexia nervosa and neurotic vomiting. *Psychoanalyt. Quart.* 10:211, 1941.

Is the hypothalamus a center of emotion? *Psychosom. Med.* 3:3, 1941.

Suggestions to O.C.D. personnel for talks on morale. III. *Mental Health Bull.* 20:1, 1942.

Psychobiologic dynamism in behavior. *Psychiat.* 5:321-347, 1942.

The hypothalamus in psychiatry. *Am. J. Psychiat.* 98:633-637, 1942.

A report of the Committee on National Defense. *Dis. Nerv. System* 3:1, 1942.

The psychodynamisms of propaganda and morale. *Dis. Nerv. System* 5:101, 1943.

Experimental neuroses and psychotherapy. *Arch. Neurol. & Psychiat.* 49:43-48, 1943.

The effects of morphine on learned adaptive responses and experimental neuroses in cats (with A. Wikler). *Arch. Neurol. & Psychiat.* 50:401-404, 1943.

Civilian morale and the professional worker. *J. Am. Dietet. Assoc.* 19:91, 1943.

Wartime industrial psychiatry. *Ment. Health Bull.* 21:1-3, 1943.

Emotional needs at different age levels. In Wood, J.F. (Ed.): *What the American Family Faces.* Chicago, Eugene Hugh Publ. Co., 1943, p. 66.

The language of phantasy. III (re-published by editorial request). In Tompkins, S.S. (Ed.): *Contemporary Psychopathology.* Cambridge, Mass., Harvard U. Press, 1943, p. 244.

Neurosis and alcohol. *Am. J. Psychiat.* 101:389, 1944.

Language, behavior and dynamic psychiatry. *Int. J. Psychoanalysis* 25:1, 1944.

Experimental neuroses and group aggression. *Am. J. Orthopsychiat.* 14:636, 1944.

Dominance, neurosis and aggression (with P. W. Siever). *Psychosom. Med.* 6:7, 1944.

Dynamic psychology of war-time communications and morale. *Dis. Nerv. System* 5:101, 1944.

The contribution of psychoanalysis to the civilian defense program. *Psychoanalyt. Rev.* 31:34, 1944.

"Counting" behavior in cats. (with D. L. Rubinfine). *J. Gen. Psychol.* 30:87, 1944.

Principles of biodynamics. *Tr. New York Acad. Sci.* 61:71, 1944.

Report of the Committee on Animal Experimentation, 1943-1944. *Psychosom. Med.* 7:46, 1944.

Psychiatry, mental hygiene and daily living. *Ment. Hyg.* 29: 650, 1945.

Biodynamics of experimental neuroses and alcoholism. *Tr. New York Academy Sci.,* Ser. II 7:61, 1945.

Alcohol as a preventive of experimental neuroses (with Marie R. Nicholson). *Quart. J. Stud. on Alcohol* 6:281, 1945.

Review of experimental catatonia. *Science* 103:28, 1946.

Analysis of the influence of alcohol on experimental neuroses in cats (with K. S. Yum). *Psychosom. Med.* 8:36, 1946.

Psychogenic vomiting. *J. Nerv. & Ment. Dis.* 103:224-233, 1946.

Problems of the neuroses: an experimental approach. *Cincinnati J. Med.* 27:73, 1946.

Una contribucion experimental al problema de la neurosis. *Arg. Arch. Neurol. Psychiat.* 12:46, 1946.

Tension in modern living: its treatment. *The Reviewing Stand* 9:6, July 20, 1947.

A note on the dynamics of suicide. *Dis. Nerv. System* 8:324-325, 1947.

Effects of cerebral electroshock on experimental neuroses in cats (with Mary Grier Jacques). *Am. J. Psychiat.* 104:92-99, 1947.

Psychiatric aspects of obstetrical nursing. In DeLee (Ed.): *Obstetrics for Nurses,* 14th Ed. Philadelphia, W. B. Saunders, 1947.

Do you know how to relax? *The Reviewing Stand* 10:3-10, 1948.

Psychological medicine and world affairs. In Harris, N.G. (Ed.): *Modern Trends in Psychological Medicine.* New York, Paul B. Hoeber, 1948.

Mental Hygiene in a world crisis. *Dis. Nerv. System* 9:210, 1948.

The neuroses (with others). In Spiegel, E. A. (Ed.): *Progress in Neurology and Psychiatry,* Vol. 3. New York, Grune & Stratton, 1948, p. 507.

Experimental masochism (with Mary Grier Jacques). *Arch. Neurol. & Psychiat.* 60:402-404, 1948.

Alcoholism. *Am. Peoples Encycl.,* Vol. 1. Chicago, Spencer Press, 1948, p. 545.

Mental hygiene. *Am. Peoples Encycl.,* Vol. 13. Chicago, Spencer Press, 1948, p. 435.

Neurasthenia. *Am. Peoples Encycl.,* Vol. 14. Chicago, Spencer Press, 1948, p. 491.

Psychiatry. *Am. Peoples Encycl.,* Vol. 16. Chicago, Spencer Press, 1948, p. 255.

Psychosomatic Medicine. *Am. Peoples Encycl.,* Vol. 16. Chicago, Spencer Press, 1948, p. 250.

Psychotherapy. *Am.Peoples Encycl.,* Vol. 16. Chicago, Spencer Prcss, 1948, p. 255.

Some practical aspects of a V.A. residency training program. *Quar. Bull. Northwestern Univ. Med. School* 23:487, 1949.

The neuroses (with R. A. Jones and others). In Spiegel, E.A. (Ed.): *Progress in Neurology and Psychiatry,* Vol. 4. New York, Grune & Stratton, 1949.

Philosophy and methodology in the training of 500 psychiatric residents. *Am. J. Psychiat.* 106:326-369, 1949.

Modern reorientation on psychoanalytic therapy. *Dis. Nerv. System* 10:3-7, 1949.

The neuroses (with Frank H. Murrin and others). In Spiegel, E.

A. (Ed.): *Progress in Neurology and Psychiatry,* Vol. 5. New York, Grune & Stratton, 1950.

A biodynamic and psychoanalytic approach to the problems of feeling and emotion. In Reymert, M.L. (Ed.): *Feelings and Emotions.* Second Mooseheart Symposium, pp. 40-75, 1950.

Experimental neuroses. *Scientific American* 82:38, 1950.

Mental hygiene: half-century mark, Pt. 2. *Today's Health* 28: 40, 1950.

Effects of direct interrupted electroshock on experimental neuroses (with Alex Arieff, Curtis Pechtel and Harold Klehr). *J. Nerv. & Ment. Dis.* 112:384-392, 1950.

The neuroses (with Thomas Tourlentes, et al.). In Spiegel, E. A. (Ed.): *Progress in Neurology and Psychiatry,* Vol. 6. New York, Grune & Stratton, 1951.

Some current concepts of sexual behavior. *Psychiat.* 14:67-72, 1951.

Can we prevent alcoholism? *The Reviewing Stand* 16:3-9, 1951.

Why you behave as you do. A health talk telecast over WGN-TV, Chicago. Published by the Illinois State Medical Society, Educational Comm., 1951.

The problem of homeostasis. *Arch. Neurol & Psychiat.* 65: 93-95, 1951.

Experimental psychiatry. *Digest of Neurol. & Psychiat.,* Series XIX, 1951.

Bibliography 1931-1942: Jules H. Masserman. *Psychiatry* 14: 123-124, 1951.

The neuroses (with Glenn A. Bacon and others). In Spiegel, E. A. (Ed.): *Progress in Neurology and Psychiatry,* Vol. 7. New York, Grune & Stratton, 1952.

Progress in psychiatry. *Am. Peoples Encycl. Year Book.* Chicago, Spencer Press, 1952.

Do lie-detectors lie? (with Mary Grier Jacques). *The Nation* 174: 368-369, 1952.

Psychiatric supplementation of the medical history and physical examination. *Dis. Nerv. System* 13: 1-8, 1952.

Therapeutic efficacy of electrocoma. *Modern Medicine,* April, 1952, pp. 135-136.

Report on European psychiatry to the World Health Organization, Geneva, Switzerland. Jan., 1952.

Experiment uber psychodynamische probleme. Psyche, eine Zeitschrift fur Tiefenpsychologie un Menschenkunde. In *Forschung and Praxis.* Sonderdruck. Heft 2. VI: 102-120, 1952-53.

Approaches experimentales des problemes psychodynamiques (translation by Maryse Choisy). *Psyche,* Supplement, 1952.

What kind of a vacation should you take? *Northwestern Univ. Reviewing Stand* 18: 1-11, 1962.

Experimental approaches to psychoanalytic concepts. *Samiska,* 6: 243-261, 1952.

The neuroses. In Spiegel, E.A. (Ed.): *Progress in Neurology and Psychiatry,* Vol. 8. New York, Grune & Stratton, 1953.

Progress in psychiatry. *Am. Peoples Encycl. Year Book.* Chicago, Spencer Press, 1953.

Experimental approaches to psychodynamic problems. *J. Mount Sinai Hosp.* 19:639-652, 1953.

Neuroses in monkeys: a preliminary report of experimental observations (with C. Pechtel). *Annals of the New York Acad. Sci.* 56: 253-265, 1953.

Behavioral changes following thalamic injury in the cat (with L. Schreiner, D. McK. Rioch and C. Pechtel). *J. Neurophysiol.* 16:234-246, 1953.

Psychoanalysis and biodynamics—an integration. *Int. J. Psychoanal.* Suppl. 34:13-43, 1953.

Contributions to European symposium on alcoholism. Copenhagen, Denmark, 1951. World Health Organization, Geneva, Switzerland, 1953.

The role of olfaction in normal and neurotic behavior in animals (with C. Pechtel). *Psychosom. Med.* 15:396-404, 1953.

Experimental neuroses. *Sci. Am. Reader.* New York, Simon & Schuster, 1953, p. 441.

Faith and delusion in psychotherapy: the Ur-delusions of man. *Am. J. Psychiat.* 110:324-333, 1953.

Music as a tool of delightful delusion. In *Music Therapy.* Lawrence, Kansas, Allen Press, 1953.

Conflict-engendered neurotic and psychotic behavior in monkeys. *J. Nerv. & Ment. Dis.* 118-408, 1953.

The neuroses (with Gloria Berkwitz, A. Pauncz, et al.). In Spiegel, E.A. (Ed.): *Progress in Neurology and Psychiatry,* Vol. 9. New York, Grune & Stratton, 1954.

Progress in Psychiatry. *Am. Peoples Encycl. Year Book.* Chicago, Spencer Press, 1954.

Music and the child in society. *Am. J. Psychother.* 8:63, 1954.

Psychoanalyse et biodynamique—une integration. *L'Encephale* 1 et 2:1-39, 121-148, 1954.

An integration of group therapeutic techniques. *Inf. Bull.* Washington, D.C., Dept. Med. & Surg., Vet. Adm., 1954, p. 4.

The conceptual dynamics of person, religion, and self. *Psychoanal. Rev.* 41:303, 1954.

Abnormalities of behavior (with Z. Gross and C. Pechtel). In Stone, C. P. (Ed.): *Annual Review of Psychology,* Stanford Annual Reviews. Palo Alto, Cal., 1954.

Can sociology be weaned from its formulae? In Hsu, F. (Ed.): *Aspects of Culture and Personality.* New York, Abelard-Schuman, 1954, p. 161.

Experimental approaches to psychodynamic problems. In Murphy, G. and Bachrach, A.J. (Eds.): *An Outline of Abnormal Psychology.* New York, Modern Library, 1954, p. 435.

Creation de névroses experimentales chez le chat par un traumatisme physiologique (with C. Pechtel and J. Cain). *Comptes r.d. Séances de la Société de Biologie* 148:2041, 1954.

Differential effects of cerebral lesions on susceptibility of animals to the induction and relief of experimental neuroses (with C. Pechtel). *Army Med. Serv. Res. Progr. Report* (1st Quarter), 1954, p. 433.

The osmatic responses of normal and neurotic monkeys (with C. Pechtel). *Ann. of the New York Acad. Sci.* 58:256-260, 1954.

Psychotherapy: a review and an integration. *Bull. Menninger Clin.* 18:162, 1954.

Moreno's "Transference, countertransference and tele." *Group Psychotherapy* 7:309, 1954.

The neuroses (with A. Pauncz, et al.). In Spiegel, E.A. (Ed.): *Progress in Neurology and Psychiatry,* Vol. 10. New York, Grune & Stratton, 1955, p. 496.

Progress in psychiatry. *Am. Peoples Encyl. Year Book,* Chicago, Spencer Press, 1955.

Differential effects of lesions of the mediodorsal nuclei of the thalamus on the normal and neurotic behavior of the cat (C. Pechtel, senior author, with L. Schreiner and M. Levitt). *J. Neurophysiol.* 11:217, 1955.

Moreno's "Interpersonal therapy, group therapy and the function of the unconscious." II. *Group Psychother.* 8:62, 1955.

Emotional reactions to death and suicide. *Am. Pract. and Digest of Treat.* 5:41. Reprinted in Liebman, S. (Ed.): *Stress Situations.* Philadelphia, J. B. Lippincott, 1955, p. 117.

Sociologic and psychologic correlates of music therapy. In *Music Therapy.* Lawrence, Kansas, Allen Press, 1955, p. 15.

The neuroses (with A. Pauncz, R. Nathan, et al.). In Spiegel,

E.A. (Ed.): *Progress in Neurology and Psychiatry,* Vol. 11. New York, Grune & Stratton, 1956, p. 327.

Progress in psychiatry. *Am. Peoples Encycl. Year Book.* Chicago, Spencer Press, 1956, p. 906.

A historical biodynamic integration of psychotherapy. In Fromm-Reichmann, Frieda and Moreno, J. L. (Eds.): *Progress in Psychotherapy.* New York, Grune & Stratton, 1956, p. 188.

Psychiatry in Latin America. I. Brazil. *Northwestern U. Quart. Bull.* 30:270, 1956.

Fundamentals of psychotherapy with special reference to respiratory diseases. In Sparer, P. (Ed.): *Personality, Stress and Tuberculosis.* New York, Intern. Univ. Press, 1956, p. 235.

Normal and neurotic olfactory behavior in monkeys (with C. Pechtel). *Tr. Soc. Biol. Psychiat.* 11:30, 1956.

Drugs and psychotherapy. In Gerty, F. (Ed.): Round-table discussion. *Psychiat. Res. Reports.* Washington, D. C., Am. Psychiat. Assoc., 1956, pp. 114-129.

How brain lesions affect normal and neurotic behavior (with C. Pechtel). *Am. J. Psychiat.* 112:865, 1956.

Neurophysiologic and pharmacologic influences on experimental neuroses (with C. Pechtel). *Am. J. Psychiat.* 113:510, 1956.

Psychiatry in Latin America. II. *Northwestern U. Quart. Bull.* 30:370, 1956.

The role of drug therapies in current and future psychiatric practice. *Psychiat. Res. Reports,* No. 4. Washington, D. C., Am. Psychiat. Assoc., 1956, pp. 95-125.

The neuroses. In Spiegel, E. A. (Ed.): *Progress in Neurology and Psychiatry,* Vol. 12. New York, Grune & Stratton, 1957, p. 515.

Progress in psychiatry. *Am. Peoples Encycl. Year Book.* Chicago, Spencer Press, 1957.

President's message. Newsletter. Acad. Psychoanal. Vol. 1, Nos. 2 & 3, 1957.

Evolution vs. revolution in psychotherapy: a biodynamic integration. *Behav. Sci.* 2:89, 1957.

Psychodynamics of aging. *Geriatrics* 12:115, 1957.

Biodynamic therapy in aging: an integration. In Masserman, J. H., and Moreno, J. L. (Eds.): *Progress in Psychotherapy,* Vol. II. New York, Grune & Stratton, 1957, p. 121.

Biodynamic therapy in the aging (editorial translation). *Imprensa Medica* 21: 275, 1957.

Psychiatry in Latin America. III. *Northwestern U. Quart. Bull.* 31: 78, 1957.

Psychiatry in Rio: the Institute of Psychologic Medicine. *Imprensa Medica.* 21:168, 1957.

Psychotherapy: an outline and an integration. II (tr. by Berenger). *Imprensa Medica* 21:217, 1957.

Experimental and historical perspectives in psychopharmacology. *Trans. Res. Conf. on Chemother.* Washington, D. C., VA, 1957, p. 20.

Humanitarian psychiatry. I. *Dept. Welfare Bull. Publ.,* Springfield, Ill., 1957.

President's message. Newletter. Acad. Psychoanal. Vol. 3-4, Sep.–Nov. 1957.

The neuroses (with A. Pauncz, et al.). In Spiegel, E. A. (Ed.): *Progress in Neurology and Psychiatry,* Vol. 13. New York, Grune & Stratton, 1958.

Progress in psychiatry. *Am. Peoples Encycl. Year Book.* Chicago, Spencer Press, 1958.

Hysteria. *Am. Peoples Encycl.* Chicago, Spencer Press, 1958.

Experimental psychopharmacology and behavioral relativity. In Hoch, P. and Zubin, J. (Eds.): *Problems of Addiction and Habituation.* New York, Grune & Stratton, 1958, pp. 110-148.

Cingulates and behavior (with M. Levitt, T. McAvoy, A. Kling, and C. Pechtel). *J. Nerv. & Ment. Dis.* 126:148, 1958.

The National Foundation for Psychiatric Research: what it is and how it concerns you. Chicago, Northwestern Univ., 1958.

Musical motions and emotional notions. In *Music Therapy.* Lawrence, Kan., Allen Press, 1958.

Say id isn't so—with music. In Masserman, J. H. (Ed.): *Science and Psychoanalysis,* Vol. I. New York, Grune & Stratton, 1958.

Psychotherapeutic progress in Latin America. In Masserman, J.H., and Moreno, J. L. (Eds.): *Progress in Psychotherapy,* Vol. III. New York, Grune & Stratton, 1958, pp. 282-310.

The amygdalae and behavior (with M. Levitt, T. McAvoy, A. Kling and C. Pechtel). *Am. J. Psychiat.* 115:14, 1958.

Evolucion y Revolucion en psicoterapia. *Actas Medico Psicologicas* 1:267, 1958.

President's message. Newsletter. Acad. of Psychoanal. Vol. 2, No. 1, 1958.

The neuroses (with A. Pauncz, et al.). In Spiegel, E. A. (Ed.): *Progress in Neurology and Psychiatry,* Vol. 14. New York, Grune & Stratton, 1959.

Progress in psychiatry. *Am. Peoples Encycl. Year Book.* Chicago, Spencer Press, 1959.

Masochism—a biodynamic review. In Masserman, J. H. (Ed.): *Science and Psychoanalysis,* Vol. II. New York, Grune & Stratton, 1959, p. 73.

Norms, neurotics and nepenthics. In Masserman, J. H. (Ed.): *Biological Psychiatry,* Vol. I. New York, Grune & Stratton, 1959, p. 90.

Science, psychiatry and religion. In Masserman, J. H., and Moreno, J. L. (Eds.): *Progress in Psychotherapy,* Vol. IV. New York, Grune & Stratton, 1959, p. 324.

Mental hygiene. *Am. Peoples Encycl.* Chicago, Spencer Press, 1959.

Behavioral pharmacology in animals. In Bradley, P. B., Deniker, P., and Raduoco-Thomas, C. (Eds.): *Neuropsychophar-*

macology. Amsterdam, Elsevier Publ. Co., 1959, pp. 97-107.

Moreno's "Transference, countertransference and tele." II. In Moreno, J.L. (Ed.): *Psychodrama.* Beacon, N. Y., Beacon House, 1959, p. 16.

Moreno's "Interpersonal therapy." II. In Moreno, J. L. (Ed.): *Psychodrama.* Beacon, N. Y., Beacon House, 1959, p. 60.

Cerebral localization: not where, but in whom (with C. Pechtel). *Am. J. Psychiat.* 116:51, 1959.

Humanitarian psychiatry. II (editor's translation). *Imprensa Medica* 23:208, 1959.

Psychiatria humanista. *Psychiatria y Psychologia Medica* (Barcelona) 4:65, 1959.

Alcohol and other drugs as preventives of experimental trauma. *Quart. J. Stud. Alc.* 20:464, 1959.

The biodynamic approaches. In Arieti, S. (Ed.): *American Handbook of Psychiatry,* Vol. II. New York, Basic Books, 1959, pp. 1680-96.

The neuroses (with A. Pauncz, et al.). In Spiegel, E. A. (Ed.): *Progress in Neurology and Psychiatry,* Vol. 15. New York, Grune & Stratton, 1960.

Progress in psychiatry. *Am. Peoples Encycl. Year Book.* Chicago, Spencer Press, 1960.

Ethology, comparative biodynamics and psychoanalytic research. In Masserman, J. H. (Ed.): *Science and Psychoanalysis,* Vol. III. New York, Grune & Stratton, 1960.

Differential responses in young vs. old animals to training, conflict and brain lesions (with C. Pechtel and L. Aarons). *Am. J. Psychiat.* 116:1018, 1960.

Preface. In Enelow, Gertrude: *Body Dynamics.* New York, Citadel Press, 1960.

Perspectives. *Trans. 4th Res. Conf. on Chemother. in Psychiat.* Washington, D. C., VA, 1960, p. 282.

Experimental approaches to psychotherapy. In Gottlieb, J. S. and Tourney, G. (Eds.): *Scientific Papers and Discussions.* Washington, D. C., Am. Psychiat. Assoc., 1960, p. 125.

Psychiatry: office problems. *Am. Practic.* 116:11, 1960.

Humanitarian psychotherapy. *Acta Psych.* 8:385-99, 1960.

Battlements and bridges in the East: a liaison with Soviet psychiatry. *Am. J. Psychiat.* 117:4, 1960.

The Czechoslovak Psychiatric Congress. In Masserman, J. H., and Moreno, J. L. (Eds.): *Progress in Psychotherapy,* Vol. V. New York, Grune & Stratton 1960, pp. 231-254.

The office therapy of psychosomatic disorders. *Arch. Gen. Psychiat.* 3:320, 1960.

A versatile multiple choice apparatus for the study of animal behavior. *J. Nerv. & Ment. Dis.* 130:547, 1960.

Drug effects on experimental neuroses in animals. In Uhr, L., and Miller, J. G. (Eds.): *Drugs and Behavior.* New York, John Wiley and Sons, 1960, p. 250.

A liaison with Soviet psychiatry, Parts I and II. *Northwestern University Quart.* Apr.-Sep., 1960.

A discussion of schizophrenia. In Auerbach, A. (Ed.): *Schizophrenia: An Integrated Approach.* New York, Ronald Press, 1960, pp. 19ff.

Comprehensive psychotherapy. *Psychosom. Med.* 1:312, 1960.

Is psychiatry a science? In Galdston, I. (Ed.): *Medicine and the Other Disciplines.* New York, Int. Univ. Press, 1960, p. 98.

The neuroses (with others). In Spiegel, E. A. (Ed.): *Progress in Neurology and Psychiatry,* Vol. 16. New York, Grune & Stratton, 1961.

Progress in psychiatry. *Am. Peoples Encycl. Year Book.* Chicago, Spencer Press, 1961.

Anxiety and the art of healing. In Masserman, J. H. (Ed.): *Current Psychiatric Therapies,* Vol. I. New York, Grune & Stratton, 1961, pp. 216-238.

Alcoholism: disease or dis-ease? *Report Am. Bus. Res. Assoc.* 19:1 1961.

Psychiatric and Psychologic Tests for Ministerial Personnel (with R. T. Palmer). *Pastoral Psychology* 12:24, 1961.

O tratamento dos pesturbacoes psicosomaticos no consultario. *Arquivas da Clinica Pinel.* 1:15, 1961.

Food acceptance in monkeys (with Curtis Pechtel and Louis Aarons). In Wortis, J. (Ed.): *Recent Advances in Biological Psychiatry.* New York, Grune & Stratton, 1961, p. 228.

Experimental approaches to psychotherapy. Congressus Psychiatricus Bohemoslovenicus cum Participatione Internationali 1959. Prof. O. Janota and Dr. E. Wolf, (Eds.). Praha, 1961, pp. 47-56.

Transference: counter and countered—a dialogue. In Leon Salzman and Jules Masserman (Eds.): *Modern Concepts in Psychoanalysis.* New York, Philosophical Library, 1962, pp. 160-172.

Psychotherapy: three objectives for the family physician. *Consultant,* Feb., 1962, pp. 12-18.

Brain stimulation, experience and behavior (with Louis Aarons and Thomas McAvoy). *Am. J. Psychol.* 118:982, 1962.

Or shall we all commit suicide? In Masserman, J. H.: *Current Psychiatric Therapies,* Vol. II. New York, Grune & Stratton, 1962, p. 273.

Behavioral adaptations after parietal cortex ablation in the neonate macaque (with L. Aarons, J. Shulman and G. P. Zimmer). In Wortis, J. (Ed.): *Recent Advances in Biological Psychiatry.* New York, Grune & Stratton, 1962, p. 347.

The contributions of experimental psychiatry to the art of healing. *Proc. Third World Congress of Psychiatry,* Montreal, 1961, Vol. 1. Univ. of Toronto & McGill Univ. Presses, 1962, pp. 25-32.

Drugs, brain and behavior: an experimental approach. *J. Neuropsychiat.* 3. Sup. 1 S104-113, 1962.

Review and comment. In Tourlentes, T.T., Pollack, S. L., and Himwich, H.E. (Eds.): *Research Approaches to Psychiatric Problems.* New York, Grune & Stratton, 1962, pp. 230-238.

Adages for aging. *Today's Health* 40: 20-23, 1962.

Emotional causes of illness: how to assess their role. *Consultant,* Nov.-Dec., 1962.

Comparative biodynamics. In Scher, J.: *Theories of the Mind.* New York, Free Press of Glencoe, 1962, pp. 15-65.

The neuroses (with others). In Spiegel, E. A. (Ed.): *Progress in NOLOGYAND Psychiatry,* Vol. 17. New York, Grune & Stratton, 1962, pp. 450-462.

An alternative to world suicide. *Chicago Medicine* 64:39, 1962.

The neuroses (with others). In Spiegel, E. A. (Ed.): *Progress in Neurology and Psychiatry,* Vol. 18. New York, Grune & Stratton, 1963, pp. 549-558.

Neuroses. In Watts, J. (Ed.): *Encyclopedia of Mental Health,* Vol. 4. New York, Watts Publ. Co., 1963, pp. 1333-1345.

Psychiatric residency training for public institutional service. *Am. J. Psychiat.* 119:1038, 1963.

Contemporary psychotherapies: a review. *Arch. Gen. Psychiat.* 8:461-464, 1962.

If tomorrow comes. . . . *Am. J. Orthopsychiat.* 33:256, 1963.

Human violence: critique and integration. In Masserman, J. H. (Ed.): *Science and Psychoanalysis,* Vol. VI. New York, Grune & Stratton, 1963, pp. 102-114.

Humanitarian psychiatry. *Bull. N. Y. Acad. Med.* 39:533-544, 1963.

Neo-analysis or neo-atavism. *Int. J. Psychoanal.* 44:384, 1963.

Is mental illness a medico-social myth? *Arch. Gen. Psychiat.* 9:175-178, 1963.

The effect of positive-choice conflicts on normal and neurotic monkeys (with Aarons, L. and Wechkin, S.). *Am. J. Psychiat.* 120:481-484, 1963.

Alcohol and neurotic behavior. In Lucia, S.P.: *Alcohol and Civilization.* New York, McGraw-Hill, 1963.

A tachistoscopic glance at recent advances in the neurophysiology of behavior. *Israel Ann. Psychol.* 1:244-254, 1963.

The contributions of experimental psychiatry to the art of healing. *Psychoanalyt. Rev.* 50:104, 1964.

Biodynamic psychotherapy. *Bulgarian Arch. of Neurol. and Psychiat.* Sophia, Bulgaria, 1964.

Review of advances in neurology and psychiatry. *Proc. of the Joint APA and Japanese Neuropsychiatric Society.* Tokyo, 1964.

The neuroses (with others). In Spiegel, E. A. (Ed.): *Progress in Neurology and Psychiatry,* Vol. 19. New York, Grune & Stratton, 1964.

The sphere of psychiatry. In Masserman, J. H. (Ed.): *Current Psychiatric Therapies,* Vol. IV. New York, Grune & Stratton, 1964.

The cry for help: a review. *JAMA* 188:149, 1964.

Altruistic behavior in the macaque. *Am. J. Psychiat.* 121: 584, 1964.

Shock to a conspecific as an aversive stimulus (with S. Wechkin and W. Terris). *Psych. Sci.* 1:47, 1964.

The world of the schizophrenic. *JAMA* 187:788, 1964.

Effects of neonate cortical ablations in the macaque (with L. Aarons, L. L. Schulman, and S. Wechkin). In Wortis, J. (Ed.): *Recent Advances in Biological Psychiatry,* Vol. VI. New York, Grune & Stratton, 1964.

Comparative and experimental contributions to the dynamics of behavior. In Masserman, J. H.: *Science and Psychoanalysis,* Vol. VII. New York, Grune & Stratton, 1964.

We know how our patients feel. *STAFF* 1:2, 1964.

First five years of the Psychiatric Training and Research Authority (with Percival Bailey). Illinois Dept. of Mental Health, Springfield, Ill., 1964.

Interrelationships of developmental, experiential and neurological determinants of behavior. In Bailey, P. (Ed.): Ill. State Res. and Training Auth., Dept. of Ment. Health, Springfield, Ill., 1964.

Recommendations on psychiatric training in Illinois Institutions. In Bailey, P., and Masserman, J. H. (Eds.): Illinois Res. and Trng. Authority, Dept. of Ment. Health, Springfield, Ill., 1964.

The neuroses (with T. Kostrubala and D. DuSold). In Spiegel, E. A. (Ed.): *Progress in Neurology and Psychiatry,* Vol. 20. New York, Grune & Stratton, 1965.

Anxiety; the protean source of communication. In Masserman, J. H. (Ed.): *Science and Psychoanalysis,* Vol. VIII. New York, Grune & Stratton, 1965.

Anxiety: aspects and answers. In Usdin, G. (Ed.): *Psychiatry in the Mid-Sixties.* Philadelphia, 1965.

East Africa: half a continent half in chaos. In Masserman, J. H.: *Current Psychiatric Therapies,* Vol. V. New York, Grune & Stratton, 1965.

The psychology of sex. In Auerbach, A. (Ed.): *Proc. of the Conf. on Sex.* U. of Calif. Press, 1965.

Historical-comparative and experimental roots of short-term psychotherapy. In Wolberg, L. (Ed.): *Short-term Psychotherapy.* New York, Grune & Stratton, 1965, pp. 23-50.

The search for the nature of communications. *The American Family in Crisis,* 3:21, Forest Hospital, Desplaines, Ill., 1965.

The teaching of psychodynamics. In Reid, J.V.O., and Wilmot, A. J. (Eds.): *Medical Education in South Africa.* Pietermaretzberg, Natal U. Press, 1965, pp. 104-109.

Man's eternal anxieties and compensating illusions. Camp

Mem. Lecture, Part I, *Ill. Med. J.*, 127:375, 1965; Part II, ibid, 127:561, 1965.

Anxiety revisited. *Am. J. Psychoanal.* 25:115-28, 1965.

Franz Alexander's techniques of therapy. *Int. J. Psychiat.* 1:2, 1965.

The study of folk psychiatry. *Int. J. Psychiat.* 1:551, 1965.

Sex and the singular psychiatrist. In Masserman, J. H.: *Science and Psychoanalysis,* Vol. IX. New York, Grune & Stratton, 1966.

Do it yourself psychotherapy for the general practitioner. *Memphis and Mid-South Med. J.* 41:79-81, 1966.

The biodynamic roots of psychoanalysis. In Marmor, J.: *Frontiers of Psychoanalysis.* New York, Basic Books, 1966.

The neuroses (with Spivy, D., Wigdahl, L., and Small, S. R.). In Spiegel, E.A. (Ed.): *Progress in Neurology and Psychiatry,* Vol. 21. New York, Grune & Stratton, 1966.

Anxiety: aspects and answers. In Usdin, G. L. (Ed.): *Psychoneurosis and Schizophrenia.* Philadelphia, J.B. Lippincott Co., 1966, pp. 32-46, 81, 87.

Discussion of Grotjahn, M.: the new technology of our ageless unconscious. *Psychoanalytic Forum* 1:14-15, 1966.

Preface. In Alexander, F., and Selesnick, S.: *The History of Psychiatry.* New York, Harper and Row, 1966.

The history of psychiatry by F. Alexander and S. Selesnick: a review. *Arch. Gen. Psychiat.,* 14:522-526, 1966.

Beatniks: up-, down-, and off-. *Arch. Gen. Psychiat,* Vol. 16, 1966.

Experimental and humanitarian approaches to the therapy of behavior disorders. *Canad. Med. J.* 95:616-621, 1966.

Psychiatry and human values. Proc. IV Intern. Congress of Psychiatry. Madrid, Spain, 1966.

Nervousness, doctor . . . *Consultant,* April, 1966, pp. 1-4.

Psychoanalysis exaggerates role of sexuality. *Frontiers of Psychiatry* 3:1-4, 1966.

The libidinous lyre. *J. Music Therapy* 2:107-114, 1966.

Experimental neuroses. *Sci. Amer.,* Mar., 1950.

Inside tips. *World Wide Abstracts* 9:2, 1966.

Report on the Fourth World Congress of Psychiatry. *Proceedings of the Council of the Am. Psychiat. Assn.,* Nov., 1966.

The timeless therapeutic trinity. In Masserman, J.H. (Ed.): *Current Psychiatric Therapies,* Vol. VII. New York, Grune & Stratton, 1967.

Fear and anxiety. In Bucklin, D. H. (Ed.): *Laboratory Biology.* Chicago, Science Research Associates, 1967.

Science and human values. In Lewis, N.D. (Ed.): *Paul Hoch Memorial Volume.* New York, Grune & Stratton, 1967.

Psychiatry in Morocco, *APA News,* Jan., 1967.

The neuroses. In Spiegel, E. A. (Ed.): *Progress in Neurology and Psychiatry*, Vol. 22. New York, Grune & Stratton, 1967.

The theatre of the absurd. APA Program Brochure, May, 1967.

Biodynamic psychology. *Psychology Today,* Oct., 1967, pp. 37-40; 55-58.

Psychoanalysis and sexuality. *Roche Reports* 3: 1-8, 1966.

Lord of the four quarters by John W. Perry: a review. *Am. J. Psychiat.,* Dec., 1966, pp. 123-126.

Karl Menninger looks at psychiatric history: a review. *JAMA* 201:222, 1967.

The techniques of psychotherapy: a review. *Med. Trip.,* Oct., 1967, p. 31.

Science, psychiatry and human values. *Proc. Fourth World Congress of Psychiatry, Psychother. and Psychosom* 1:703-707, 1967.

Hippies and their future. *U. S. News & World Report* 63:58-63, July, 1967.

Focus on Jules Masserman. *Roche Reports* 9:10-13, Feb., 1967.

Hippies. *Northwestern Review* 3:26-31, 1967.

The neurotic cat. *Psychology Today* 1:37-58, 1967.

East and West: psychiatric theory and therapy. Fairview Fdn., Chicago, 1967, p. 18.

Social relationships and aggression in rhesus monkeys (with S. Wechkin and M. Woolf). *Arch. Gen. Psychiat.* 18:210-213, 1968.

Science, human values and psychiatry. *Psychother. and Psychosom.* 158:1-10, 1968.

The biodynamic roots of psychoanalysis. In Marmor, J. (Ed.): *Modern Psychoanalysis: New Directions and Perspectives.* New York, Basic Books, 1968.

The investigation of psychotherapy by A. B. Goldstein and S. J. Dean: a review. *Am. J. Psychiat.,* 1968.

Dialogue with Erik Erikson by R. I. Evans: a review. *Mental Hygiene,* 1968.

Beatniks. *Ala. J. Med. Sci.* 5:74-79, 1968.

The art of the ballet: motion and emotion. APA Brochure, Boston, Mass. Annual Meeting, 1968.

The game of fashion. *Roche Reports* 5:1, 1968.

Alliances and aggressions among rhesus monkeys. In Masserman, J. H. (Ed.): *Science and Psychoanalysis,* Vol. XII. New York, Grune & Stratton, 1968.

Comparative and clinical approaches to biodynamic therapy. In Masserman, J. H. (Ed): *Science and Psychoanalysis,* Vol. XII, New York, Grune & Stratton, 1968.

The beatnik, up-, down-, and off-.II. Theory into practice. Ohio State U. 7:38-42, 1968.

Tribute to Paul Hoch: science, human values and psychiatry. In Strahl, M. O. and Lewis, N. D. (Eds.): *Complete Psychiatrist: The Achievements of Paul H. Hoch, M.D.* Albany, N. Y., State U. of New York Press, 1968, pp. 698-706.

The vagaries of youth. *Austral. J. Forensic Psychiatry,* 1968.

Biodynamic psychiatry: academic address to the Australia-New Zealand College of Psychiatry. *Austr. J. Psychiat.,* 1968.

Experimental approaches to behavior disorders. *J. Biol. Psychol.* 10:39-47, 1968.

Debatable conclusions. *Int. J. Psychiat.* 6:281, 1968.

The neuroses (with L. Wigdahl, et al.). In Spiegel, E. A. (Ed.): *Progress in Neurology and Psychiatry,* Vol. 23. New York, Grune & Stratton, 1968.

The vagaries of American youth. *Austral. J. Forensic Psychiatry,* 1969.

The neurotic cat. *Readings in Psychiatry Today.* Del Mar, Cal., CRM Books, 1969, p. 132.

Alcoholism—disease or dis-ease? a review. *Business Report,* 1969.

The neuroses (with N. Borelli, et al.). In Spiegel, E.A. (Ed.): *Progress in Neurology and Psychiatry,* Vol. 24. New York, Grune & Stratton, 1969.

With how much ease can we call alcoholism a disease? *Report on Alcohol* 27:17-27, 1969.

Asymptotic systems of survival. In Gray, W., Duhl, F.V. and Rizzo, N.D. (Eds.): *General Systems Theory.* Boston, Mass., Little, Brown & Co., 1969.

Others in press.

Films

Teaching motion picture films distributed internationally by the Psychological Cinema Register, State College, Pennsylvania. (Fully subtitled, silent and black and white, unless otherwise specified.)

F1. Effects of Stimulation and Destruction of the Hypothalamus on behavior, 508 feet, 1937-40.

F2. The Hypothalamus and the Heart, 60 feet, in color, 1939.

F3. The Role of the Hypothalamus in Emotion, 626 feet, 2 reels. 1940-43.

F4. Experimental Diminution of Neurotic Behavior, 423 feet. 1941-44.

F5. The Dynamics of an Experimental Neurosis, 4 reels. 1941-42.

F6. Active Readjustments in Therapy, 394 feet. 1941-44.

F7. Conditioned Feeding and Experimental Neuroses in Cats, 504 ft. 1941-44.

F8. Effects of Frustrations and Conflicts, 359 ft. 1941-44.

F9. Inter-cat Relationships in a Manipulative Feeding Situation, 200 feet. 1942.

F10. The effects of Morphine on Neuroses, 407 feet. 1942.

F11. Dominance, Neurosis and Aggression, 698 feet, 2 reels. 1942-43.

F12. The effects of Morphine on Learned Adaptive Behavior and Experimental Neurosis in Cats, 1 reel. 1943.

F13. Neurosis and Alcohol, 612 feet, 2 reels. 1943.

F14. Dynamics of Competition, 330 feet. 1943-44.

F15. Alcohol as a Preventive of Experimental Neurosis, 400 ft. 1945.

F16. Effects of Electroshock on Neuroses, 700 feet, 2 reels. 1945.

F17. Effects of Electroshock Therapy on Experimental Neuroses, 600 ft. 1945.

F18. Experimental Masochism (with Mary Grier Jacques), 200 ft. 1946.

F19. Hypothalamic Cardiac Control, 100 ft. (Col) 1946.

F20. Effects of Direct Interrupted Electroshock on Experimental Neuroses (with Alex J. Arieff, and Harold Klehr), 700 ft. 1947.

F21. Experimental Neuroses in Monkeys (with C. Pechtel), 450 feet. 1948.

F22. Penrod: The Evolution of Behavior Patterns in an Infant Macaque (with I Bernstein and L. Aarons), 450 ft. 1956.

F23. Discrimination of Oddity: Abstract Behavior in Monkey and Ape (with I. Bernstein and L. Aarons), 450 ft. 1957.

F24. Osmatic Behavior in Normal and Neurotic Monkeys (with C. Pechtel), 350 ft. 1957.

F25. Technique of Temporal Lobectomy in Neonate Macaques (with L. Aarons), 250 ft. 1964.

F26. Effects of Neonate Parietal Lobotomy and Temporal Lobectomy on Development and Behavior (with L. Aarons), 400 ft. 1964.

F27. Effects of Neonate Brain Lesions on Discriminative Learning (with L. Aarons), 650 ft. 1964.

F28. Alcoholism, 800 ft., color and sound. Charles Pfizer Laboratories, 235 E. 42nd St., New York, N. Y., 10017, 1965.

F29. Delayed Sensory Feedback (with Marvin Wolf), 400 ft., color and sound. Chicago, 1968.

F30. Irregularly Delayed Experimental Closure in the Rhesus Monkey, 600 ft., color and sound. Chicago, 1969.

F31. The Fourth International Congress of Psychiatry, 800 ft., color and sound. The Fairview Hospital Foundation, Chicago. 1969.

F32. Techniques of the Psychiatric Interview. I: General Videotape, 1 hour. Downey Veterans Hospital, Downey, Illinois, 1969.

F33. Techniques of the Psychiatric Interview. II: Schizoid Paranoia. Downey Veterans Hospital, Downey, Ill., 1969.

F34. Symposium on the musical "Hair" (with Karl Menninger, Howard Rome and L. Jolyon West). Fairview Hospital Foundation, 1969.

F35. Exemplification of Behavior in Monkeys, 400 ft., color, subtitles, 1969.

INDEX OF SUBJECTS

INDEX OF NAMES

Thanks are due to Miss Savilla Laird, my invaluable secretary for eighteen years, for the collation of the index, and to Miss Laird and Mrs. Joan Warmbrun of the Center for Advanced Study in the Behavioral Sciences for typing the manuscript. I am also indebted to Mrs. Georgiana Yates for the careful correction of proofs.

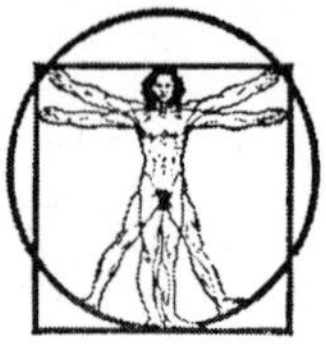

The Americanization of the Unconscious

by JOHN SEELEY

If sociology and psychoanalysis are to advance, the practitioners of these disciplines must encounter each other, argues John Seeley, Professor of Sociology at Brandeis University. "Each discipline has immense explanatory power. Each illuminates and makes intelligible a vast range of otherwise disjointed and seemingly unrelated events. Each, moreover, addresses itself not simply to such 'random' events, but to those both most crucial for the view man has of himself, and most critical for any rational hope of human betterment . . . If either account is substantially neglected, we are clearly condemned to timeless continuation of the misery, destruction, and folly that is the record of history and life-history."

In the author's view, it is no longer profitable to speak of the *psychological,* the *social,* or the *ontogenetic* as if we had hold of three problems, three fields, and three "levels" of logical analysis. "It is not that these things—personality, society, human development—are causally related; it is that they are logically related, for the simple reason that they are different ways of stating the same thing. The worst intellectual heresy of the day (a genuine 'scandal' in the medieval sense) is to pretend that they are separate and, in a way yet to be discovered, causally related. If we say, for instance, that alteration in family behavior affects the behavior of members of the family, we are talking sheer animism: altered family behavior *is* altered family *member* behavior. We are talking about identities, not causal sequences.

"To this joint and common, theoretical and practical enterprise, psychoanalysis brings a great deal that is unique and indispensable for the welfare of both concerns. So," says Seeley, "does the activity that has gone under such varied labels as applied psychology and applied sociology. Both disciplines, like any other unreconstructed patient, bring a crushing burden of useless and counteruseful views, habits, investments, cripplings, blindnesses, nonorders, and disorders, but it is precisely out of engagement with such sad mixes of assets and liabilities that we have learned most of what little we do know about man, ourselves and each other. I suggest we stop playing autistically in our corners and encounter each other."

Contents: I. THE REVOLUTIONS: PSYCHIATRIC AND SOCIOLOGICAL: 1. The Americanization of the Unconscious, 2. The Psychiatrist as Reluctant Revolutionary, 3. Psychiatry: Revolution, Reform, and "Reaction", 4. Social Values, the Mental Health Movement, and Mental Health, 5. The Future of Psychiatry, 6. The Sociological Revolution; II. THE PSYCHOANALYTIC STANCE OF SOCIAL SCIENCE: 7. Psychoanalysis: Model for Social Science, 8. Social Psychology, Self, and Society, 9. Personal Science, 10. The Problem of Social Problems, 11. Social Science: Some Probative Problems, 12. Applied Sociology as a Vocation, 13. Phylogeny and Ontogeny of Applied Sociology, 14. The Making and Taking of Problems; III. SOCIETY IN PSYCHODYNAMIC PERSPECTIVE: 15. The Shaping of Human Nature, 16. Society, Social Pathology, and Mental Ills, 17. Hostility in Modern Society, 18. Progress from Poverty, 19. Crestwood Heights: A Transaction, 20. "Lex Salutis, Salus Legis . . .", 21. The Law of the Retardate and the Retardation of the Law, 22. Parents—The Last Proletariat?, 23. Education: What For? 24. The Facts of Life, 25. Mental Health and the Secondary School, 26. Education for Mental Health: An Experiment, 27. The Forest Hill Village, "Human Relations Classes", 28. A Controlled Experiment, 29. Guidance and the Youth Culture, 30. Guidance: A Plea for Abandonment, 31. "Planning for Mental Health"—Paradise Stormed, 32. Adolescence: The Management of Emancipation in History and Life History; IV. EPILOGUE: 33. The Beneficial Encounter.

465 pages **$8.95**

SCIENCE HOUSE, 59 4th Ave., New York, N.Y. 10003

Psychoanalytic Treatment of Schizophrenic and Characterological Disorders

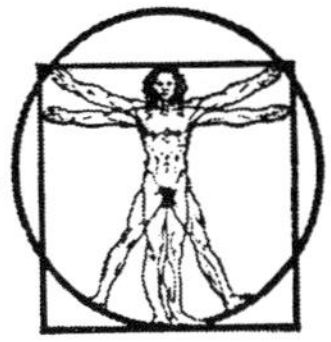

by L. BRYCE BOYER and PETER L. GIOVACCHINI

The authors examine the question of what is analyzable and the conceptual basis of the analytic process. They conclude that clinical phenomena show that we can extend our concepts of what is considered psychoanalytically treatable.

The authors reject the usual cliches of fragile ego, shaky defenses, and psychotic core. Their perspective is ego psychology which they feel furnishes an observational approach that is particularly pertinent to the study of patients with characterological problems, whereas concentration upon the id and psychodynamic factors has greater explanatory significance for the psychoneuroses.

This is a thoughtful and provocative book that will be of interest to anyone with a clinical interest in the treatment of characterologic and schizophrenic disorders.

Contents: Preface 1 and Preface 2: I. Introduction; II. Historical Development of Psychoanalytic Psychotherapy of the Schizophrenias: Freud's Contributions. Background Information; III. Historical Development of Psychoanalytic Therapy of the Schizophrenias: Contributions of the Followers of Freud; IV. Office Treatment of Schizophrenic Patients: The Use of Psychoanalytic Therapy With Few Parameters. Introduction; V. The Psychotic Identifications in Schizophrenia: The Technical Problem; VI. Psychoanalytic treatment of Character Disorders: Introduction; VII. Some Elements of the Therapeutic Action in the Treatment of Character Disorders; VIII. Further Theoretical and Clinical Aspects; IX. Epilogue; Bibliography.

384 pages **$8.00**

The Effects of Psychotherapy

by HANS J. EYSENCK

Is psychotherapy effective? "Not in any demonstrable way," answers Hans J. Eysenck, Professor of Psychology at the Institute of Psychiatry of the University of London. In this book he surveys the major outcome studies on the effectiveness of psychotherapy. Summarizing the published research data he concludes, "the therapeutic effects of psychotherapy are small and do not in any demonstrable way add to the non-specific effects of routine medical treatment, or to such events as occur in the patients' everyday experience."

Eysenck's shocking judgment on psychotherapy is applauded by some of the 17 discussants in this volume and contested by others. For example: Lawrence Kubie, "I do not believe that his own investigations or any of those he quotes have even faced the technical problems which must be solved before such investigations can be carried out." Joseph Wolpe, "Its arguments are mainly unanswerable and its major conclusions unimpeachable." In the debate presented here the methodological problems in evaluating psychotherapy and the various interpretations of published research data are made clear.

Contents: THE EFFECTS OF PSYCHOTHERAPY by Hans J. Eysenck: DISCUSSIONS: Elizabeth R. Zetzel; Jerome D. Frank; Christian Astrup; Joseph Zubin; Paul Meehl; D. Muller-Hegemann; Edward Glover; J. T. Barendregt; Ignacio Matte-Blanco; Hans H. Strupp; Joseph H. Handlon; Henry A. Davidson; Joseph Wolpe; Lawrence S. Kubie; Ray Hyman and Louis Berger; Robert Kellner; Stuart Rosenthal: REPLY by Hans J. Eysenck.

100 pages **$6.00**

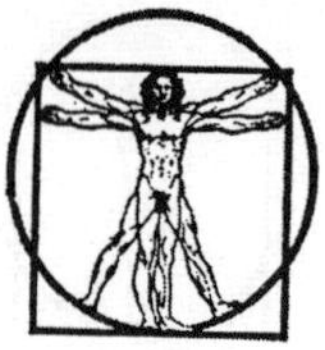

Essays in Self-Destruction

edited by EDWIN SHNEIDMAN

Essays in Self-Destruction delves into the dark side of man. The suicidal aspects of human behavior are explored in this volume by experts who have systematically studied the phenomena of self-destruction in its very process.

But suicide is not the sole province of these writings. They deal in fascinating detail with all of the partial deaths to which man is prone, a wide range of self-damaging and self-negating behavior, taking in all of the diminishing, reductive, truncating, and inimical patterns of life encountered in the study of the human personality. Indeed, it is the basic credo of this book that the study of self-destructive behavior is the study of human personality.

Contents: FOREWORD by Karl A. Menninger; I. LITERARY AND PHILOSOPHIC ESSAYS: 1. Dead to the World: The Passions of Herman Melville, 2. Shakespeare's Suicides, 3. Death as a Motive of Philosophic Thought, 4. Buddha and Self-Destruction, 5. Values and Value-Conflict in Self-Destruction, 6. Can a Philosophy Make One Philosophical?; II. SOCIOLOGICAL AND ETHNOGRAPHIC ESSAYS: 7. Death in American Society, 8. Practical Sociological Reasoning, 9. Suicide and Loss in Social Interaction, 10. The Search for Help, 11. Japanese Adolescent Suicide and Social Structure, 12. Suicide as a Public Health Problem; III. PSYCHOLOGICAL AND PSYCHIATRIC ESSAYS: 13. Self-Destruction and Sexual Perversion, 14. The Components of Personal Despair, 15. Sigmund Freud on Suicide, 16. Self-Poisoning, 17. Crisis, Disaster and Suicide, 18. The Psychology of Fatal Accident, 19. Suicide Among Police; IV. TAXONOMIC AND FORENSIC ESSAYS: 20 Multiple Determinants of Suicide, 21. The Forensic Pathologist and the Multi-Disciplinary Approach to Death, 22. The Suicidal Life-Space, 23. Can a Mouse Commit Suicide?, 24. Sleep and Self-Destruction; INDEX.

438 pages **$12.50**

The State of Psychiatry

Essays by AUBREY LEWIS, Vol. 1

The State of Psychiatry marks the retirement of Aubrey Lewis, perhaps the most influential figure in English psychiatry in the 20th century, from the Professorship of Psychiatry at the University of London and the directorship of the Institute of Psychiatry, Maudsley Hospital.

In this book Professor Lewis reviews the psychiatric past, surveys the transitional stage psychiatry has now reached, and looks forward to the attainable future. He pays a great deal of attention to disputed areas of psychiatric practice and inquiry; how psychiatrists should be chosen and educated; what concepts and methods are required for the furtherance of psychiatry, and what part social treatment and psychological treatment should play. The essays in this volume go far in communicating the clarity of thought and disciplined reasoning characteristic of Lewis' personal encounters.

Contents: HISTORY: 1. The Story of Unreason, 2. Phillippe Pinel and the English, 3. J. C. Reil's Concepts of Brain Function, 4. Henry Maudsley: His Work and Influence, 5. Sigmund Freud: 1856–1939, 6. Jung's Early Work, 7. Melancholia: A Historical Review; EDUCATION: 8. Psychiatric Education: Background and History, 9. The Education of Psychiatrists, 10. Psychiatric Education and Training; ESSAYS AND ADDRESSES: 11. Philosophy and Psychiatry, 12. Health as a Social Concept, 13. Between Guesswork and Certainty in Psychiatry, 14. The Study of Defect, 15. Agents of Cultural Advance, 16. Ebb and Flow in Social Psychiatry, 17. Medicine and the Affectations of the Mind, 18. The Psychology of Shakespeare.

298 pages **$12.50**

SCIENCE HOUSE, 59 4th Ave., New York, N.Y. 10003

A Study of Interpersonal Relations

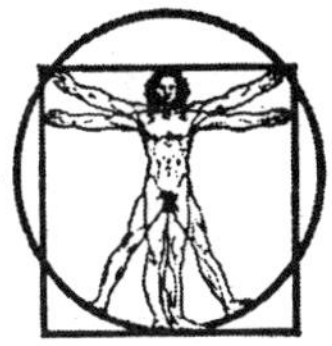

edited by PATRICK MULLAHY

A collection of outstanding contributions by a group of pioneers in the scientific study of man as a social being, this volume lays the groundwork for a radical challenge to current thought and technique in psychiatry. It probes many of the values which, in our Western culture, have come to be regarded as eternal and immutable criteria of mental health and mental illness. The views expressed here point to the social order itself, rather than to the frustration of fixed biological needs and drives, as the ultimate matrix of functional disorder.

Interpersonal psychiatry, Patrick Mullahy maintains in his introduction to this volume, cannot begin to be properly evaluated until it is thoroughly understood. This collection of papers, many of them classics, should engender a deeper, more comprehensive interest in interpersonal psychiatry. Despite the progress made in psychiatry, psychology, and social science in the years since this collection was first printed, most of the papers remain as fresh, as exciting, and as valuable as the day they were written. They provide a frame of reference which, in varying degrees of comprehensiveness and depth of insight, has been increasingly adopted as its significance has gradually dawned on the minds of students of human behavior.

Contents: SUBJECTS AND CONTRIBUTORS: ERNEST G. SCHACHTEL: On Memory and Childhood Amnesia; ERNEST BEAGLEHOLE: Interpersonal Theory and Social Psychology; JANET RIOCH: The Transference Phenomenon in Psycho-Therapy; HAROLD LASSWELL, Person, Personality, Group Culture; HARRY STACK SULLIVAN: Introduction to the Study of Interpersonal Relations; Notes on Investigation, Therapy, and Education in Psychiatry and Their Relations to Schizophrenia; Therapeutic Investigations in Schizophrenia; FRIEDA FROMM-REICHMANN: Recent Advances in Psycho-Therapy; Remarks on the Philosophy of Mental Disorders; CLARA THOMPSON: Cultural Pressures in the Psychology of Women; The Role of Women in this Culture; Changing Concepts of Homosexuality.

507 pages **$9.50**

Inquiries in Psychiatry

Essays by AUBREY LEWIS, Vol. II

This second volume of Aubrey Lewis' collected works illustrates the intrinsic fascination of psychiatry as an endeavor and demonstrates how papers written in the scientific tradition, without rancor, without empty posturing, but with attention to detail, can contribute so very much.

Contents: CLINICAL PSYCHIATRY: 1. The Experience of Time in Mental Disorder; 2. The Psychopathology of Insight; 3. Melancholia: A Clinical Survey of Depressive States; 4. Melancholia: A Prognostic Study; 5. States of Depression: Their Clinical and Aetiological Differentiation; 6. Problems of Obsessional Illness; 7. Obsessional Illness; 8. A Study of Cretinism in London; 9. Aspects of Psychosomatic Medicine; SOCIAL PSYCHIATRY: 10. Neurosis and Unemployment; 11. Social Causes of Admission to a Mental Hospital for the Aged; 12. Vocational Aspects of Neurosis in Soldiers; 13. Social Psychiatry; 14. The Offspring of Parents both Mentally Ill; 15. Fertility and Mental Illness; 16. Demographic Aspects of Mental Disorder.

326 pages **$12.50**

The Psychology of Suicide

by EDWIN SHNEIDMAN, ROBERT LITMAN and NORMAN FARBEROW

In 1955 the authors organized the Los Angeles Suicide Prevention Center. Since then they have authored or edited, separately and jointly, some seventy-five publications, including four books, all of which show a continual pursuit of fresh ideas and new clinical and intellectual adventures relating to the understanding and prevention of suicide.

This volume is a sampler of their writings. It conveys their insights in classification, diagnosis, and evaluation of self-destruction, their experience in the organization of suicide prevention, and their treatment of potentially suicidal patients.

Contents: I. THEORY AND TAXONOMY: 1. Orientations Toward Death, 2. Suicide, Sleep and Death, 3. Sleep and Self-Destruction, 4. The Logic of Suicide; II. ADMINISTRATION AND ORGANIZATION: 5. The Los Angeles Suicide Prevention Center, 6. Suicide Prevention Around the Clock, 7. The Role of Non-Professional Volunteers in a Suicide Prevention Center, 8. How to Prevent Suicide, 9. Some Recent National Developments in Suicide Prevention; III. STATISTICS AND DEMOGRAPHY: 10. Some Comparisons between Genuine and Simulated Suicide Notes, 11. Suicide and Age, 12. TAT Heroes of Suicidal and Non-Suicidal Subjects, 13. Statistical Comparisons between Attempted and Committed Suicides, 14. A Socio-Psychological Investigation of Suicide; IV. DIAGNOSIS AND EVALUATION: GENERAL: 15. Emergency Evaluation and Self-Destructive Potentiality, 16. Procedures and Techniques in Evaluation and Management of Suicidal Persons, 17. Suicide: A Clinical Manifestation of Acting Out, 18. Suicide: Symptom of Lethality; V. DIAGNOSIS AND EVALUATION: SPECIFIC CLINICAL GROUPS: 19. Evaluation and Treatment of Suicidal Risk Among Schizophrenic Patients in Psychiatric Hospitals, 20. Suicide Among General Medical and Surgical Hospital Patients with Malignant Neoplasms, 21. Suicide Among Patients with Diagnosis of Anxiety Reaction or Depressive Reaction in General Medical and Surgical Hospitals, 22. Suicide Among Patients with Cardiovascular Illnesses, 23. Case History and Hospital Factors in Suicides of Neuropsychiatric Hospital Patients; VI. THERAPY AND TREATMENT: 24. Some Aspects of the Treatment of the Potentially Suicidal Patient, 25. The Suicidal Crisis in Psychotherapy, 26. Immobilization Response to Suicidal Behavior, 27. Management of Acutely Suicidal Patients in Medical Practice, 28. Suicide Prevention in Hospitals, 29. When Patients Commit Suicide; VII. FORENSIC AND PROFESSIONAL ISSUES: 30. Investigations of Equivocal Deaths, 31. Sample Investigations of Equivocal Suicidal Deaths, 32. Medical-Legal Aspects of Suicide, 33. Police Aspects of Suicide, 34. Frederic v. United States, 35. Suicide: Trauma and Taboo, 36. Suggestions for Revision of the Death Certificate; VII. BIOGRAPHY AND LITERATURE: 37. Sigmund Freud on Suicide, 38. The Deaths of Herman Melville; IX BOOK REVIEWS: 39. A Look into the Dark, 40. A Puzzle Remains Perplexing, 41. Pioneer in Suicidology, 42. Hope as Help, 43. Tragedy Compounded: INDICES.

$15.00

Psychiatry in the Communist World

edited by ARI KIEV

For the first time, material on psychiatric theory and practice in most of the Communist world is brought together in one volume. Of particular interest is the varying extent to which Marxist-Leninist theory is interwoven with psychiatry; the way psychotherapy is viewed as a process of re-educating the central nervous system by extinguishing pathologically conditional connections and forming healthy new ones; and the great number of treatment and rehabilitative measures which are utilized on a large scale; e.g., the compulsory treatment of alcoholics.

Contents: 1. Introduction; 2. Hungary; 3. Mainland China 4. Czechoslovakia; 5. Bulgaria; 6. Poland; 7. Yugoslavia; 8. East Germany; 9. Soviet Union; 10. Rumania; 11. Epilogue; 12. References; 13. Index

$10.00

Treatment of Schizophrenia

A Comparative Study of Five Treatment Methods

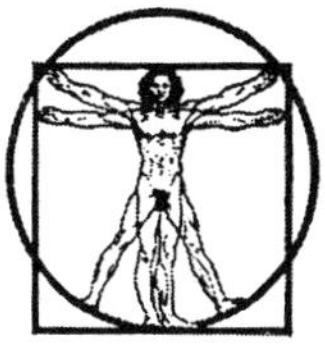

by PHILIP R. A. MAY, A. HUSSAIN TUMA, and LUTHER S. DISTLER

This is an extensive study of five different treatment modalities for schizophrenic patients: ataraxic drugs alone; individual psychotherapy alone; the combination of individual psychotherapy and ataraxic drugs; electroshock; and plain, reasonable care without the addition of any of these "specific" treatments.

In the past century there has been considerable progress in the understanding of schizophrenia, and a diversity of treatment methods has been developed. The sobering fact is that until this report there has been no firm evidence that any of these methods is more effective than any other. The results of this long and carefully run experiment show that: Drug therapy is the most effective single form of treatment for the general run of schizophrenic hospital patients. The value of psychotherapy alone for the hospitalized schizophrenic patient has been greatly exaggerated, for it adds little or nothing to conservative milieu therapy. Insight is a secondary development in the process of recovery; restitution leads to insight and not vice-versa. Electro-convulsive shock therapy is not as desirable as drug or psychotherapy plus drug. And milieu therapy alone is relatively ineffective. Evidently a thoughtful reappraisal of our whole thinking about the psychotherapy of the schizophrenic patient is in order.

$12.50

The Contributions of Harry Stack Sullivan

edited and with an introduction by PATRICK MULLAHY

Since the first edition of this book, several volumes of Sullivan's lectures have appeared. These have broadened the base of information available for knowing and evaluating his achievements. Yet a great many misunderstandings of Sullivan's ideas still exist. These papers, which are relatively nontechnical and contain concise explications of most of his important conceptions, will clarify some of these misunderstandings and contribute toward a more profound grasp of interpersonal theory.

Contents: SULLIVAN'S CONCEPTIONS: I. Patrick Mullahy, The Theories of Harry Stack Sullivan: II. Alfred H. Stanton, Sullivan's Conceptions; SULLIVAN AS A CLINICIAN: III. Clara Thompson, Sullivan and Psychoanalysis; IV. Mary J. White, Sullivan and Treatment; SULLIVAN AND THE SOCIAL SCIENCES: V. Gardner Murphy and Elizabeth Cattell, Sullivan and Field Theory; VI. Leonard S. Cottrell and Nelson N. Foote, Sullivan's Contribution to Social Psychology; VII. Charles S. Johnson, Sullivan's Contribution to Sociology; Bibliography.

238 pages **$6.95**

SCIENCE HOUSE, 59 4th Ave., New York, N.Y. 10003

SCIENCE HOUSE, 59 FOURTH AVENUE, NEW YORK, N.Y. 10003

Please send me the book(s) listed below. I understand that you will pay packing costs and postage if payment is enclosed with this order.

Title/Author **Price**

....

....

....

....

Bill me and add shipping costs ☐ ☐ Check enclosed in full payment $........

Name____________________ Address____________________

City________________ State________________ Zip________

SCIENCE HOUSE, 59 FOURTH AVENUE, NEW YORK, N.Y. 10003

Please send me the book(s) listed below. I understand that you will pay packing costs and postage if payment is enclosed with this order.

Title/Author **Price**

....

....

....

....

Bill me and add shipping costs ☐ ☐ Check enclosed in full payment $........

Name____________________ Address____________________

City________________ State________________ Zip________

SCIENCE HOUSE, 59 FOURTH AVENUE, NEW YORK, N.Y. 10003

Please send me the book(s) listed below. I understand that you will pay packing costs and postage if payment is enclosed with this order.

Title/Author **Price**

....

....

....

....

Bill me and add shipping costs ☐ ☐ Check enclosed in full payment $........

Name____________________ Address____________________

City________________ State________________ Zip________